Charles Seale-Hayne Library

University of Plymouth

(01752) 588 588

LibraryandITenquiries@plymouth.ac.uk

Aspects of Consciousness

Aspects of Consciousness

Volume 4
Clinical Issues

Edited by
Robin Stevens
Department of Psychology
Nottingham University
Nottingham, England

1984

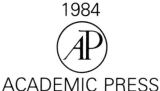

ACADEMIC PRESS
(Harcourt Brace Jovanovich, Publishers)
London   Orlando   San Diego   New York
Toronto   Montreal   Sydney   Tokyo

ACADEMIC PRESS, INC. (LONDON) LTD.
24-28 Oval Road,
London NW1 7DX

United States Edition published by
ACADEMIC PRESS, INC.
Orlando, Florida 32887

British Library Cataloguing in Publication Data

Aspects of consciousness.

   Vol. 4, Clinical issues
   1. Consciousness
   I. Stevens, Robin
   153   BF311

Library of Congress Cataloging in Publication Data

Main entry under title:

Aspects of consciousness.

   Vol. 4 edited by Robin Stevens.
   Includes bibliographies and indexes.
   Contents: v. 1. Psychological issues.--v. 2. Structural
issues.--[etc.]--v. 4 Clinical issues.
   1. Consciousness. 2. Consciousness--Physiological
aspects. 3. Awareness. 4. Self-perception. 5. Cognition
disorders. I. Underwood, Geoffrey. 2. Stevens, Robin.
BF311.A73   153   79-41233
ISBN 0-12-708804-0 (v. 4)

PRINTED IN THE UNITED STATES OF AMERICA

84 85 86 87   9 8 7 6 5 4 3 2 1

Contributors

Numbers in parentheses indicate the pages on which the authors' contributions begin.

Carl B. Dodrill (103), *Department of Neurological Surgery, University of Washington School of Medicine, Seattle, Washington 98104, U.S.A.*

Peter Eames (1), *St. Andrew's Hospital, Northampton NN1 5DG, England*

J. A. C. Empson (207), *Department of Psychology, The University, Hull HU6 7RX, England*

Andrew Mayes (65), *Department of Psychology, University of Manchester, Manchester M13 9PL, England*

Robin Stevens (167), *Department of Psychology, Nottingham University, Nottingham NG7 2RD, England*

James A. Thompson (41), *Department of Psychiatry, Middlesex Hospital, London W1N 8AA, England*

Malcolm P. I. Weller (117), *Friern Hospital, Whittington Hospital, Royal Northern Hospital, and Royal Free Hospital School of Medicine, London, England*

David Wood (229), *Department of Psychology, Nottingham University, Nottingham NG7 2RD, England*

Roger Ll. Wood (1), *St. Andrew's Hospital, Northampton NN1 5DG, England*

Preface

Alteration or disruption of consciousness is often found in various clinical conditions. It is usually, but not always, the consequence of a brain disorder. Over the years such matters have been informally addressed by many clinicians, but now they are being discussed more formally, here and elsewhere. One reason for this is that derangements of consciousness are of theoretical interest; another may be the current emphasis in psychology on mental states and cognition.

Clinicians are primarily concerned with practicalities, such as the effects of brain damage on consciousness or the aberrations in consciousness that arise from the effects of various drugs and toxins. But an understanding of consciousness requires more than an elaboration of the states of sleep, wakefulness, and coma. Thus, if we are to understand the causes and consequences of abnormalities of consciousness, a detailed analysis is needed of the many aspects of consciousness and of the relationships among awareness, mental activity, and personal action.

Since mentalism is respectable once again in psychology, the questions that arise regarding mental activity, the psychological substrate of consciousness, and self-awareness have been debated openly in the pages of journals and various books (including the earlier volumes of this treatise). This is a desirable development because psychologists are now concerned with questions that their colleagues in related disciplines, and the informed nonprofessional for that matter, would consider to be of importance toward an understanding of the richness and complexity of our mental life. However, a better understanding of consciousness is also important in dealing with our mental health, and the contributors to this volume have written with this aim in mind.

When consciousness is discussed within a biological framework, as was true of the contributions to Volume 2 of this treatise, or within the context of clinical disorders, then clearly it is assumed that consciousness is the product of a physicochemical system. Consciousness is a metaphysical state that is either an epiphenomenon of the action of the whole brain or restricted portions of it, or it is an emergent property of a biological mechanism of a certain complexity. A dualistic view of consciousness, akin to the Cartesian line on the mind–brain problem, must view an individual's stream of consciousness as a parallel psychic state that is not a direct product of brain. This position is uncongenial to most psychologists, biologists, and clinicians. Moreover, it is not particularly helpful to those dealing with derangements of consciousness.

The approach taken by the contributors to the present book is that consciousness is the result of physical events within the nervous system. Thus, disorders of consciousness are also likely to be reflected within these physical processes, and, as a corollary, the reestablishment of "normal" consciousness can sometimes be engineered by action on these same physical processes. This is a powerful argument in favor of a monistic view of consciousness and the brain. However, it does not preclude the use of psychological treatments for disorders of consciousness. Although consciousness may be the product of the brain, it is surely well established that mental activity and brain activity are, in a sense, reflexive. One acts on the other, which in turn reacts on the first. Thus, the treatment of disorders of consciousness, such as those following brain damage, psychiatric disturbance, or sensory loss, could well be "psychological" in some circumstances.

The contents of this volume are broader in scope than might be expected from a cursory consideration of clinical issues regarding consciousness. But the topics that one would expect to be covered are included. Thus, the effects on consciousness of brain damage in adults are discussed by Eames and Llewelyn Wood, and brain damage in children is reviewed by Thompson. A more specific discussion, directed at the effects of organic disorders on human memory, is provided by Mayes. Concluding the first section of the book is an analysis by Dodrill of the neuropsychological implications of epilepsy.

The next two chapters deal with psychiatric disorders. The first, by Weller, discusses the thought disturbances created by schizophrenia and questions the way it is diagnosed. The second, by Stevens, appraises current ideas on anorexia nervosa, a disorder that raises questions about self-awareness. No discussion of clinical issues relevant to consciousness would be complete without an examination of sleep disorders, and Empson's chapter considers these, together with their treatment. The concluding chapter by Wood poses interesting questions about the role of language in consciousness and the state of consciousness in the congenitally deaf person.

It is hoped that this volume will be of value for two main reasons. First, it provides specific information relevant to several issues where consciousness is altered by organic or psychological "defects" or both. Second, it should sensitize the reader to the range of disorders where altered consciousness might be expected. If it also makes those who deal with patients more critically aware of the way in which various illnesses cause changes in mental processes, then its purpose will have been served.

Nottingham   *Robin Stevens*
December 1984

Contents

1 Consciousness in the Brain-damaged Adult
PETER EAMES AND ROGER LL. WOOD

2 Consciousness in the Brain-damaged Child
JAMES A. THOMPSON

Contents

7 Sleep and Its Disorders
J. A. C. EMPSON

8 Consciousness and Deafness
DAVID WOOD

Contents of Volume 1

Psychological Issues

EDITED BY GEOFFREY UNDERWOOD AND ROBIN STEVENS

Contents of Volume 2

Structural Issues

EDITED BY GEOFFREY UNDERWOOD AND ROBIN STEVENS

Contents of Volume 3

Awareness and Self Awareness

EDITED BY GEOFFREY UNDERWOOD

1 Consciousness in the Brain-damaged Adult

PETER EAMES

and

RODGER LI. WOOD

The Kemsley Unit,
St. Andrew's Hospital,
Northampton, England

1 General Aspects

1.1 Terminology

There can be few words as confusing as the word *consciousness*. Even within the chapters of this treatise (see especially Volumes 1 and 2), it is apparent that the word has to do service for a wide variety of meanings, both amongst different people and for the same people at different times. So our first task must be to establish some definitions for this chapter. Physicians, surgeons, and clinical psychologists deal daily with disorders of "consciousness," and have a real need for many of the terms they have come to use. Often enough these conform to everyday usage, so no great apology is made for failing to follow terminology put forward by any particular psychological theorist.

In trying to tease out the important strands in the idea of consciousness, a principle of considerable importance is that of dissociability: if a phenomenon can be shown to vary independently of other phenomena, this is rather powerful evidence for the view that the phenomenon is based on a separate brain mechanism (or perhaps set of mechanisms). Clinical disorders are the best source of evidence of this sort, and we shall draw extensively upon them in our analysis.

Whereas for most psychologists the main use of the word *consciousness* is to refer to awareness of information about the environment (e.g., as in "consciousness as a control process"—see T. H. Carr, Chapter 6, Volume 1 of this treatise), for clinicians the standard use is for reference to the *state* of con-

Aspects of Consciousness
Volume 4. Clinical Issues

sciousness, a state which is inferred in the individual from observable behavioural evidence. Typical expressions are "state of consciousness," "level of consciousness," and "clouding of consciousness." The state of being conscious is contrasted, on the one hand, with the state of being *asleep* and, on the other hand, with the state of being *unconscious* or *comatose*. (Semantic problems arise because there is evidence for two rather different continua, the one being normal, the other pathological; yet there do not seem to be adequate terms to differentiate them.) The main alternative to the word *consciousness* for this state is the term *arousal*. A major objection to this is that the term already carries an independent meaning: arousal of a wide range of physiological mechanisms (skin conductance level, for example), even to quite high levels, may be seen either in full, clear consciousness, or in coma, or indeed, in sleep. (See, fot example, M. J. Apter, Chapter 3, Volume 1 of this treatise.) Another alternative, *alertness*, is used to describe variations in the conscious state, but offends logic if one wishes to describe variations in the degree of *un*consciousness. We shall use *alertness* for the former purpose, and, more generally, we shall use the word *consciousness* to refer only to the *state* aspect.

For the phenomenon of *being conscious of something* (including the set of ideas about *consciousness as a control process*), we prefer the rather ordinary word *awareness*. Although awareness is obviously intimately connected with ideas of *content of awareness*, and the two are often lumped together, at least in terms of brain mechanisms (Plum and Posner, 1982), we consider that evidence shows that the two are dissociable.

The last area generally subsumed under the word *consciousness* is the great Cartesian problem of "awareness of being aware." Purely for reasons of verbal economy, we refer to this as *self-awareness*. However, it will figure relatively little in this discussion, since it remains an area in which, scientifically at least, there is very little understanding, explanation, or even acceptable conceptualisation.

1.2 States and Mechanisms

Attention, memory, perception, drive, and *control process* are terms (and indeed concepts) of great importance in understanding the psychological disturbances which occur in brain-damaged adults. We do not consider them to be themselves aspects of consciousness, but because of the constant interactions of such functions with consciousness and awareness, they need to be examined in some depth. For the most part, such interactions occur in all directions. For example, a high level of alertness increases perceptual accuracy; increased impact of stimuli (whether by virtue of intensity or because of particular significance to the individual) raises the level of alertness.

A number of clinical states demonstrate the dissociability of consciousness from content of awareness. There is content of awareness in dreams (though whether there is, in fact, awareness seems an unanswerable question). The state of akinetic mutism, which may be produced by very small lesions in the diencephalon, is one of full behavioural alertness in the absence of any evidence of awareness (Cairns, 1952). The same is true of persistent vegetative state (PVS), sometimes known as coma vigile or appalic state (a derivative of *pallium,* which refers to the cerebral contex); yet here there is anatomical evidence for absence of content (rather than of awareness itself) in the widespread, often total destruction of the cerebral cortex, and thus of perceptual analytical power: there is simply no information of which to be aware. Attention and memory mechanisms clearly function in sleep (though presumably not in coma), since stimuli of different degrees of significance to the individual (e.g., his name and a neutral name) produce different degrees of increase in the level of consciousness (Oswald *et al.,* 1960).

Considering the effects of brain damage on these various phenomena, it would be helpful to catalogue the brain areas subserving them. Unfortunately, we cannot go far towards this ideal at present. There is overwhelming evidence that consciousness is controlled by mechanisms in the upper brain stem, and that different mechanisms are involved for the consciousness–sleep and consciousness–coma continua (Moruzzi and Magoun, 1949; Jouvet, 1972; Moruzzi, i972). On the other hand, there must be parallel or alternative mechanisms, since the state of unconsciousness can be reversible in spite of the irreversibility of the lesion producing it (Beck *et al.,* 1969). Moreover, brief loss of consciousness sometimes follows acute lesions of the dominant hemisphere: this is seen in some strokes, and, more "cleanly," in some patients undergoing the Wada test. (The Wada test is a procedure in which neuropsychological functions are examined during the injection unilaterally into a carotid artery of amylobarbitone (amobarbital), the most usual purpose of the test being to establish which hemisphere is dominant for language—see Wada and Rasmussen, 1960.)

Although a wide range of lesions may result in akinetic mutism (Cairns, 1952), including reversible ones (Cairns *et al.,* 1941), the minimal causal lesions are necessarily in the diencephalon, close to the walls of the anteroinferior part of the third ventricle. Here, it appears that the state is reversible only as far as the lesion is reversible. The same applies to the state of absence of content of awareness seen in PVS.

More intriguing (because nothing at all is known of the mechanisms which may be disturbed) are the clinical disturbances of awareness seen in psychotic states (especially schizophrenia). Some patients give very clear accounts of a state which deserves the description "self-awareness of a lack of content of awareness"—the phenomena known as "poverty of thought" and "thought blocking," for example. Others complain of confusingly increased content of awareness. We accept, of course, that the latter (and therefore perhaps the former too) is best understood in terms of attention mechanisms, but nevertheless, the phenomena provide further evidence of dissociation between the major aspects of consciousness.

There are, of course, great difficulties in assessing the presence or absence of awareness itself (as distinct from content of awareness). However good the reporter may be, there is a major problem in the fact that, almost always, one must rely on retrospective reports, and these cannot adequately distinguish between absence of awareness at the time, and failure to remember it later. However, some hypnotic phenomena (for example, the temporary "abolition" of a number or letter) do support the dissociability of awareness itself. Hypnotic phenomena are part of a range of what are variously referred to as altered or alternative states of consciousness (Silverman, 1968; see also R. G. Ley and M. P. Bryden, Chapter 8, Volume 2, this treatise). Some hypnotic phenomena are mainly of scientific and philosophical interest—meditational and ecstatic states, for example. Others, such as hypnotic and dissociative (hysterical) states, are of particular clinical interest. Although it is difficult (if not impossible) to obtain clear introspective descriptions of these states, nevertheless, at the purely observational level they do appear to involve at least variations in awareness, in the presence of full alertness and evidence of normal potential content. For example, patients with hysteria may show, by the high degree of organisation of their behaviour, that all environmental cues are being processed normally, yet they may be unaware of their own behaviour and often unaware of specific information which, nevertheless, they show evidence of using in the control of their behaviour.

1.3 Brain Damage

1.3.1 Types of Damage

Brain damage is a much abused term, tending to be used loosely to describe any upset of brain function. We restrict our use of it to insults to the brain which result in some permanent physical change. Our clinical experience has been very largely with adults, and so we are here considering the effects, on consciousness and on awareness, of acquired physical damage to the substance of the fully developed brain.

There are four main types of insult which need to be distinguished, because they produce rather different patterns of damage and different effects on consciousness and on awareness.

a. Stroke

Stroke is a term used to denote any lasting disturbance of brain function resulting from disruption of cranial blood supply. Cerebral artery thrombosis (clotting within the artery) and embolism (blockage of the artery by some piece of debris in the circulation) cut off the blood supply (and therefore prevent arrival of oxygen and nutrients, and removal of toxic metabolites) to a circumscribed area of brain tissue supplied uniquely by the affected artery. This leads to the death of tissue, which is called infarction. Rupture of an artery will do the same, but, in addition, there is physical destruction of the brain in the area of the rupture caused by the physical and chemical effects of the sudden injection of a quantity of blood. There may then be more widespread damage, too, if blood enters the cerebrospinal fluid spaces, since many brain areas subjacent to the spaces may be affected. Moreover, the intracranial pressure may rise and produce general compression effects, and also retard the entry of blood into the cranium through the proper channels. In these circumstances the pattern of a combination of localised and diffuse damage may resemble that produced by trauma to the head.

b. Head Injury

Head injury does not disturb consciousness if the head is stationary at the moment of impact, and remains so thereafter. (A classic example would be the injury to Phineas Gage described by Harlow, 1868.) In the vast majority of head injuries, however, there is a sudden transfer of kinetic energy: either the head is hit by a rapidly moving object, and is thus caused to accelerate in space, or the head is moving rapidly and is very suddenly brought to a halt. The brain is roughly tethered within the skull in a way which allows little back-and-forth or side-to-side movement, so that the main effect of such a transfer of kinetic energy is to set up extremely rapid rotational oscillations of the brain, the axis being the brain stem. Thus, the main insults to the brain are from the enormous shearing forces inflicted upon the fibre systems of the brain stem and diencephalon and from waves of high pressure, moving centrifugally towards the cortical surface, which cause diffusely scattered lesions whose greatest density tends to be at the junction of the cortical grey matter with the subjacent white matter. (In each case, the lesions caused are partly direct shearing of fibres, and partly tiny haemorrhages.) In addition, there may be contusions (bruises) of the cortical surface at the points of impact against the inside of the skull, there may be localised areas of destruction from penetration by skull fragments, and there may later be bleeding from surface or deep blood vessels which leads to large clots, which compress both surrounding brain and (because the system is enclosed within the unyielding skull) the brain stem.

c. Encephalitis

Encephalitis is the term used for infections and inflammations of the brain substance. All such conditions involve patchy infiltration of brain substance by inflammatory cells, and often tiny blood vessels are also inflamed and may therefore rupture or become blocked, thus producing tiny areas of permanent damage. Inflammation also involves exudation of fluid within the brain tissue, which increases pressure, often in local areas, and which thus may damage nerve and supporting cells. This sort of patchy process may occur in one or a few localised areas of the brain, or in many widely scattered areas, so that the overall pattern is often patchily diffuse. If the patient survives, the inflammatory process gradually subsides and clears, but often leaves equally patchily diffuse areas of permanently damaged brain.

d. Diffuse Insults

Finally, a distinctive pattern of very diffuse damage is produced when the brain as a whole is deprived of blood supply (ischaemia), oxygen (hypoxia), or glucose (hypoglycaemia). Typical circumstances which produce these results are persistently low blood pressure (as in cardiac arrest or severe shock), inadequate oxygenation of blood (as in anaesthetic accidents or carbon monoxide poisoning), and insulin overdosage. There are some differences in detail, but in general terms the areas of brain which suffer most from such insults are those parts of the cerebral cortex that form the boundary zones between areas of supply of the different major cerebral arteries (posterior parietal, posterior and inferior temporal, and orbitomedial frontal regions of the brain). In addition, certain deep structures, especially the basal ganglia, are usually affected.

1.3.2 Effects of Damage

Obviously, damage to any particular area of the brain will disrupt any particular function that area may have. The clearest examples are the severe language disorders (dysphasias) produced by lesions of the temporoparietal and posteroinferior frontal regions of the dominant hemisphere, and the unilateral paralyses produced by contralateral lesions of the posterior frontal region. The more diffuse the lesion, or the more complex the pattern of lesions, the more complex and widespread will be the disturbances of function.

In the present context, it is important to note the general features of the four types of insult referred to in the preceding section.

a. Cerebral Infarction (Classical Stroke)

Cerebral infarction produces localised neurological abnormality (paralysis, dysphasia, loss of sensation, and so on), but does not usually disturb consciousness (unless the vertebrobasilar arteries, which supply the brain stem, are involved, in which case loss of consciousness is the rule). Sometimes, but by no means always, infarction of part of the dominant hemisphere may be accompanied by transient loss of consciousness. Whether this is produced, as is sometimes claimed, by the cortical lesion, or from disturbance of brain stem function resulting from the unusual pattern of blood supply, is uncertain. Its inconstancy invites the latter explanation. Obviously, loss of an area of brain will limit to some extent the potential content of awareness, but there is no evidence that the fact of awareness is in any way affected.

b. Cerebral Haemorrhage

If the cerebral haemorrhage involves only a small area of bleeding, its effects may be no different from those of infarction. (Indeed, volumes have been written on the difficulty of distinguishing between the two conditions clinically—see Marshall, 1968.) But a large volume of blood (which destroys surrounding brain tissue and also leads to a sudden rise in intracranial pressure, and thus to distortion of the brain stem) will usually produce a quite sudden loss of consciousness, recovery from which is clinically very similar to recovery from head injury.

c. Head Injury

Head injury associated with transfer of kinetic energy, of almost any degree of severity, alters consciousness. That it is the acceleratory force which is responsible is demonstrated by the preservation of consciousness in nonacceleratory head injury (however severe), but also by the fact that "whiplash injury" (the very sudden flexing and extending of the head on the neck which results from sudden jolts) regularly causes "concussion" (with loss of consciousness and transient amnesia) without any actual blow to the head. In the great majority of cases, consciousness is regained within a month of head injury, however severe this may have been. (This is judged not only on the basis of behavioural criteria, but also, for example, on the basis of the reappearance of typical sleep–waking cycles in the EEG.) The state which follows depends very much on the severity of the brain injury, varying from normality to PVS. However, there is a small proportion of patients in whom actual coma may last for many months. Neuropathological evidence (see Adams and Graham, 1972) suggests that they have suffered immediate direct damage to the upper brain stem. They are a particularly important group because, whilst they usually have severe physical handicaps from other brain stem damage, ultimately they often have relatively undisturbed intellect and awareness.

d. Encephalitis

Encephalitis may or may not affect consciousness: if upper brainstem structures are directly affected by the process, then consciousness is certainly diminished or lost; if the process is very widespread or diffuse in the brain, sufficient to produce significant brain swelling, then, just as with any other cause of brain swelling, brain stem functions (and therefore consciousness) may be affected by physical distortion. At times, the onset of the clinical illness may in fact be marked by epilepsy with loss of consciousness. Sometimes, however, there is little reduction in the level of consciousness, but there are clear abnormal changes in the content of awareness, and in particular such illnesses are often accompanied by hallucinations. After recovery from the acute illness, the clinical picture is dominated by the effects of loss of function of permanently damaged areas, and these will obviously affect the content of awareness. But, as after head injury, if the patient survives, consciousness itself invariably returns.

e. Diffuse Lesions

Diffuse lesions always cause an initial loss of consciousness. Since the whole brain is affected by the metabolic insufficiency, there is no need to postulate any mechanism other than disturbance of brain stem mechanisms. Usually, emergence from coma is much less distinctly identifiable than after head injury, and it is quite prolonged. Indeed, some degree of reduced alertness is usually recognisable for many months after a severe insult of this sort. Moreover, there are often disturbances of the content of awareness, resulting from severe perceptual disorders, which persist for years. Such disorders are often neurologically relatively subtle, reflecting the fact that the boundary zones are mainly in areas subserving high-order neuropsychological functions. Our recent experience (unpublished) suggests that the insults also lead, very often, to a disturbance of awareness of the kind qualitatively indistinguishable (so far) from that of severe hysterical states.

f. Transient Disturbances

The course of the disturbances of consciousness so far described has the pattern of a maximum degree initially, with subsequent improvement with the passage of time. Although during the course of improvement there are often fluctuations (perhaps connected with the diurnal variations associated with normal or disturbed sleep–waking cycles), the general trend is always towards improvement. There is, however, an entirely separate class of disturbances of consciousness which may result from any of the insults mentioned above. These are the transient disturbances produced by epileptic activity. Any brain lesion may disturb mechanisms which ordinarily control the electrical activity of the brain and prevent the development of inappropriate or spontaneous discharges. Such control mechanisms operate both at the local cortical level and on the great modulatory systems of the brain stem and diencephalon. Disturbances may thus result either in strictly localised abnormal discharges (producing "focal epilepsy," discrete disturbances of behaviour or experience), or in abnormal discharges which propagate generally throughout the brain (producing "generalised epilepsy," which is characterised by loss of consciousness and, usually, generalised convulsion). Of course, a focal discharge may be propagated to central mechanisms and lead to a secondary generalised discharge. In either case, the generalised discharge may be full, or may be restricted and thus produce only a partial disturbance of consciousness. In the vast majority of cases, epileptic discharges are paroxysmal—that is, sudden in onset and brief in duration. Rarely, though, there may be very long-lasting continuous abnormal discharges, known clinically as status epilepticus. When these involve full generalised discharges, the patient remains unconscious, and convulsions recur with brief interludes of motor inhibition. However, examples are known of continuous "partial" generalised discharges which may produce clinical states of persisting confusion or "clouding of consciousness" (Niedermeyer and Khalifeh, 1965). The fact that such states may be accompanied by no signs of drowsiness may be advanced as one piece of evidence for a qualitative difference between the consciousness–sleep and the consciousness–coma continua. However, the possibility exists that such states represent more or less specific disturbances of awareness, rather than of consciousness.

1.4 Attention and Memory

1.4.1 Attention

The existence of a content of awareness depends very much upon the state of consciousness. This is because content relies on the controlled processing of information, which influences in turn the selection of stimuli and behavioural responses (Posner, 1975). Underwood (1978), describing the selective control of behaviour, develops this idea by expanding the Atkinson and Shiffrin (1968) use of the term *control process* as something "under the direct volitional control of the individual" to refer to the more general concept of attention (e.g., "Attention may be viewed as the major control process in the passage of information into and out of the memory system and, indeed, through the human information processing system as a whole").

Problems of attention are a central characteristic of the severely brain injured. Until recently attention problems have been neglected, with emphasis being given to measuring the impairment of memory after brain injury (Newcombe, 1982; Wood, 1983), probably because there has been no generally agreed upon definition of attention. However, three senses of the term predominate in the psychological and biological literature, which describe three *processes* of attention (Posner, 1975; van Zomeren, 1981): alerting (this is termed by the authors *alertness,* which we have already reserved as a term applying to variations in the level of consciousness), selection, and effort.

a. Alerting

Alerting describes a level of awareness of the existence of information. It is what Sokolov (1963) called an ''orienting response'' and has two components. The first is *arousal,* which is a phasic, short-lived, and reflex response to input, and the second is *activation,* a tonic, long-lasting, and involuntary readiness to respond (Posner, 1975; McGuinness and Pribram, 1980). Posner sees these two components, which are involved in maintaining a level of awareness, as also particularly implicated in and linked to a *state* of consciousness: ''An organismic state which affects general receptivity to input of information.'' (As we have seen, there exist clinical states of apparently full alertness in which, nevertheless, the individual does not ''orient'' to any stimuli in the environment, and we take this as evidence of distinctness between the interacting functional systems underlying the two processes.)

b. Selection

The second attentional process affecting content involves the ability to select, from the potential content of awareness, information which is important to existing behaviour. The selected item is more likely to affect awareness, memory, or behaviour than are other items presented simultaneously. When the basis of selection is a simple, physical property of the stimulus, which does not depend upon its prior identification (for example, its location), selection is said to involve ''stimulus set.'' When the basis of selection does depend on prior identification by the nervous system (e.g., ''select consonants rather than vowels''), the term *response set* is used (Broadbent, 1971). This differentiation appears to discriminate between different levels of procesing or controlled attention, an idea that has received support from those models of memory which rely on information-processing strategies (e.g., Craik and Lockhart, 1972). Such models provide a convenient way of explaining cognitive impairment following brain injury, and this will be discussed in a later section.

c. Conscious Effort

The third process involves the maintenance of an attentional set, in order to be able to monitor changes in the environment, thus allowing the individual to adapt behaviour according to the available and selected cues. This sense of attention has been related to the degree of conscious effort invested by the individual in the processing of information, and involves what one is aware of perceiving at a given moment, and what consequently will have an increased likelihood of being available for later recall. When an individual begins to attend to a stimulus in a way that could be called effortful or "conscious," there occur clear behavioural and physiological changes (Khanman, 1973). It also appears that, under certain conditions, a specific brain mechanism may be correlated with this subjective experience, and that this brain mechanism produces what van Zomeren and Deelman (1978) describe as "tonic changes of alertness, which occur slowly and involuntarily, and are mostly explained as resulting from physiological changes in the organism."

1.4.2 Memory

The disturbances of attention described above affect the efficiency of the channelling of controlled processing of information into awareness. This interferes in turn with the reliable storage of information, influencing even more the content of awareness. Thus, we establish the relationship between storage of information and consciousness. This is particularly true of certain aspects of short-term memory, described as "working memory" (Baddeley and Hitch, 1974), because it seems to be a particularly active stage of information storage, which involves processing of information for meaningfulness and permanent storage.

One process associated with short-term memory is rehearsal. This is the cycling of information through the memory store to help maintain information while it is being processed, and to transfer information about the rehearsed items to long-term memory. It is debatable whether rehearsal is a form of conscious processing or not. Sperling (1967) suggested that it was a conscious event whereby we implicitly or subvocally repeat items to ourselves or use mental representations of sounds in order to analyse and store information from short-term memory. Evidence for this idea was obtained from the rate at which subjects rehearsed a series of letters to themselves 10 times. By comparing the subvocal rehearsal rate to the rate when using overt vocal speech, it was found that the two rates were about the same (usually about three to six letters per second) (Landauer, 1962).

Craik and Watkins (1973) distinguished two types of rehearsal which differed in their effects on long-term memory storage. The first type involved "maintenance rehearsal," which was used only to maintain items in short-term memory by renewing them before they could be forgotten: this had no effect on long-term storage. The second type was "elaborative rehearsal," which not only maintained items in short-term memory, but enhanced their storage in long-term memory. This conforms to the Craik and Lockhart (1972) information-processing model of memory, which incorporates different levels of processing: maintenance rehearsal would represent processing at a shallow acoustic level, whilst elaborative rehearsal corresponds to deep, meaningful processing in which the rehearsed items are associated with one another and generally enriched through contact with an established store of knowledge.

Descriptions of working memory make many references to information processing at different levels of awareness, which closely resemble descriptions of attentional processing. Baddeley and Hitch (1974) suggest that working memory has a limited capacity, and this has obvious similarities to the concept of attention as a limited capacity system. Therefore, maintaining items in memory can be viewed as an attentional process, and the storage of information will compete for capacity with any other attentional process.

2 Clinical Aspects

Section 2 presents an overview of the various disturbances of consciousness and awareness. A tentative classification of their clinical aspects and behavioral manifestations is presented in Table 1.

TABLE 1
A Tentative Classification

Disturbances of consciousness
   Primary
      Coma
      Confusion
      Reduced alertness
      Transient (epilepsy)
   Secondary
      Drive disorders
Disturbance of awareness
   Primary
      Akinetic mutism
Disturbances of the content of awareness
   Primary
      PVS
      Dissociative states
      Transient (epilepsy)
      Lateralisation
   Secondary
      Dyshedonias (e.g., anhedonia, euphoria)
      Attention disorders
      Memory disorders
Disturbances of self-awareness
   Primary
      Disorders of insight

2.1 Disturbances of Consciousness

2.1.1 Coma

The extension of knowledge and understanding of disturbances of consciousness seems often to stem from pooled experience. This is, of course, essential when phenomena can be demonstrated only by statistical means, since large numbers of observations are needed. A problem which has bedevilled research in the area of coma over many generations has been the absence of any objective and reliable criteria for the definition of coma. This has restricted advance not only in the understanding of coma itself, but also in the ability to predict the significance and probable consequences of any particular coma. Traditionally, this field has been littered with a host of adjectives and varietal nouns (for example, "profound coma," "semicoma," "stupor"), which have depended on entirely subjective and unstandardisable judgements. It is by no means uncommon to find in the literature, alongside explicit statements of the essential continuity of various "stages" of coma, rather vague instructions on how to identify the lines between "stages." There seems to have been a practical failure to recognise that, in any continuum, lines can be drawn only arbitrarily, and that arbitration depends necessarily on the existence of fixed standards. It was not until 1974 that this nettle was grasped firmly and decisively. Teasdale and Jennett (1974) published a simple scale which yields a total numerical score (now universally known as the Glasgow Coma Scale score) from which it is possible to specify (arbitrarily, of course, but with great reliability) a degree of reduction of the level of consciousness from a norm. Because it was designed for practical clinical use, the greatest merits of this scale have been its simplicity and its reliability, whether applied by a first-year student nurse or by a professor of neurosurgery (Teasdale *et al.*, 1978). The scale has met with an unusually high degree of acceptance in centres all over the world (though, perhaps predictably, not universal acceptance), and its impact on the extension of understanding of the essential and predictable qualities of coma has been dramatic. For the first time this scale allowed the collection of huge amounts of data in a collaborative study between centres in Britain, Holland, and the United States, which, with the aid of computer analysis, has turned the business of predicting eventual outcome from assessment within the first few days of coma into a remarkably fine (though, of course, not perfect) science (Jennett *et al.*, 1979). At a more mundane level the scale has allowed the gradual development of a genuine uniformity in the classification of injuries into arbitrary "degrees of severity," from which emerge helpful indications of the sorts of problems that need to be anticipated in any particular recovering patient.

Similar problems attend the prediction of outcome from nontraumatic coma, and much the same sort of approach to finding solutions has been followed by a group working in the United States and Britain, following a large group of patients subjected to extensive initial investigation (Bates *et al.*, 1977).

2.1.2 Confusion

In the process of recovery, coma is succeeded by a period of "confusion." How prominent and lengthy this period is depends to a large extent on the nature of the injury. Thus, it tends to be brief after stroke, longer than, but to some extent proportional to, coma after head injury, and often much longer than coma, though very variable and fluctuating, after the more diffuse lesions. The concept of "confusion" is not an easy one. Certainly it is characterised by a failure to retain new information, yet qualitatively it is very different from other amnesic states. For one thing, it involves a variable inability to access long-established information (in other words, a failure of long-term memory). Often direct observation gives evidence of a fluctuating level of alertness (but this is not always so). Most importantly, yet often most elusively, it involves confusion of different times and different places, often varying from minute to minute, with the same sort of quality (which, granted, is mostly subjectively judged) that most of us have experienced on coming awake suddenly from a dream. There is a general, though not very accurate, relationship between the severity of an injury (and therefore the length of coma) and the degree of the confusional state: after 2 or 3 weeks in coma following head injury, a patient may spend 2 or 3 months in a variably, but often dramatically obviously, confused state; on the other hand, it is fairly commonplace to observe a concussed rugby player who, from the distance of the touchline, appears to be functioning normally, yet who in conversation shows subtle signs of confusion—and who will later have no memory for quite a large chunk of time. In the great majority of cases, once the confusional state subsides (which tends to occur gradually to an observer, yet seems to be quite sudden to the individual), functional memory is grossly intact, and the period of confusion stands out in retrospect as a period for which no memories exist (though there may sometimes be isolated islands of brief memories). At this point, the period of confusion becomes known as the period of posttraumatic amnesia. Of course, if the injury has also produced severe deficits of memory function, then the only way of identifying the point of change from posttraumatic confusion is to observe its occurrence, since an individual with a severe memory disorder is in no position to look back and identify the reappearance of continuous memory.

Because there is a more or less reliable relationship between the duration of coma and the duration of posttraumatic confusion, because (until the coming of the Glasgow Coma Scale) measurement of coma duration has generally been a vague business, and because the patient himself can, often even years later, give a fairly accurate estimate of posttraumatic amnesia, the duration of posttraumatic amnesia has been used more than any other measure of severity of injury (Russell, 1971).

Phenomenologically, there are many similarities between posttraumatic confusional states and the confusional states resulting from severe acute infections (like the delirium of pneumonia in preantibiotic days) or from intoxication. Thus, not only are there the confusions which arise from the misplacement in time or place of bits of information, but also perceptual distortions, illusions, and even hallucinations are common, and physical overactivity is often encountered. Although there seems in general to be a lowering of the "level of consciousness," there are also some features which seem to reflect an excessive *heightening* of consciousness (or at least of "arousal"). Probably the best studied state of confusion has been the toxic confusional state produced by overdosage with anticholinergic drugs, the best known example being deadly nightshade poisoning, in which there is a combination of overactivity in brain stem arousal mechanisms with inefficient and distorted cortical activity. Since sedative drugs which selectively reduce alertness can be relied upon to intensify confusion, this seems to be further evidence for a dissociation between consciousness on the one hand, and mechanisms which drive activity levels on the other. When damage to the brain is relatively diffuse (after the diffuse insults or after head injury), it is likely that the confusional state depends as much on physical disruption of cortical activity as on the reduced level of alertness which represents the gradual recovery of mechanisms which maintain consciousness.

2.1.3 Reduced Alertness

That this is so seems to be confirmed by the fact that, once the confusional state has settled, there remains, often for many weeks after even relatively mild injury, evidence of persisting, though very gradually resolving, reduced alertness. Thus, patients usually complain that, in order to achieve their habitual levels of activity and performance, they need much increased stimulation from the environment (which, of course, includes prompting and "chivvying" by other people). One of the most universal complaints after head injury, which may linger for months, is an increased sense of fatigability: quite long-lasting exhaustion can follow from periods of activity which would normally be taken in stride. There often seems to be a purely physical element in this (which may be related more to "drive mechanisms" than to alertness), yet the most common complaint, even amongst individuals whose work and life habits are much more physical than intellectual, is that it is mental activity which most readily induces fatigue.

One of the main problems in teasing out the nature of particular phenomena after brain injury is that most such injuries (with the main exception of stroke) produce lesions very diffusely in the brain, so that many brain systems are affected simultaneously. A step towards finding a way around such problems is to focus attention on relatively mild injuries and their effects. After severe head injury, disturbances of attention and of memory occur which usually persist for many years, and, in some patients at least, outlast problems of fatigability, and at least overt appearances of reduced alertness. Such problems are regularly described by the patient as difficulties of "concentration." On the other hand, when both day-to-day functioning and formal testing reveal little or no abnormality of attention or memory, the same complaint of difficulty with "concentration" is usually made during the same time period over which fatigability and "lack of go" are mentioned. This seems to suggest that, after mild injury, concentration difficulties may be a function of the same reduced level of alertness (Gronwall and Wrightson, 1974).

2.1.4 Transient Disturbances

A description of underlying mechanisms of epileptic disturbance appears in Section 1.3.2f. The clinical import of such disturbances after brain injury is that they tend to occur against a background of gradual improvement in the enduring levels of alertness, but are susceptible to specific treatment. The need, therefore, is to recognise them when they occur, since otherwise the indication for specific treatment may be missed. The key feature is that they are paroxysmal in pattern. However, it is also helpful to know that epileptic disturbances often appear after a delay of some weeks or months following brain injury: obviously, nerve cells which have been destroyed cannot be the origin of electrical disturbance, and this delay suggests that some aspect of the healing process may be crucial. In particular, some neuropathologists have tended to focus on the possibility that the gradual contraction of scar tissues may produce physical distortion of nerve cell envelopes, which induces electrical instability.

2.1.5 Drive Disorders

The physiological bases and indeed, the conceptualisation of drive remain ill characterised, and the literature on drive and drives is still dominated by arguments over the question of whether there is some underlying "general drive factor" or only a collection of "specific drive factors." Clinical experience leaves little room for doubt, however, that many patients after brain injury (and particularly after head injury and the very diffuse insults) have their overall behaviour pattern dominated by a lack of activity, interest, initiative, and perseverance, and the combination seems most easily described as a reduction of drive. Such patients invariably appear underalerted, and show a tendency to drowsiness and somnolence. In a number of such patients we have been able to show (Eames, in preparation) what appears to be a quite specific effect of systematic vestibular stimulation in increasing not only the level of alertness, but also general activity level, initiative, and so on. In these patients, attempts to increase perceptual stimulation through other means (mainly the general stimulation of a busy programme of activities and accompanied by much prompting and reward) appears to have only short-lasting effects on alertness, and none on the other features; in other patients, who show manifest reduced alertness but also spontaneous interest in some restricted activities, a generally stimulating setting produces visible improvements, whereas vestibular stimulation does not. Although such studies are at an early stage, they do suggest that some brain injuries have specific effects on a general drive mechanism, creating a reduction of activity which can have secondary reducing effects on alertness.

2.2 Disturbance of Awareness

Akinetic Mutism

Cairns *et al.* (1941) appear to have coined the phrase *akinetic mutism,* and Cairns (1952) further explored its significance. (The phenomenon is particularly well reviewed by Plum and Posner, 1982, pp. 7–8, 24–26.) It is known in the French literature as *coma vigile* (vigilant coma). The essence of this state is that the patient appears fully alert but exhibits virtually no spontaneous movement or speech; in those patients who show this state as a reversible or intermittent disturbance of brain function, there is no evidence of any subjective experience during periods of akinetic mutism, but there is virtually normal cognitive functioning at other times. There is, of course, no way of knowing whether such individuals are unaware of their environment in this state, or whether the lesion responsible simply prevents the formation of memories. (On the other hand, individuals with Korsakoff's psychosis quite clearly display evidence of experience, yet, if they recover, have no memory for those experiences.) But since the reversible cases show that the lesion responsible can be anatomically very restricted, and that perceptual and cognitive mechanisms are intact, it does at least seem possible that the deficit is purely one of a mechanism which allows information into awareness. A piece of evidence which might argue against this possibility is that a similar external appearance is seen in individuals in catatonic states, following which patients give clear evidence of complete awareness.

2.3 Disorders of the Content of Awareness

2.3.1 Persistent Vegetative State (PVS)

Unfortunately, much the same sort of external appearance is seen in patients who suffer severe and widespread damage to the brain, in particular to the cerebral cortex. In the distant past, such patients were often described as being in "permanent coma," although (long before the appearance of the Glasgow Coma

Scale) it had become apparent that coma is never permanent. The French appear to have used the term *coma vigile* to describe akinetic mutism and this state. Another common term has been *apallic state,* derived from the term *pallium* (meaning "mantle"), and it implies the complete destruction of the cerebral cortex. Jennett and Plum (1972) proposed the term persistent vegetative state (PVS), which has a great deal of merit from the clinical point of view. (It has, unhappily, encouraged the media to disseminate distress by describing people in such states as "vegetables.") If the cortex is destroyed, then clearly there can be no perceptual analysis of the environment, nor can there be internal manipulation of information (thinking); in other words, there can be no content of awareness. Clinically, however, there is a problem: after very severe head injury, for example, patients emerge from coma (in the absence of specific brain stem lesions), after some 2 to 4 weeks, into PVS; but many such patients gradually show further improvement, and, indeed, some individuals make quite good cognitive recoveries over the course of the succeeding months or years, so that obviously "persistent" does not necessarily mean "permanent." The clear implication is that the cerebral cortex can be functionally disconnected without necessarily being destroyed. Lesser degrees of cortical destruction may remove the possibility of awareness of particular types of perceptual or conceptual information. Thus, complete destruction of cortical language areas leads to a clinical state in which many aspects of functioning are intact, but no communication is possible, and the individual, though alert, moving, and even largely self-caring, appears to be completely inaccessible to interpersonal interactions.

2.3.2 Dissociative States

The phenomenon of hysteria has fascinated mankind for millennia. (For recent comprehensive views see Merskey, 1979, and Roy, 1982.) The external appearance of an abnormality of function or behaviour can, of course, be produced by a brain lesion. It may also be produced by quite deliberate "acting," and this is usually referred to as "malingering." The essence of the problem of hysteria is that similar appearances can be produced without the individual's being aware of the deliberate act, and also by, perhaps, rather different mechanisms which can produce abnormalities incapable of being "malingered," yet involving no pathological disturbance of brain function (as far as is known). This is not the place for an extensive discussion of the validity of the concept, but we should point out that we take the view that the evidence indicates that hysterical (or "dissociative") states are qualitatively different from malingering, and that they depend on brain mechanisms which are not susceptible to direct, voluntary control by the individual. Dissociative mechanisms are able, quite selectively, to block awareness of restricted sets of information. At one level, for example, in the instance of paralysis and loss of sensation from an entire limb, it is possible to interpret the clinical state in terms of an aberration of selective attention, and some persuasive attempts have been made to account for this on the basis of central sensory gating mechanisms (Ludwig, 1972). In other hysterical states, it may be perfectly clear that the behaviour is produced deliberately, but that the planning and effort of doing so are themselves not available to awareness, and the individual can, so to speak, justifiably claim innocence. It has long been known that brain injury is a rather frequent antecedent of hysterical states (see Whitlock, 1967). Our own experience with patients with severe brain injuries strongly suggests that very severe dissociative states may in fact be induced (regardless of premorbid personality), particularly by the very diffuse lesions, and we are in the process of trying to analyse this situation: at this stage there appears to be a very strong association between these severe dissociative states and damage to the striatum.

2.3.3 Transient Disorders

Some epileptic disturbances take the form of paroxysmal episodes of distortion of perceptions, which can seriously disturb and falsify the content of awareness. Probably the best known example is an experience which also appears regularly in "normal" individuals, indeed, it is probably a universal experience, particularly during adolescence. This is the phenomenon of *déjà vu*. The essence of the phenomenon is that the perceptual experience in progress at the time of the episode is invested with an overwhelming feeling of familiarity, such that the individual feels utterly certain (for just a brief moment) that he has had precisely the same experience before. Epileptic disturbances arising in or near the limbic part of the temporal lobes are particularly often associated with *déjà vu* experiences. The complementary experience (a total strangeness of even the best known environment, known as *jamais vu*) appears extremely rarely, if ever, in normal individuals, but again is met with in some cases of temporal lobe epilepsy. It appears that localized discharges can give rise to a whole perceptual atmosphere. Other examples are depersonalisation (in which the individual feels unreal in a real environment), derealisation (in which the individual feels real in an unreal environment), and micropsia or macropsia (in which the environment is perceived as small and distant, or large and close). Although the individual is clearly and accurately aware of the details of his environment, the whole experience is distorted in such a way as to suggest that the dysfunction involved is in modulatory mechanisms.

2.3.4 Lateralised Disturbances

There is a curious but well-defined group of disturbances of awareness affecting one or the other side of the body. Some of these have been characterised as disturbances of "body schema" (see Weinstein, 1969), but some do not fit this description, yet seem to be part of the same spectrum. The feature which all of these disturbances seem to have in common is that they are produced by lesions specifically in the parietal cortex. These phenomena range from somatosensory or visual "inattention" (in which stimuli may be normally perceived on either side of the body, or in either visual field separately, but the stimulus contralateral to the affected hemisphere is not perceived if both sides are stimulated simultaneously), through "neglect" (in which one side of the body is persistently neglected), to the fully fledged picture of "hemiasomatognosia" (where the patient denies that one-half of his body actually belongs to him, and may go so far as to try to throw his own arm or leg out of the bed). Traditionally, these effects have been described as affecting the nondominant hemisphere (i.e., the hemisphere not principally involved in language). However, it is now apparent that the same phenomena follow lesions of the parietal cortex of the dominant hemisphere, but are often much more difficult to demonstrate because receptive language function is sufficiently disturbed to make it impossible to rely on the patient's responses to the questions and commands, Dimond (1980, Chapter 14) helpfully surveys this topic. He seems to believe that the disorder is one of awareness itself (he uses the word *consciousness,* but the context makes it clear that he is referring to what we prefer to call *awareness*), though he points out that others interpret such disorders in terms of abnormalities of the channelling of information into awareness.

In a small number of patients, we have seen what at first sight may be a related problem. These have all been patients with severe head injury and unilateral hemiparesis (i.e., a one-sided limb weakness with some spasticity, though not of total or very severe degree). Although none showed any evidence of sensory inattention or other sensory deficit, nevertheless each tended to "ignore" the paretic side in automatic movement patterns; at the same time, each was able to show almost normal movements of the affected side when these were carried out under concentrated conscious control. It is rather difficult to implicate sensory or perceptual factors in such a disturbance, the more so because none of these patients had significant or clinically testable disturbances of other aspects of parietal lobe function. In terms of functional mechanisms which have been described thus far, perhaps the most likely candidate, the disturbance of which might explain this phenomenon, is the "corollary discharge" or "efferent copy": the suggestion is that any learned motor pattern is put out not only as a direct command-producing movement, but also in a parallel (or "corollary") discharge, which forms the basis of fully learned or "automatic" patterns of movement.

2.3.5 Secondary Disturbances

Secondary disturbances means disturbances of entirely other brain systems, which disturb, therefore, functions separate from awareness, but which nevertheless have significant impacts upon the content of awareness. The major disorders in this category (Table 1) are those of attention and memory, and these are of such great importance that they are dealt with in a separate section (Section 3).

Here, it seems appropriate to discuss the two main types of dyshedonia, anhedonia and euphoria. The vast literature on brain stimulation reward (for a comprehensive review see Rolls, 1975) clearly supports the view that there are brain systems which underlie the perception of pleasure and pain. If this is so, it might be expected that some brain lesions at least could produce clinical states in which the ability to feel pleasure (or, indeed, pain) would be disturbed. Because of the patchy, diffuse, and unpredictable pattern of brain lesions produced by head injury, it would not be surprising if such problems appeared in this condition, and this does, indeed, seem to be the case. The very diffuse insults, which often affect the deep structures (especially the diencephalon) in a more predictable way, also seem to be associated with this sort of problem. A reduction in hedonic responsiveness inevitably reduces the incentive value of potential behavioural goals, and thus reduces motivation. It also reduces, presumably, the impact of a wide variety of stimuli (if not all). The potential effects on alertness are clear.

On the other hand, euphoria (a persistent and therefore often inappropriate inner feeling of happiness and outer appearance of cheerfulness) is often associated with a general fatuousness following severe head injury. Frequently this is associated with classical features of frontal lobe dysfunction, but not always. From other neurological conditions in which this feature appears (notably in multiple sclerosis), euphoria is known to be producible by lesions in the high midbrain; however, there are well-known connections between the midbrain and the limbic parts of the frontal lobes, so that it is difficult to know where the relevant lesions are most likely to be after head injury.

These disturbances of affect do not appear, at least in any specific way, to alter cognitive aspects of the content of awareness, but they certainly alter the emotional tone, or atmosphere, rather as the epileptic distortions of perception do.

3. Attention and Memory Disorders

3.1 Differential Effects of Types of Brain Damage

On the whole, the various forms of stroke have little effect on modulatory cognitive processes, although one very specific exception to this is the rare occurrence of small infarctions (usually produced by embolism) in the thalamus, which produce a general reduction in the sharpness of memory function, a specific but variable deficit of nominal dysphasia (the inability to name objects), and some other abnormalities of language function which interfere with verbal memory. All of the other forms of injury under discussion are likely to produce abnormalities of both attention and memory. This is presumably not a result of the actual diffuseness of lesions, but because diffuse processes are the more likely to cause lesions in vital areas.

3.2 Attention

3.2.1 Brain Injury and Attentional Capacity

The information-processing system appears to be particularly vulnerable to the effects of brain injury (Norrman and Svahn, 1961; Miller, 1970; Gronwall and Sampson, 1974; van Zomeren and Deelman, 1978). Not all the attentional processes described in Section 1 are equally affected, however, and it is clear that attention is not some kind of unitary phenomenon (Underwood, 1978; R. Stevens, Chapter 2, Volume 2, this treatise), and there is a need to consider different aspects of the attentional system individually.

Worden (1966) and Lezak (1976) suggest that problems of attention should be diagnosed on the basis of observations of the behaviour and experience of humans. Diller and Weinberg (1972) argue that it is only by comparing various observations of behaviour that it becomes possible to discriminate between global deficits of attention and those that are more discrete or specific to one perceptual modality. This is certainly the case as far as brain-injured patients are concerned. Problems of information processing or attentional control are usually described in such behavioural terms as "poor concentration," "short attention span," and "distractibility." These attention deficits have been described in the head-injury literature since Mayer (1904) first commented on the problems that traumatically brain-injured patients had in concentrating on simple and interesting activities. Goldstein (1939) commented on distractibility, suggesting that a "forced responsiveness' to stimuli was one of the most characteristic features of the brain-damage syndrome. McGhie (1969) gave support to this by stating that the most common form of attentional deficit to be associated with brain damage was "the failure of the normal inhibitory processes resulting in distractibility."

It is important to discriminate between "short attention span" and "distractibility." They may appear to be similar at the behavioural level, but there is some indication that they involve quite different information-processing characteristics. A patient who has a short attention span is unable to maintain a focus of attention and therefore passively shifts attention to extraneous stimuli when maintenance lapses. The distractible patient, on the other hand, appears unable to inhibit extraneous stimuli, with the result that he cannot prevent the orienting response from occurring. Put more simply, the former problem involves being unable to attend, the latter problem involves being unable *not* to attend.

It is not easy to explain the difference in information-processing terms. Distractibility appears to involve a disinhibition of orienting response in which the patient is unable to avoid directing his attention to every novel stimulus that occurs in the environment. This could be due to overarousal, which increases receptiveness to stimulation. This in turn would interfere with efficient stimulus selection (Broadbent, 1971). Broadbent suggested that if we hold a particular attentional set (e.g., a position in space or a sensory modality) it is theoretically possible for a peripheral gate to be set up which might allow in stimuli from one source and not from another. This kind of stimulus selection might become impaired in an overaroused state because an overactive phasic component could increase the reflexive response tendency, whilst the increased tonic aspect of alerting reduces even further any voluntary control the person may have over a discriminative response to external signals.

Whereas the distractible patient is unable to select efficiently, and screen out unimportant stimuli, the patient with a short attention span lacks the degree of conscious effort necessary to maintain an attentional set. Although he may not easily be distracted by extraneous noise, he fails to show a level of vigilance, probably as a result of some selective attentional deficit, which is a central rather than a peripheral feature of information processing (Miller, 1970; Gronwall and Sampson, 1974). This approximates to Broadbent's second basis upon which selection could be made, that of response- or memory-dependent selection. In this case, selection is made on the basis of identification of a new stimulus, through contact with stored information (e.g., "select the letters and ignore the colours"). Thus, a patient with a short attention span would be less efficient in these vigilance aspects of stimulus selection, and would allow more nontarget stimuli to slip through into awareness, breaking up the already fragile attentional set, which would lead to complaints of poor concentration and slowness in responding to stimuli.

3.2.2 Brain Injury and Information-processing Strategies

Shallice (1972) proposed that the concepts of awareness may be identified with an information-processing stage in which different "action systems" compete for dominance. In its simplest terms, this can be restated by saying that a consequence of processing one signal is widespread inhibition in the processing of other signals. Although this may be the case, it does not tell us whether inhibition or suppression of some signals, while allowing the processing of others, is a controlled process involving awareness, or not. The model of information processing proposed by Shiffrin and Schneider (1977) attempts to answer this, and offers a good framework for understanding information-processing problems experienced by the severely brain injured.

Shiffrin and Schneider proposed two kinds of cognitive processing, a conscious form of processing, which they describe as "controlled," and an effortless procedure, which they describe as "automatic" processing. Controlled processing is required to cope with novel information. The individual needs to focus his full attention on the stimulus, and make a conscious effort to encode the new information in terms of a phonemic or semantic structure. This process continues (if the stimulus is repeated) until it is learned and can be processed in what appears to be an automatic way. An example of this is learning to drive a motor car. At first one has to make a conscious effort at coordinating the various responses required in the complex movement of, for example, turning right at a junction. This involves looking in the mirror, changing gear, depressing brake and clutch alternately with accelerator, moving the steering wheel, and so on. Initially, each of these movements requires individual attention, and is performed in a dysfluent way. As the procedure becomes learned, each unit of thought or movement merges into the next so that the total response is performed in an almost continuous, fluent, and effortless automatic manner.

Controlled processing is thus a conscious (or aware) mode of operation that relies heavily on attention and is limited by the individual's capacity to cope with the amount of new information available at any given time and also the speed with which the information is presented. Automatic processing, on the other hand, occurs without conscious control and proceeds without stressing the capacity of the information-processing system. It does not demand attention, and proceeds to a level of abstraction determined by prior learning. Because one gives little effort or attention in the automatic mode, it allows an individual to expand his processing capacities—for example, when one has learned to drive, it is possible both to drive and to listen to the radio at the same time, whereas before, the radio would have been an unwelcome distraction in the learning process.

This "two-process" model has the advantage of describing how different kinds of attentional impairment can affect performance. Shiffrin and Schneider propose two basic forms of attention disorder which can interfere with information processing. The first is described as a "focussed attentional deficit" (FAD), which occurs when a learned response to a particular stimulus is replaced by an unfamiliar response. For example, if, as a result of training, we learn to exhibit response A to stimulus X, then response A will gradually become a largely automatic response whenever X occurs. If, however, we are told to replace response A with a new response B every time X occurs, then we have to stop before making the usual response, making a conscious effort to inhibit response A in favour of the now appropriate response B. A FAD is therefore said to occur whenever automatic processing of information is interrupted by the subject's having to produce a new response which conflicts with the one which has previously been trained. Van Zomeren and Deelman (1982) give an example of this by describing a man who, after buying a new car, found that, compared with his old car, many of the controls were on the opposite side of the steering wheel.

Thus, he had to change from the largely automatic mode of response when driving, to a more conscious, controlled mode, to remind himself where the new controls were and to inhibit a previously overlearned response, which might turn on the windscreen wipers instead of indicating left.

The other disorder of attention recognised by Shiffrin and Schneider was described as a "divided attentional deficit" (DAD). It mainly involves the controlled aspects of information processing. Because it is a limited ability, a DAD occurs whenever controlled processing fails to accommodate all the information necessary for optimal task performance. This occurs because the available processing capacity must be divided over several different, yet related, cognitive operations involved in the task performance. Deficits of this kind are common in everyday life. Van Zomeren and Deelman give an example of a DAD experience which occurs when one has to deal with a large amount of new information, such as might be given if one asked a stranger the way to an address in an unfamiliar part of town. The complicated list of instructions is more than most people can process within a specified time, and, inevitably in such situations, one must repeat the request for directions farther down the road. The earlier example of learning to drive also illustrates a DAD: the inexperienced driver cannot cope with such a variety of response alternatives, with the result that performance is slow and hesitating, with frequent errors, until, as a result of training, the actions become automatic.

The series of studies made by Shiffrin and Schneider to support this "two-process" model indicates that controlled processing, which relies on awareness and controlled aspects of attention, is much more vulnerable to FADs and DADs than is automatic processing, which is a largely effortless process requiring minimum attention. This helps to explain why, after brain injury, many patients describe problems of concentration, lack of stamina for mental activity, and a tendency to make errors in day-to-day behaviour that are quite uncharacteristic of their premorbid state. Following head injury, many behaviours that were once automatic appear to require a more conscious effort and a greater degree of attentional control than was previously necessary. This involves a certain irony. By virtue of the brain injury itself, patients find problems concentrating or switching attention from one stimulus to another. As a result of injury, however, they are forced to revert from what was once a largely automatic mode of processing to a form of controlled processing for many of their day-to-day behaviours. Because controlled processing embodies most of the characteristics of the attentional processing system (e.g., limited capacity, selectivity, and so on) the inevitable result is that most patients encounter a variety of problems, not only those mentioned earlier, but also blunting and slowing down of thought processes and reaction times.

Reason (1979) gives an explanation of day-to-day behaviour errors which parallels many of the Shiffrin and Schneider ideas, and which appears to explain the difficulties presented by the head-injured patient. Like Shiffrin and

Schneider, he describes the different levels of conscious control necessary for different behaviours. During the learning phase of an activity, the unskilled performer relies heavily on the feedback available from a task and hence consciously attends to the activity (controlled processing). Once the action is learned, the individual's performance is controlled by a series of "pre-arranged instruction sequences," which act independently of feedback information (automatic processing) and leave the individual free to concentrate on other aspects of the same or different tasks. Reason suggests that "critical decision points" occur even in familiar and well-practised activities. If such a point occurs when actions or situations are common to two or more behavioural sequences, then failure to attend correctly to the behavioural alternatives may result in a completely inappropriate behaviour. The level of complexity of a particular behaviour, and the predictability of the environment, will obviously influence the frequency with which these "attentional switches" need to occur.

The two-process model of Shiffrin and Schneider, and the "actions not as planned" ideas of Reason, both describe an automatic mode of processing which is a reliable, effortless, process that functions up to a level determined by prior learning. Controlled processing, however, is a more vulnerable process, subject to FADs and DADs. Van Zomeren et al., (1983) argue that any analysis of attention deficits after brain injury must ask at least two questions: is automatic processing still efficient and effortless? Is controlled processing disturbed to an abnormal degree by DADs and FADs? In a review of the available data, they failed to find any "strong evidence" for FADs. Various selective attentional tasks, involving choice reaction time measures with or without an irrelevant stimulus, showed that distraction had a disproportionate effect on the patients. This cannot be explained as a FAD, however, since the subjects had never been trained to react to the irrelevant stimulus, and could therefore not be considered as operating in the automatic mode on these tasks. They conclude that the distraction effect is best explained as a DAD, that is, by a slowing down of consciously controlled processing. Time seems to be a critical factor for the occurrence of DADs. But the concept of DADs relies not only on speed but also on controlled strategies, and these controlled strategies have been found to be influenced disproportionately by two variables, the number of stimulus alternatives, and the stimulus–response compatibility.

In support of the first variable, Miller (1970) showed that the more alternatives a patient has to respond to, the slower the response time will be. Miller concluded that the effect of a head injury must be to slow down decision making, and therefore information processing, a conclusion later reached by Gronwall and Sampson (1974) and van Zomeren and Deelman (1976). The latter study found that the amount by which information processing was slowed down was proportional to the length of coma after injury. The effect of stimulus–response compatibility is to increase the degree of controlled processing and therefore task difficulty. Reason (1979) describes this as a discrimination failure, which accounts for the significant number of errors in the behaviour of normal individuals during the performance of simple day-to-day activities. Discrimination failures are defined as the misclassification of input "usually due to a confusion (because of their similarity) between the perceptual, functional, spatial and temporal characteristics of stimulus objects."

Attention deficits produced by a slowing down in the execution of consciously controlled strategies inevitably produce deficits in other cognitive activities. The "slowing-down-of-information-processing" model would predict that head-injured patients would perform worse than normal on a variety of cognitive tasks in which processing time is important. Deelman (1977) showed this was the case when comparing timed intelligence tests to intelligence tests without a time limit. Mandelberg (1975) seems to find the same effect in the difference between verbal and performance parts of the Wechsler Adult Intelligence Scale when the scale was administered to head-injured patients.

3.3 Memory Disorders

A. Mayes, in Chapter 1, Volume 2, this treatise, refers to a "central distinction" about how information comes to be stored in human memory. On the one hand, we have information processing, which is regarded as a flexible activity over which we exert considerable voluntary control. On the other hand, we have the memory stores, which are the structural aspects of memory, providing the constraints within which our processing capacities must operate. These memory stores hold information for a period of time while it is processed by means of pattern recognition and rehearsal, the information-processing systems which act on material in those structures.

Attention plays a central role in the processing of information throughout memory (Atkinson and Shiffrin, 1968; Underwood, 1978). When information first arrives for processing, it is assumed to be held in large modality-specific stores from which it is rapidly lost unless it is attended to. Items which are attended to are transferred into a short-term or "primary" memory store. This is a postattentional store, and has limited capacity, which means that items can be maintained in this store only by rehearsal (by paying attention to them). It is reasonable, therefore, to suggest that the evidence already provided, describing deficits of attention capacity following brain injury, and their effect on the information-processing systems, would interfere with memory by disrupting the processing of information rather than by damaging some hypothetical structures (memory stores). A DAD, for example, may have a serious effect on memory function. Individuals with DADs would be limited in the amount of information they were able to cope with, and because they were unable to store all the information presented to them, they would forget or confuse such information. This would help to explain the reports of head-injured patients who describe being unable to cope with a shopping list, or who fail to remember instructions, or become confused when more than a small number of units of information are presented to them. Such patients do not actually *forget* such information: if they are prompted, they remember it quite easily. The problem, therefore, is not so much the forgetting of information as the failure to remember it. This is probably because the information is not being processed properly, or has become confused with (or is subject to interference by) other information present at the same time. In head injury, at least, there is a strong prima facie case for memory impairment to be interpreted as an acquisition problem, in which information is not processed and organised properly for later recall. This appears to affect spontaneous recall: the individual forgets that he has something to remember, rather than actually losing information altogether.

Whilst there may be an attractive case for brain injury's affecting the processing of information, there is an equally persuasive argument to suggest that damage to memory structures also leads to significant loss of recallability. There has been a distinct tendency to equate memory structures with memory stores. This may be an erroneous assumption, however, because those neuroanatomical structures which are implicated in memory may serve the same function as the lateral geniculate nuclei in the processing of visual information: this would mean that they were centres for the decoding and organisation of information for further processing, rather than storehouses for information per se.

The argument for memory impairment as a consequence of damage to memory structures arises because of occasions when the memory loss may be material specific, as in the case of unilateral temporal lobe lesions (Milner, 1966). Studies of the effects of brain injuries of this kind have been possible because of the use of anterior temporal lobectomy as a surgical treatment for temporal lobe epilepsy. The resection of the temporal lobe typically includes the anterior 6 cm of the temporal lobe and the underlying structures (uncus, amygdala, and parts of hippocampus and parahippocampal gyrus). These structures form part of the complex limbic system, which has been considered as an important set of structures for memory storage, and defects of memory associated with surgical lesions in this area have specific characteristics according to the side of operation. Lesions of the left temporal lobe result in a disturbance of verbal memory, with impairment of learning and recognition of verbal material, whether orally or visually presented, and regardless of whether retention is measured by recognition, free recall, or rate of associative learning (Milner, 1962; Milner and Kimura, 1964). Weingartner (1968) found a verbal learning deficit with dominant hemisphere lesions, despite the visual presentation of the materials. However, this has not been the finding of Luria and Karasseva (1968) or Warrington and Shallice (1969), who argue that patients with dominant hemisphere lesions may have difficulty with verbal memory for all forms of auditory material, but have little or no difficulty with the same material presented visually. There is, therefore, some debate about whether memory loss following a unilateral lesion is simply material specific, or material *and* modality specific (Walsh, 1978). Memory disorders produced by such unilateral lesions could be regarded as a selective disturbance of awareness for the processing of material or modality-specific information, because certain structures necessary for the consolidation of that information are damaged.

Often, however, brain injury is not in the form of circumscribed surgical lesions, but of more widespread or distributed lesions, which may produce impoverishment of many aspects of memory so that the patient becomes incapable of any effective thought process. The best known syndrome of this kind is Korsakoff's amnesia, often produced by bilateral damage to the structures of the mesial parts of the temporal lobes (though sometimes seen following quite small lesions of midline diencephalic structures). With the more widespread lesions producing the Korsakoff syndrome, memory and awareness are more radically affected, because the extent of the memory loss may be so profound that a patient has to make do with two "islands" of awareness. One incorporates the here and now. Patients usually have a fairly clear sensorium and are cognisant of what is happening in their environment. They are unable to retain such information for more than a few minutes, however, nor do they seem able to use such information to anticipate future events. Their awareness is therefore isolated in a brief temporal context from which they are unable to escape. The other "island" of awareness is far removed from the here and now, and consists of retained memories, which have been established many years before some critical time in the development of their amnesic syndrome. It appears, therefore, that the amnesic patient has a temporal restriction of awareness, in which his experiences of the immediate present can relate only to experiences of the distant past, without any bridges (at the verbal or cognitive level at least) between the two.

An even more fascinating example of the relationship between awareness and memory is seen following head injury, during the period of posttraumatic confusion (see Section 2.1.2). Most studies of learning and memory after head injury have concentrated on memory deficits after the end of the period of confusion (Brooks, 1984). These invariably show that head-injured patients perform significantly worse than controls on a variety of tests involving recall, recognition, and relearning of both verbal and nonverbal material—a very widespread deficit. Given the evidence for an information-processing disturbance described earlier in this section, it appears reasonable to attribute most of the impairments of memory to deficits of attention, and to a loss of efficiency of information processing (van Zomeren *et al.,* 1983).

Some studies have commented on the nature of memory performance in the posttraumatic confusional phase (Whitty and Zangwill, 1966; Russell, 1971).

The essential feature of this period is that, yet again, a patient's awareness is restricted to a short interval of time. Recognition memory is rarely affected, and patients can usually recognise members of their family, and indeed are aware of their surroundings and may even respond normally on measures of short-term memory. They are unable to retain information during this period, however, and characteristically show a failure to recall information from one interval of time to another, for example, failing to remember that relatives who visit in the afternoon also came to visit in the morning. Whitty and Zangwill describe a patient who performed normally on measures of short-term memory, and yet the following day was not only unable to remember the tests, but unable to remember the examiner who administered them. It appears, therefore, that we may also be able to describe this kind of memory loss as due to an impairment of the temporal aspects of awareness, intimately related to attentional control of information processing, with the result that new information is lost to the system because it is not effectively rehearsed or organised according to one or another of the processing strategies that are normally under our attentional control.

4 Treatment Issues

The preceding attempt at an analysis of disturbances of "consciousness" yields what may be some helpful pointers to methods of approaching treatment. The general picture which emerges is one of a number of probably distinct mechanisms, which determine whether or not the individual is conscious and, if so, whether he is aware, and of what he may be aware. In addition, a number of other equally distinct mechanisms interact with these more primary ones, and thus in an indirect way may affect the state of consciousness, or the experiences of awareness. The most productive way of exploring possibilities for treatment, then, is to examine each of the elements which seem to be involved for possible ways of enhancing relatively undisturbed functions, so as to reduce the deficits in more disturbed ones. Since any form of treatment needs to justify itself, we should note that decreased alertness and decreased awareness, or its content, both serve to diminish the immediacy and therefore the quality of experience: people who have once been "normal" and then acquire damage to the brain almost always perceive themselves as different and diminished; although the usually stated aim of rehabilitation is to restore *function* as far as is possible within any permanent restraints of brain damage, we consider that effort should also be directed towards trying to restore the *quality of the experience,* since this is as much an integral part of human existence as is functioning. A slightly different, though related, purpose of treatment is to try to maximise the *rate* of recovery, since it does seem likely that any means of treatment hastens a return to full alertness and awareness is likely to enhance other aspects of recovery.

4.1 Epilepsy

Before exploring the theme of the previous paragraph, it may be helpful, lest it be forgotten, to point out that epileptic disturbances are usually quite specifically treatable with anticonvulsant drugs. As was mentioned earlier, the first necessary condition for this is to recognise that a disturbance is likely to have an epileptic basis. Clearly this is not the place for any extensive discussion of the details of such treatment, but there is one particular aspect that bears strongly on the present discussion. In using anticonvulsants, especially in conditions where consciousness and awareness are already diminished and vulnerable, it is particularly important to be aware of the potential sedative effects of many anticonvulsant drugs. Indeed, it is only in the last 10 years, in practical terms, that the choice has included two very efficient drugs which have minimal or no adverse effects on alertness. It is obviously extremely important to avoid the Pyrrhic victory of abolishing occasional transient disturbances of consciousness, only to replace them by a persistent lowering of alertness.

4.2 Coma and Reduced Alertness

Because the evidence strongly suggests that consciousness is maintained largely by the brain stem reticular formation, and because all sensory inputs give branching inputs to that system, there has been, in recent years, a growing practice in acute centres dealing with head injury (and other causes of coma) of attempting to hasten the return of consciousness through systematic programmes of "sensory stimulation." This practice has become quite widespread in the United States, where all sorts of assaults on the sensorium have been used, from frequent stimulation of the skin with objects of a variety of textures, through frequent passive manipulation of the limbs, the playing of loud tape recordings of the victim's relatives or friends, and flashing of multicoloured lights, to the most aggressive of all, namely regular attempts at vestibular stimulation through irrigation of the external ear with ice cold water. At the same time, there has been a countermovement promoting the use of gentle tape recordings of "ordinary daily noises," designed as much to minimise the grossly abnormal environment of an intensive care setting as to provide extra "sensory stimulation." No evidence appears to have been put forward from which to judge whether either of these approaches has any effect on coma duration. Indeed, there are theoretical reasons for doubting this: correlations between coma duration and long-term outcome appear to be paralleled by the relationship with the degree of diffuse damage caused at the time of injury, and it is impossible to see how the degree of such damage could be altered retrospectively. On the other hand, duration of coma seems to be related to the degree of reversible physical disturbance of the upper brain stem, and one would anticipate that extra inputs would have little effect, simply because they would not arrive at a mechanism capable of responding. Those who favour an organised but "normalising" sort of sensory stimulation, however, do not claim to be altering coma duration, but do claim (albeit anecdotally) to reduce the degree of agitation during the later stages of, and recovery from, coma, and this certainly seems a useful therapeutic aim.

Once consciousness is recovered, any degree of reduced alertness diminishes functioning in a number of ways, as we have seen: it reduces the readiness and speed of responses and of cognition in general, and in a qualitative way it reduces the impact and clarity of the content of awareness, thus also reducing the value of awareness as a vehicle for difficult problem solving (or controlled processing). It has generally been agreed (though again no actual evidence seems to exist on this point as far as man is concerned) that the more general environmental stimulation is limited, the less efficient is the performance of the individual. Perhaps because of contributions of particular behavioural characteristics from particular sorts of lesions (most of all, the "catastrophic reactions" to which individuals with right frontal and some other right hemisphere lesions are disposed, in which excessive stimulation leads to a complete breakdown of behaviour patterns), the general view is that moderate amounts of environmental stimulation, coupled with adequate rest periods, produce the best enhancement of performance. Many go on to assume that recovery rate and perhaps even scope are also enhanced, but there is no real evidence for this in man. (There is, however, some degree of evidence in animals: Braun, 1978, and Finger, 1978.) Apart from this, there seems to be no established way of usefully increasing alertness after brain injury. There is a variety of "stimulant drugs" available, none of which seems to have any useful effect, since what they seem to stimulate is arousal rather than alertness, and as often as not this has deleterious effects upon behaviour and experience. We ourselves have been surprised to find an absence of effect on alertness from the application of very consistent contingent reward for behavioural evidence of alertness. We have already mentioned that specifically and systematically increasing vestibular input has only a brief and transient effect on alertness (and therefore on slowness and on cognitive efficiency).

4.3 PVS and Dissociative States

As far as attempts at increasing the content of awareness in PVS and in dissociative states is concerned, there is again little to say. As has already been noted, PVS may be a permanent state, or there may be very slow and gradual recovery of some degree of function, and of evidence of mental life. If the patient is allowed gradually to slip into a setting of minimal external stimulation, it may well be that any such recovery may pass unnoticed, but certainly there exists no evidence to suggest that stimulation in itself can alter the underlying state of affairs. In dissociative states, it does seem possible to produce quite dramatic alterations in functioning and in expressed content of awareness through the intravenous administration of a barbiturate (or similar anaesthetic drug) combined with a stimulant drug (typically methamphetamine) (in other words, using a traditional method of "abreaction"). Where the patient is amenable to such an approach, hypnosis seems also capable of producing similar effects. However, these are transient changes, and we know of no approaches which can produce more lasting effects.

4.4 Manipulating Secondary Disorders

For the time being, then, it would seem that therapeutic approaches directed at primary abnormalities have very little to offer. Luckily, it is possible to achieve much more success, at least with some patients, by attempting to modify the functioning of other systems which interact with the primary ones. In particular, we have found that treatment methods aimed at drive and attention can produce gradual but lasting and quite extensive improvements in alertness and awareness.

4.4.1 Drive

As a result of observing beneficial (though transient) effects of trampolining on alertness in one patient, we tried the effect of a very simple method of applying systematic vestibular stimulation in a particularly underalerted and driveless individual. The method used was simply spinning the patient in a "secretary's chair" for periods of several minutes, once or twice a day. The first feature of interest (which is, in a way, a sine qua non for this treatment) was that the patient showed none of the usually expected responses to this manoeuvre—pallor, sweating, nausea, and subsequent giddiness and gross unsteadiness. At first we thought there was no useful effect, but by the end of about 10 days of such treatment, it became apparent that the patient was generally and persistently more alert and interested in his surroundings. As long as the daily treatment was continued, his drive level and alertness remained high; once it was stopped, no change was seen for between 1 and 2 weeks, but then there was a gradual falling off of activity and interest, back to baseline levels. Sustained changes in each direction could be produced by stopping or restarting the treatment schedule. We have since had similar experiences with a number of further patients, and in Section 2.1.5 some of the reasons are given for considering this as likely to be a primary effect on drive, with secondary effects on alertness and awareness.

4.4.2 Attention Training

Cognitive retraining appears to be a rapidly developing interest among clinical neuropsychologists, and in particular there is a great deal of activity in developing microcomputer techniques for the retraining of various aspects of attention and memory (Trexler, 1982). So far, there is little hard evidence to show the effectiveness of such training techniques, and the evidence which exists is often of an unreliable kind. However, it does appear that the procedures used for the retraining of cognitive function based on information-processing theory are more soundly based than are many of the strategies used in memory retraining (visual imagery training, mnemonics, PQRST methods), which have not been shown to be clinically effective, are extremely labour intensive, and rely on just those information-processing strategies which the patient is unable to generate.

Having been repeatedly disappointed with the results of memory-training procedures, we have concentrated on methods of trying to retrain attention. Initially, in trying to feel our way, we relied on simple electronic games (Simon and Home Computer versions of arcade games). From this we developed to various uses of the Possum trainer (with schedules requiring the subject to select, by button press, those symbols in a moving display which matched a statically displayed symbol), progressively introducing interference, and adding an auditory vigilance task, at first alone and later simultaneously. Eventually we moved on to the use of microcomputer programmes which, of course, allow the elaboration of tasks much more directly tailored to the needs of our patients, and to the wide range of starting and progressed levels of skill. At present, the attention-training programme centres on two tasks, one presenting an attentional problem which involves readiness, speed, and also visual scanning, the other incorporating a trail-learning task as well as an attentional one.

Early attempts (Wood, 1983) to improve attentional control, reduce distractibility, and increase attention span have proved remarkably successful, with improvements recorded not only on the individual training tasks, but also on independent outcome measures like behavioural recordings of attention to task in therapy sessions, rating scale assessments of general behaviour, and general performance as measured by token earnings in a structured token economy. Thus, there appears to be a generalisation of the treatment effect, which does not seem to result from other approaches to the retraining of cognitive functions which have been reported (e.g., Wilson, 1983).

4.4.3 Memory

Powell (1981) argues, and our clinical experience supports his view, that memory responds more effectively to training through behaviour modification techniques than to training which relies on purely cognitive strategies. It is often the case that brain-injured patients with memory impairment are able to use cognitive strategies to improve memory only when they are repeatedly reminded to use them or, indeed, reminded of the details of the techniques, since they simply forget, and therefore do not use the strategies spontaneously in the course of day-to-day living. The use of behavioural methods to improve memory has a basic logic when one remembers that in normal individuals memory is never perfect, and most of us need to rely on some form of aide memoire at some time or another. Writing something down in a note book, on the back of the hand, or elsewhere; tying a knot in one's handkerchief, or transferring one's watch from one wrist to the other, are behavioural habits frequently used by the normal population (Harris, 1980). This shows that people are quite used to the idea of memory aids, and the best therapeutic progress seems likely to be achieved by building upon the aids which people spontaneously use. These are behavioural habits which can be inculcated by means of structured sessional behaviour modification techniques, thus bypassing the problem of learning the techniques cognitively.

5 Conclusions

We suggest that consciousness and awareness are disturbed by injuries to the brain systems which subserve them, and that recovery of these systems depends upon the degree to which damage is reversible. Once recovery of damage is complete, there seems to be little that can be done to improve functioning by direct attack on the damaged mechanisms, but the overall functions (consciousness and awareness) can nevertheless be improved by some measures designed to enhance other brain systems which interact with the primary ones. In particular, there do appear to be ways of enhancing drive and attention, which may quite radically alter the overall functioning of the individual, including his alertness and his ability to use awareness to control and optimise the processing of information. Perhaps the most difficult question to answer would be whether such methods also improve the quality of experience, but obviously this is a goal worth working towards.

References

Adams, H., and Graham, D. I. (1972). The pathology of blunt head injuries. *In* "Scientific Foundations of Neurology" (Eds. Macdonald Critchley, J. L. O'Leary and Bryan Jennett), pp. 478–491. Heinemann, London.

Atkinson, R. C., and Shiffrin, R. M. (1968). Human memory: A proposed system and its control processes. *In* "The Psychology of Learning and Motivation" (Eds. K. W. Spence and J. T. Spence), Vol. 2. Academic Press, London and New York.

Baddeley, A., and Hitch, G. (1974). Working memory. *In* "Recent Advances in Learning and Motivation" (Ed. G. H. Bowers), Vol. 8, pp. 47–49. Academic Press, London and New York.

Bates, D., Caronna, J. J., Cartlidge, N. E. F., *et al.* (1977). A prospective study of nontraumatic coma: Methods and results in 310 patients. *Annals of Neurology,* **2,** 211–220.

Beck, E. C., Dustman, R. E., and Makoto Sakai (1969). Electrophysiological correlates of selective attention. *In* "Attention in Neurophysiology" (Eds. C. R. Evans and T. B. Mulholland) pp. 396–416.

Braun, J. J. (1978). Time and recovery from brain damage. *In* "Recovery from Brain Damage" (Ed. S. Finger). Plenum, New York and London.

Brooks, D. N. (1984). Cognitive deficits after head injury. *In* "Closed Head Injury." Oxford University Press, London.

Broadbent, D. E. (1971). "Decision and Stress." Pergamon, London.

Cairns, H. (1952). Disturbances of consciousness with lesions of the brain and diencephalon. *Brain,* **75,** 109–146.

Cairns, H., Oldfield, R. C., Pennybacker, J. B., *et al.* (1941). Akinetic mutism with an epidermoid cyst of the third ventricle. *Brain,* **64,** 273–290.

Craik, F. I. M., and Lockhart, R. S. (1972). Levels of processing: A framework for memory research. *Journal of Verbal Learning and Verbal Behaviour,* **11,** 671–684.

Craik, F. I. M., and Watkins, M. J. (1973). The role of rehearsal in short term memory. *Journal of Verbal Learning and Verbal Behaviour,* **12,** 599–607.

Deelman, B. G. (1977). "Memory deficits after closed head injury." Paper presented at The International Neuropsychology Society (European) Conference, Oxford.

Diller, L., and Weinberg, J. (1972). Differential aspects of attention in brain damaged persons. *Periphery and Motor Skills,* **35,** 71–81.

Dimond, S. J. (1980). "Neuropsychology." Butterworth, London and Boston.

Fingers, S. (1978). Lesion momentum and behaviour. "The Recovery from Brain Damage" (Ed. S. Finger). Plenum, New York and London.

Goldstein, K. (1939). "The Organism." American Book Company, New York.

Gronwall, D., and Sampson, H. (1974). "Psychological Effects of Concussion." Aukland University Press.

Gronwall, D., and Wrightson, P. (1974). Delayed recovery of intellectual function after minor head injury. *Lancet,* **2,** 605–609.

Harlow, J. M. (1868). Passage of an iron rod through the head. *Publ. Mass. Med. Soc. Boston,* **2,** 327–346.

Harris, J. (1980). Memory aids people use: Two interview studies. *Memory & Cognition,* **8,** 31–38.

Jennett, B., and Plum, F. (1972). The persistent vegetative state: A syndrome in search of a name. *Lancet,* **1,** 734–737.

Jennett, B., Teasdale, G., Braakman, R. *et al.* (1979). Prognosis of patients with severe head injury. *Neurosurgery,* **4,** 283–288.

Jouvet, M. (1972). The role of monoamines and acetylcholine-containing neurones in the regulation of the sleep-waking cycle. *Reviews of Physiology,* **64,** 1–165.

Khanman, D. (1973). "Attention and Effort." Prentice Hall, Englewood Cliffs.

Landauer, T. K. (1962). Rate of implicit speech. *Perception and Motor Skills,* **15,** 646–657.

Lezak, M. D. (1976). "Neuropsychological Assessment." Oxford University Press, New York and London.

Ludwig, A. M. (1972). Hysteria: A neurobiological theory. *Archives of General Psychiatry,* **27,** 771–777.

Luria, A. R., and Karasseva, F. A. (1968). Disturbances of auditory speech memory in focal lesions of the deep regions of the left temporal lobe. *Neuropsychologia,* **6,** 97–104.

McGhie, A. (1969). "Pathology of Attention." Penguin, London.

McGuinness, S., and Pribram, K. (1980). The Neuropsychology of Attention: Emotional and Motivational Controls. *In* "The Brain and Psychology" (Ed. M. C. Wittrock). Academic Press, New York.

Mandelberg, I. A. (1975). Cognitive recovery after severe head injury, No. 1 (Serial Testing on the W.A.I.S.). *Journal of Neurology Neurosurgery and Psychiatry,* **38,** 1127–1132.

Marshall, J. (1968). "The Management of Cerebrovascular Disease." Churchill, London.

Merskey, H. (1979). "The Analysis of Hysteria." Bailliere Tindall, London.

Meyer, A. (1904). The anatomical facts and clinical varieties of traumatic insanity. *American Journal Insanity,* **60,** 373–441.

Miller, E. (1970). Simple and choice reaction time following head injury. *Cortex,* **6,** 121–127.

Milner, B. (1962). Laterality effects in audition. *In* "Interhemispheric Relations and Cerebral Dominance" (Ed. V. B. Mountcastle). Johns Hopkins Press, Baltimore.

Milner, B. (1966). Amnesia following operations on the temporal lobes. *In* "Amnesia" (Eds. C. W. M. Whitty and O. L. Zangwill). Butterworth, London.

Milner, B., and Kimura, D. (1964). "Dissociable Visual Learning Defects after Temporal Lobectomy in Man." Paper read at the 35th Annual Meeting of the Eastern Psychological Association, Philadelphia.

Moruzzi, G. (1972). The sleep-waking cycle. *Reviews of Physiology,* **64,** 1–165.

Moruzzi, G., and Magoun, H. W. (1949). Brain stem reticular formation and activation of the EEG. *Electroencephalography and Clinical Neurophysiology,* **1,** 455–473.

Newcombe, F. (1982). The psychological consequences of closed head injury assessment and rehabilitation. *Injury,* **14,** 111–136.

Niedermeyer, E., and Khalifeh, R. (1965). Petit mal states: An electroclinical approach. *Epilepsia,* **6,** 250–262.

Norrman, B., and Svahn, K. (1961). A follow-up study of severe brain injuries. *Acta Psychiatrica Scandinavica,* **37,** 236–264.

Oswold, I., Taylor, A. M., and Treisman, M. (1960). Discriminative responses to stimulation during human sleep. *Brain,* **83,** 440–453.

Plum, F., and Posner, J. B. (1982). The diagnosis of stupor and coma. Davis, Philadelphia.

Posner, M. (1975). "Psychobiology of Attention" (Eds. M. Gazzaniga and C. Blakemore). Academic Press, New York.

Powell, G. (1981). "Brain Function Therapy." Gower, London.

Reason, J. (1979). Actions not as planned. *In* "Aspects of Consciousness" (Eds. G. Underwood and R. Stevens) Vol. 1. Academic Press, London and New York.

Rolls, E. T. (1975). "The Brain and Reward." Pergamon, Oxford.

Roy, A. (1982). "Hysteria." Wylie, Chichester and New York.

Russell, W. R., and Smith, A. (1961). Post-traumatic amnesia in closed head injury. *Archives of Neurology,* **5,** 4–17.

Shallice, T. (1972) Dual functions of consciousness. *Psych. Review,* **79,** 383–393.

Shiffrin, R. M., and Schneider, W. (1977). Controlled and automatic human information processing, II perceptual learning, automatic attending and a general theory. *Psychological Review,* **84,** 127–190.

Silverman, J. (1968). A paradigm for the study of altered states of consciousness. *British Journal of Psychiatry,* **114,** 1201–1218.

Sokolov, Y. N. (1963). Perception and the conditioned reflex. *Ann. Review, Physiol.,* **25,** 545–580.

Sperling, G. (1967). Successive approximations to a model for short term memory. *Acta Psychologica,* **27,** 285–292.

Teasdale, G., and Jennett, B. (1974). Assessment of impaired consciousness and coma: A practical scale. *Lancet,* **2,** 81–84.

Teasdale, G., Knill-Jones, R., and van der Sande, J. (1978). Observer variability in assessing impaired consciousness and coma. *Journal Neurology Neurosurgery Psychiatatry,* **41,** 603–610.

Trexler, L. E. (1982). "Cognitive Rehabilitation, Conceptualisation and Intervention." Plenum, New York.

Underwood, G. (1978). Attentional selectivity and behaviour control. *In* "Strategies of information processing (Ed. G. Underwood). Academic Press, London.

van Zomeren, E. (1981). "Reaction Time and Attention after Closed Head Injury." Ph.D. Thesis, University of Groningen, Netherlands.

van Zomeren, E., and Deelman, B. G. (1976). Differential effects of simple and choice reaction after closed head injury. *Clinical Neurology and Neurosurgery,* **79,** 81–90.

van Zomeren, E., and Deelman, B. G. (1978). Long term recovery of visual reaction time after closed head injury. *Journal of Neurology Neurosurgery and Psychiatry,* **41,** 452–457.

van Zomeren, E., Brouer, F., and Deelman, B. G. (1983). "Attention deficits: The riddles of selectivity, speed, alertness" (Ed. D. N. Brooks). Oxford University Press.

Wada, J., and Rasmussen, T. (1960). Intracarotid injection of sodium amytal for the lateralisation of cerebral speech dominance: Experimental and clinical observations. *Journal Neurosurgery,* **17,** 266–282.

Walsh, K. (1978). "Neuropsychology: A Clinical Approach." Churchill and Livingstone, London and New York.

Warrington, E. K., and Shallice, T. (1969). The selective impairment of auditory verbal short term memory. *Brain,* **92,** 885–896.

Weingartner, H. (1968). Verbal learning of patients with temporal lobe lesions. *Journal of Verbal Learning and Verbal Behaviour,* **7,** 520–526.

Weinstein, E. A. (1969). Disorders of the body scheme in organic mental syndromes. *In* "Handbook of Clinical Neurology" (Eds. P. J. Vinken and G. W. Bruyn), Vol. 4. North Holland, Amsterdam.

Whitlock, F. A. (1967). The aetiology of hysteria. *Acta Psychiatry Scandinavian,* **43,** 144–162.

Whitty, C. W. M., and Zangwill, O. L. (1966). "Amensia." Butterworth, London.

Wilson, B. (1983). Success and failure in memory training following cerebral vascular accidents. *Cortex,* **4,** 581–595.

Wood, R. Ll. (1983). Management of attention disorders following brain injury. *In* "Management of Memory Disorders" (Eds. N. Moffat and B. Wilson). Croon Helm, London.

Worden, F. G. (1966). Attention and Auditory Electrophysiology. *In* "Progress in Physiological Psychology" (Eds. E. Stellar and J. Sprague), Vol. 1. Pergamon, New York.

2 Consciousness in the Brain-damaged Child

JAMES A. THOMPSON

Department of Psychiatry,
Middlesex Hospital,
London, England

1 Introduction

Whilst the relationship between mind and brain has been a source of speculation for at least 2000 years, the last one hundred years have seen a tremendous acceleration of investigation and conjecture on this subject, and some explanation must be ventured for this increased interest in the brain and its workings. One reason may have been that the fascinating behaviour of brain-injured patients seemed to offer a window into the mind, in which consciousness could be conceived of as a physical state of the brain. This view of consciousness assumed that certain brain mechanisms had to be in proper functioning order for the subject to be able to attend to the world and control his interactions with it.

A reductionist spirit inspired the search for "centres" in the brain, each of which was to be related to a particular deficit and, by implication, to a particular skill in uninjured brains. Also, the last one hundred years have provided a crop of patients who, while young and healthy, have sustained missile wounds of the brain in warfare. These subjects have had cerebral injuries which were more easily localisable than naturally occurring injuries, and which could be considered to have occurred in otherwise healthy tissue. Precision in the localisation of lesions assisted the search for "centres," but left unresolved another problem. This was that in most cases inferences about brain from behaviour were made harder by the extra parameter of the unknown effects of a lesion. A malfunctioning system was rarely easier to understand than one that was working properly.

The concept of consciousness may be used as a description of states of arousal and attention, as awareness and perception of self, and as a process whereby mental operations are controlled. In the first sense, there is a behaviourally defined gradient from unconsciousness through transitional states of sleep, drowsiness, and hypnagogic reverie to fully alert vigilance. This gradient has neurophysiological correlates such as EEG patterns which can be linked to brain stem and subcortical function. This concept is relevant to the understanding of the brain-damaged child in two ways. First, the duration of loss of consciousness can give an estimate of the severity of a traumatic head injury. Second, alterations and fluctuations in full consciousness may be a consequence of such injuries. In the second sense, consciousness as awareness and perception of self is less easy to quantify, since individual differences will always exist in self-descriptions and self-perceptions. An oblique approach is to draw inferences from behaviour about self-esteem and self-image. In the third sense, consciousness as a control process is probably best conceptualised as span of apprehension or working memory and, as such, lends itself fairly easily to psychometric examination.

The underlying assumption in the use of the above concepts of consciousness in the context of brain damage is that consciousness is essentially a physical state of the brain. The developmental aspects of brain function have been even harder to study by the method of making inferences from the deficits of brain-injured subjects to the cerebral organisation of uninjured subjects. Naturally occurring brain damage in children is beset with all the methodological problems of the adult samples, plus the additional complication of normal developmental processes. Not only are the injuries caused by diseases difficult to localise, but they must often be inferred from the very behaviour which one is attempting to link with brain function. In addition, while the adult has a series of fairly stable skills, which afford some ways of assessing his postinjury abilities, the child is still in the process of establishing his competencies, and, since the pace of change is often so fast, postinjury comparisons are made more difficult. Traumatic injuries make it possible to be precise about the lesions in many cases, but the problems of developmental change remain.

Research findings indicate that fairly predictable deficits, though of a general kind, can be expected to follow cortical injury in adults. Children, on the other hand, seem capable of a considerable power of recovery and plasticity of cortical function. Studies of subjects who had received cortical injuries between infancy and adulthood help to trace a developmental history of brain function. Before that can be done some issues need to be resolved.

2 How Does One Localise an Injury and Measure its Extent?

The problem of localising a cortical lesion is considerable, and the very nature of the brain makes it impossible in most cases to say more than that the major damage occurred in a certain area. In the case of an abcess, for example, although it is clear that damage had occurred at one point, the normal functioning of the brain may have been disrupted over a wider area although no obvious injury may be apparent. To a large extent these problems can be diminished by the study of traumatic injuries only. These do not have a long time course and are, on the whole, easier to localise on neurosurgical examination. Being specific about the extent of the lesion can be difficult, since the length of the dural tear may have little relation to the length of the lesion as it goes deeper into the brain. Although some neurosurgeons measure and record the length, breadth, and depth of the injury, this is by no means a universal practise. Some reports merely give a size description without any reference points.

Another problem is the possibility of a contrecoup lesion in cases where the cranium has received a very strong blow. There is no real way of detecting such injuries whilst they remain minor. However, open head injuries are far less likely to show generalised effects than closed head injuries, and they present the most restricted forms of damage to the brain.

Studies of cortical function inevitably run up against the problem of making decisions as to how lesions are to be classified for the purposes of analysis. Size, type, site, and age at injury are obvious factors, each of which carries its own difficulties. In particular, site and size may not be known. However, even if the locus of the lesion is clear, it is not clear how each of these is to be classified. The usual division into anatomical lobes may not correspond to functional reality. Further, some effects may be due to hemispheric influences over and above effects of a particular lobe. An argument could be made for bilateral classifications, such as those wherein the frontal lobes are contrasted with the rest of the cortex.

Division by hemispheres has a long tradition in neuropsychology. Hughlings Jackson (1874/1932) spoke of the left as the "leading" hemisphere, in which propositional language was formulated, ascribing to the right hemisphere the task of visual processing. Such a division is the first step in data analysis, usually as part of a two-way analysis of variance with lobe of injury as the other factor. This is the basic procedure utilised in the analyses further described below.

3 Mechanisms of Brain Damage

Brains may be damaged in various ways, which may range from generalised effects such as from carbon monoxide poisoning to the more specific effects of, for example, a steel shaft driven into the skull. Any study of the localisation of cognitive functions in the cortex must attempt to collect subjects with as discrete and as circumscribed a series of lesions as possible.

Traumatic injuries, as mentioned above, are generally easier to localise than diseases of the nervous system. These traumatic injuries may result in the loss of cerebral tissue, as well as the interruption of neural pathways between undamaged areas. However, other injuries, less easily detected, may take place as an overall effect of the impact on the skull. The blow may knock the brain against the skull, causing contusions on the surface, and may twist and shake the brain so that internal stresses and shears may take place. These injuries are generally hard to detect in surviving subjects, and are identified at postmortem examination. Strich (1969) has asserted

> There is no doubt that degeneration of nerve fibres occurs in the cerebral hemispheres and brain stem as a result of trauma. Furthermore, there can be little doubt now that it occurs frequently, and in cases of mild as well as severe head injury. The evidence available at present strongly suggests that this degeneration is the consequence of tearing or stretching of nerve fibres, due to mechanical forces acting at the time of the accident. (p. 503)

Strich studied the brains of five patients who had received apparently uncomplicated head injuries, yet had remained in a state of severe dementia with gross neurological abnormalities until they died some months later. These patients had become unconscious immediately after their accident and showed severe neurological abnormalities and a decerebrate or decorticate posture when examined. They did not, however, show raised intracranial pressure. Although the grey matter was almost unaffected, there was widespread degeneration of nerve fibres in the white matter of the brain. There was histological evidence of interrupted nerve fibres in acute cases, and torn blood vessels were demonstrated in relation to small haemorrhages in the cerebral hemispheres and brain stem. Strich found the degeneration difficult to explain except on a mechanical basis.

Strich observed that in all cases of protracted coma studied (a series of over 50 subjects) there was no instance when postmortem revealed lesions confined to the brain stem—all had extensive hemispheric damage as well. When an axon is interrupted, easily visible masses of axoplasm—retraction balls—form at both cut ends of the nerve within hours. The presence of these retraction balls thus indicates ruptured axons.

The direction in which nerve fibres run seems to have a bearing on whether a blow to the head will injure them or not. Large numbers of retraction balls may be seen in the descending tracts of the pons, in one case, whereas the adjacent transverse fibres in the same case appear normal. This would accord with the theoretical formulations of Holbourn (1943), who pointed out that of all possible forces which might damage a highly incompressible but easily distortable substance like brain tissue, stresses and strains set up during rotation are the most injurious. These forces exert stresses in relation to fibre direction, and since hemispheres are mirror images and not exact replicas, under certain conditions a fibre tract might be damaged in one hemisphere and spared in another. Strich noted that in her cases the corpus callosum was always involved, and the anterior commissure and the fornices were frequently damaged.

It must be realized that only severe injuries which cause death are seen by the pathologist, and mild trauma cases may well survive a lifetime, which would not be followed by postmortem examination. This is, of course, particularly true of children who survive their injuries. Indeed, R. D. Adams, commenting on Strich's (1969) work (p. 526), stated "We should be cautious about extrapolating from the partial pathological pictures obtained from the examination of a few cases of protracted coma to the more common general state of concussion and traumatic paralysis."

One way by which this problem might be resolved would be the production of concussion in primates, who could then be subjected to postmortem examination.

4 Induced Concussion

Cerebral concussion has been defined by Ward (1966) as "the loss of consciousness and associated traumatic amnesia which occurs as the consequence of head trauma in the absence of physical damage to the brain." Defined in this way, concussion is essentially a reversible process, and an interruption of function without permanent physical damage.

The general pattern of recovery after severe head injury has been described by Hooper (1969). The patient falls unconscious and remains for a while in an unresponsive, immobile coma. Emerging from this state of paralytic unconsciousness, the patient successively passes through stages of stupor, confusion with or without delirium, and finally an almost lucid phase with automatism before becoming fully alert. It would seem that there is a hierarchy of recovery— awareness of stimuli comes first, then motor and sensory recovery, then the restoration of memory and other cognitive functions.

Ommaya and Gennarelli (1974) feel that this pattern of recovery supports the idea of "a greater vulnerability of the cortex and particularly of the limbic and fronto-temporal cortices which occupy zones of great structural irregularity and variation in tissue density." In their view one of the essential problems in the study of consciousness is to determine which of the effects are reversible, and which mechanisms are involved in disturbances of consciousness.

Although falling unconscious is the most dramatic and easily detectable effect of a blow to the head which can be related to an essentially reversible effect on the brain stem, any description of the mechanisms of head injury must explain how traumatic disturbance of consciousness or alertness relates to other effects of trauma on neural function and structure, particularly the traumatic amnesias. (p. 634)

They conducted their investigations by subjecting 24 squirrel monkeys to high-velocity head acceleration, administered by a device to a helmeted subject, thus avoiding any open head injuries. Half of the monkeys received the acceleration in a straight line ahead mode, while the other half had their head rotated forwards and down 45° by the acceleration. In addition to clinical examination of the animals, the effects of these procedures were measured by recording the somatosensory evoked response at the skull surface to median nerve stimulation at the wrist, and the animals were sacrificed within 24 hr so that the location of any resultant lesions could be established.

All the animals in the rotated group exhibited paralytic coma, while none of the other group suffered traumatic unconsciousness. A greater number of gross primary lesions distributed in a diffusely widespread symmetrical manner occurred in the rotated group, whilst only a few asymmetrically placed focal lesions developed in the other group. Rotation seems necessary for concussion to occur, and focal damage can be produced (by the straight line ahead method) without loss of consciousness. Ommaya and Gennarelli (1974) comment:

> These facts, coupled with the association of diffuse surface as well as deeper lesions with cerebral concussion only in the rotated group, support our hypothesis that cerebral concussion of a severity great enough to produce paralytic coma requires shear strains occurring in widespread and diffuse manner involving the cerebral cortex and deeper structures with brain stem involvement being primarily a reversible affair. (p. 643)

The authors propose that there is

> a graded set of clinical syndromes following head injury wherein increasing severity of disturbance in level and content of consciousness is caused by mechanically induced strains affecting the brain in a centripetal sequence of disruptive effect on function and structure. The effects of this sequence always begin at the surfaces of the brain in mild cases and extends inwards to affect the diencephalic–mesencephalic core at the most severe levels of trauma. (p. 638)

This hypothesised system assumes a decreasing effect as the shear strains reach the centre of the brain mass, and the degree of associated irreversible structural damage will depend to a great extent on the material and structural properties of these tissues. Paralytic coma will not develop until the well-protected mesencephalic alerting system of the brain is reached and disconnected. Those parts of the cortex covered by smooth surfaces, such as the occipital lobes, should suffer least, whereas those areas covered by rough surfaces, such as the frontal poles, the temporal lobes, and the orbital cortex should suffer most. It would seem that a patient cannot go into coma without receiving some damage to these areas.

It remains to be seen to what extent findings in monkeys can be extrapolated to man. Not only are the brain mass/skull size ratios different, but it is also the case that the location and extent of lesions will be affected by the locations of bony protrusions, dural partitions, vascular anatomy, and other sources of interfaces between tissues of different densities. However, it seems likely that the major findings, that of a gradient of severity from periphery to centre and that of the

implication of rotational components in paralytic coma, can possibly be extended to man.

5 Damage to Children's Brains

It is clear that experiments of this sort cannot be performed on humans, and that the possible sites of injury in a concussed person must generally remain a matter for conjecture. This is also true of age differences, since children who survive head injuries take longest to come to postmortem, and it is difficult to say how injuries to children differ in their effects from those sustained by adults. Some of the possible differences have been suggested by Graft (1975).

> The flexible, incompletely fused bones of the child's skull confer both advantages and disadvantages as a form of protection against injury compared to the rigid skull of the adult. Injury due to acceleration of the brain within the skull is minimized by the elasticity of the bones which serve to absorb a much greater part of the force generated on impact. However, this same flexibility of the skull with underdeveloped bony buttresses at the base, combined with the much shallower convolutions on the surface leads to a much greater deformation of the brain on impact and shearing forces are set up within the brain substance leading to secondary degeneration of nerve fibres which have been stretched or torn. The maximum shearing forces take place in those parts of the brain which are fixed, and the brain stem, being tethered, often bears the brunt of damage due to this mechanism. (p. 446)

It is clear that full effects of an impact to the skull are very difficult to specify and localise. Certainly a blow to the head may cause injury at sites other than the main skull fracture. However, these injuries cannot be accurately localised on the basis of the original impact itself, and must await precise localisation at postmortem.

6 Intelligence and Learning

The main feature to emerge from work done on the cognitive effects of adult cortical lesions is the lack of a systematic approach to the subject. Study after study tends to add to an accumulation of details which never integrate into a coherent picture, because each investigation has made its own assumptions and has followed its own procedure. However, one finding which stands out to some extent is the insensitivity of intelligence tests to the effects of cortical injury. At the simple level one must argue that intellect is a function of the brain, and that damage to the brain should make its impact on intelligence. However, IQ scores are often unaffected by even quite extensive injuries.

These null results prompt two questions. First, if they do not fail on this measure, can a task be found that will "make silent lesions speak"? Second, what is it about brain functions which allows the brain to retain relatively un-disturbed levels of intelligence despite a reduction in the available mass of functioning tissue?

The attempt to answer the first question leads to a fascinating series of experiments, in which a particular incapacity is linked uncertainly to the functioning of a particular cortical area—for example, map reading is impaired by parietal lesions. It is the nature of these investigations that they follow individual hares down ever narrowing lanes, and rarely attempt an overall picture. Answers to the second question are more difficult to find. It seems that one can only conclude that it is a capacity of brain to reduplicate functions, and that undamaged areas "rally round" and stand in for the functions of injured zones.

An attempt must be made, however, to establish some consistent findings, and there is certainly plenty of evidence for one finding—asymmetry of function in the brain. The fact that the left hemisphere subserves language and the right visuospatial abilities hardly constitutes a blueprint of cortical function, but it offers at least one reasonably consistent finding to be traced through a developmental approach to brain damage.

7 Effects of Early and Late Injury

Hebb (1942) outlined the major differences in effect between early and late brain injury and hypothesised that early injury had a less selective and more generalised effect than late injury. Arguing from the observation that in mentally handicapped, presumably brain-damaged children vocabulary scores were depressed, whereas this was not the case for brain-damaged adults, Hebb proposed the hypothesis that "an intact cerebrum is necessary for the normal development of certain test abilities, but not for their retention at a nearly normal level. In other words, more cerebral efficiency or more intellectual power is needed for intellectual development than for later functioning at the same level" (p. 286). This distinction between the development and the retention of abilities has great potential in the study of age-related effects, and the supporting evidence is tenuous though plausible.

Faced with a complex situation, the subject sees it in a new way and makes a new response—not more responses or harder responses. Now often in such modifications of behaviour it is the first steps which demand intellectual capacity. Learning to solve a problem demands more intellectual effort than solving more problems of the same kind. (p. 286)

The dichotomy is between reason and practise, invention and repetition, synthesis and skill.

The general features of this theory are that an individual who is injured at any age will suffer a reduction in his power to develop new abilities, and that this limitation is more important to the developing child, who thereby suffers a reduction in learning capacity, whereas the adult can coast along on previously acquired skills. Hebb's definition of intellectual power is therefore "capacity to develop a test ability in the absence of any previous relevant experience." In the case of second-language learning, it is fairly clear that the degree of first-language competence will have a major effect, but it is less easy to specify what the carry-over will be between more disparate intellectual skills.

A test score at any time will therefore contain an unknown blend of experience and native wit. Given a wide enough range of experience during development, similarities in the rates of development of abilities will argue for an underlying innate general level of ability. Hebb found that, during development, test abilities correlated "rather well," supporting general ability as a working concept. However, after the age of 20, and after brain injury or schizophrenia, abilities very independently, and it is no longer possible to pick any test at random as an index of this general ability. Only vocabulary retains its position as an indicator of former general ability.

What effects would this view of intelligence have on the study of the relationship of intelligence to the human brain? One effect would be to recast the plasticity/specificity dichotomy into a continuum, and assume that at different ages different skills would be composed of different combinations of these underlying intelligences. Any task might require a proportion of total cortical mass and a proportion of specific cortical zones for its successful completion. "In the analysis of cerebral function the question becomes what abilities are localized, and for what abilities must we take into account mass action and equipotentiality of function?" (p. 290). A partial answer to this question might be given if certain assumptions are made: first, that tests which require the same amount of undifferentiated cortical mass will correlate; second, that tests which tap idiosyncratic cortical zones will be relatively unrelated to any of the other tests. These assumptions would relate total cortical mass to "g" and specific cortical zones to "s." The larger the proportion of variance accounted for by the first general factor in a component analysis, the larger the importance of total cortical mass.

8 Testing for Brain Damage

Research in the field of *brain damage,* a term as precise as *body damage* (Herbert, 1964), has tended to concentrate on the problem of selection rather than description. The aim of this research appears not to be the analysis of the performance of those who are known to be brain damaged, but to attempt to establish that children with problems of one sort or another may have some degree of brain injury. Study after study has hunted for a brain-damage litmus, some concatenation of tests, measures, scores, discrepancies, or ratios that will pluck out children with damaged brains from a population which is making varying use of its intact cerebrums.

It is often unclear what the aims of such studies can be. Many brain-damaged children will be visibly so on examination—for them no master test is needed. For those in whom there is a presumption of damage, what will confirmation or disconfirmation contribute to their treatment? No therapy can follow unless one understands the conditions and stimuli which will facilitate change. And if children are assessed on the basis of their problems, then having an intact brain no more excludes them from the need of care than having a damaged brain excludes them from the hope of improvement.

The attention which has been paid to the will-o-the-wisp of a brain damage test has resulted in an imbalance in the literature which must be followed if it is reviewed at all. This preference for diagnosis over treatment was criticised by Meyer (1957), who felt that psychologists should not only detect abnormalities, but formulate explanations, test these, demonstrate conditions which alter the abnormality, and aim for a cure. "The widely held view that the consequences of brain injuries are irreversible has prevented progress in this field" (p. 105).

The central interest in this study are the claims that have been made for the WISC as a brain-damage indicator, a purpose for which it was not designed. The full scale IQ itself has not been championed an an indicator—the range of intelligence in the injured groups tends to be too wide for this to be feasible. Possibly postinjury decrement might be a more useful variable, but this will only rarely be available.

The most popular index based on the Wechsler scales was the "verbal-minus-performance" measure, which relied on the notion that verbal items were more resistant to deterioration than performance items. Field (1960) showed that discrepancies of 20 points or more occurred in 10% of normal 10 year olds, and neither Norris (1960) nor Rowley (1961) could substantiate the claims made for this index. McFie (1961b) was similarly unable to find support for the verbal-minus-performance index, finding that age of injury was a crucial variable, since it was only in postinfantile injuries that the deficits approximated to the adult injury pattern. Heller (1963), studying Wechsler scores for both adult and child referrals to a psychiatric hospital, found that the incidence of discrepancies between verbal and performance scores was no higher than that found in the normal population, and that the correlation between these subscales was as high as that found in normals—lending no support to the view that a group of subjects with a potential overrepresentation of brain-damaged patients would show a high proportion of verbal–performance discrepancies. Fisher and Parsons (1962) failed to find any convincing evidence that the ratios computed from combinations of Wechsler–Bellevue weighted subtests scores proposed by Hewson (1949) were of any use in selecting out subjects with brain damage.

Herbert (1964) in his review of the available tests states "there is no satisfactory valid and reliable diagnostic test of childhood brain-injury" (p. 211). His methodological criticisms included inadequate standardisation, frequent over-representation of subnormal children in the samples studied, failure to point out that there may be considerable overlap in the scores of brain-damaged and brain-intact children even though their mean scores are significantly different, failure to control for visual field defects, failure to estimate how well the tests discriminate between brain-damaged and neurotic, as opposed to normal, children, failure to estimate the reliability of the tests, particularly when they involve subjective estimates, and failure to relate the sensitivity of the tests to the base rates.

This catalogue of failures in part obscures the more important question as to what function an efficient test of brain damage would serve. In terms of the treatment of the child it would be without any practical consequences, and in terms of understanding cortical function it would raise more questions than it would answer. The more interesting and more clumsy question might be "What sort of lesion, in which part of the brain, sustained at what age by what sort of child has what effect?" Herbert remarks "When factors such as age, previous personality, envionmental background, locus and type of injury, are known to be important determinants of the effects of cerebral insults, the common emphasis on brain pathology as the sole independent variable producing symptoms is seen to be unacceptable" (p. 210). Herbert comes to the conclusion that

Psychologists could make a more valuable contribution by the development and application of tests which describe the various psychological deficits resulting from brain-injuries and which have implications for the academic and social training of the child, rather than by evolving diagnostic tests of dubious clinical value. (1964, p. 212)

9 Effects of Lesions Sustained in Childhood

A developmental approach to the consequences of cortical lesion in children comes up against several problems. First, children are more difficult to assess than adults. They are still learning and accumulating strategies of thought, and tests often catch them halfway through the creation of a cognitive skill. Second, because of the rate of development, postinjury intervals are potentially of more importance. Most of the work on cortical injury in childhood has not been designed to meet these objections. Too often mention is made of, for example, "verbal skill" without an explanation of the implications of having tested children and adults on completely different items. Real comparability of material is difficult to achieve across widely differing ages, and this complicates the assessment of posttraumatic abilities.

As previously noted, consciousness can be seen as a gradient from simple reflex activity, purposeless movements, purposeful movements but no speech, the ability to utter phrases, uninhibited action, and speech with disorientation and amnesia for current events, through to full orientation and alertness.

Many of the early studies concentrated on the effects of injury on intelligence, and it is only in more recent years that schooling and behaviour have been systematically investigated. McFie (1961a) reported on intelligence test results of 14 patients with infantile hemiplegia who had undergone hemispherectomy and a further nine who had undergone partial removal of damaged tissue. The wide range of ages and abilities, as well as the retrospective nature of the study, meant that assessments were made on a variety of intelligence tests, though each patient was retested on the same instrument postoperatively.

Overall, the group gained 8 IQ points postoperatively as compared to the partial removal group who lost 3 points. This striking gain may be due to practise effects, lower levels of anticonvulsant medication, and reduced interference from the now-removed malfunctioning cerebral tissue. Only this last factor would account for the difference between the two groups. Inspection of the background data on these patients revealed that the age of injury had a major effect on eventual outcome. Those subjects who had sustained infantile injuries gained 10 points on average, whereas those injured over the age of 1 lost 1.5 points, a difference which was significant at the 1% level. Curiously there are no significant differences between hemispheres, though those with a left hemispherectomy gained 4.5 points more than the right hemispherectomy group. Neither age at operation nor preoperative intelligence appear to influence the final outcome.

Only six patients completed the Wechsler–Bellevue scale, obtaining on average a 4.5-point lead of performance scores over verbal, a suggestive but nonsignificant difference. Postoperative gains, in general, favoured performance. These same patients, all with infantile injuries, failed on both Weigls's sorting task and the sentence learning test, but were able (in four out of five cases) to obtain the maximum score on Memory for Designs, a pattern of abilities generally found among left hemisphere injuries, even though four out of the six cases had in fact undergone right hemispherectomy.

The suggestion would seem to be that in a situation in which there was a major reduction in available cortex at a very early age performance skills occupied more cortical space than verbal abilities, which were thereby reduced in power. Conversely, it could be argued that the reduced cortex lacks specialisation of function, and that the apparent differences of ability between verbal and nonverbal skills are artifacts of task complexity, and that it is simply easier to remember a design than to learn a sentence.

McFie gathered a further 42 unoperated children in whom there was evidence of right hemisphere injury and distributed them according to age at injury and

TABLE 1
Verbal and Performance Impairment after Right
Hemisphere Injury

Wechsler scale	Relative loss	
	Infantile	Juvenile
Verbal	34	8
Performance	9	14

type of cognitive impairment, adding them to the hemispherectomy group, with results which are summarized in Table 1.

Verbal impairment is more common with early injury, performance impairment more likely with later injury, differences which are statistically highly significant. It suggests that in these patients there may be a critical period for the establishment of language mechanisms, such that children with later injuries go on to achieve verbal skills, whereas those with early injuries do not. It is not immediately clear why early damage to the nonlanguage hemisphere should be associated with later dysphasia. Commenting on these results McFie states

By the end of the first year, it appears likely that the conventional partition of functions into right and left hemispheres has begun, and that subsequent injury to a hemisphere does not entirely dislodge its functions to the other side, with the result that removal of a hemisphere removes a certain amount of functioning tissue. (1961a, p. 248)

The remaining hemisphere must now do the work of two, and it is testimony to the difficulty of this requirement that the intelligence quotients of the group are skewed toward the subnormal range of abilities. Verbal skills seem to bear the brunt of this reduction in overall intellectual capacity, and this imbalance is surprisingly even more true of the right than the left hemisphere. In his review of earlier published work McFie noted that the mean postoperative intelligence quotient of the 12 cases was 63, and that in the majority of cases verbal abilities were poorer than nonverbal ones, an observation confirmed in the study under discussion. One question, however, remains unanswered: "Is there evidence of a critical age at which the apparent relative impairment of language function is replaced by the usual pattern of impairment according to hemisphere affected?" (1961a, p. 242).

McFie (1961b) studied the intelligence test results of 40 children with localised cerebral lesions acquired after the first year of life. No differences in overall intellectual ability were found to be significant when the group was divided according to side and lobe of lesion; neither was there a significant, nor indeed consistent, effect of the age at which the injury had been sustained. Inspection of the Wechsler scores for the 30 subjects who had been tested on this scale failed to reveal any significant differences between hemispheres, the suggestive differences being for the most part similar to those found in adults. Lower scores on Digit Span and Similarities occurred with left hemisphere lesions, lower scores on Picture Arrangement and Block Design with right hemisphere injuries, and Picture Completion scores remained unaffected by lesions in either hemisphere. This much is in keeping with the adult pattern, but the right hemisphere deficit on Digit Symbol and the general impairment on Vocabulary seem to be a specific characteristic of childhood injury. The Memory for Designs test was hardest for patients with right parietal injuries, and harder for all the right-sided injuries than for the left, as in the adult case. The apparent sensitivity of Vocabulary to childhood injuries agrees with the findings of Hebb (1942) and indicates that vocabulary is a skill in the making, whereas memorization of designs, at least for the material used in this study, appears to be an established ability little affected by cortical injury. However, it is not possible to draw further conclusions from this study, since the subject sample is small and the ages at which the lesions were acquired are not given. It presents, however, an extremely interesting field for further investigation, and holds out the possibility of achieving results which would sketch out the patterns of cortical cognitive development.

Studies on the intelligence of children with cerebral palsy (Rutter, Graham, and Yule, 1970) show that over many separate investigations about a third of children with cerebral palsy were found to have an IQ below 55 and about a fifth had mild retardation (IQ range from 55 to 69). The children in the sample actually studied achieved a mean IQ of 78, which was considerably different from that of the epileptic children, IQ 102, and those whose lesion was below the brain stem, whose mean IQ was even higher at 107. A particularly interesting aspect was that whilst those with hemiplegia had a slight overrepresentation in the lower intelligence range, the diplegics had more, and those with bilateral hemiplegia even more representation. This would suggest that with severe lesions there was a fairly close association between motor and intellectual impairment. There was little suggestion that cerebral palsy caused a particular type of intellectual impairment, since the only significant feature of the Wechsler scores was a slight but significant superiority of verbal over performance skills.

Scholastic ability was particularly impaired, and even when expected reading levels were controlled for intelligence, 41% of the sample had specific reading retardation, as compared to 4% of the normal population. It is hard to avoid the conclusion that the cortical structures necessary for reading have been damaged and that this is the reason for their disability. Their school attendance is not so poor as to offer an explanation for their difficulties, since many children with even poorer attendance can read and write considerably better.

10 Effects of Localised Cortical Injury in Childhood

A study of 282 subjects who had sustained focal cortical lesions in childhood (Thompson, 1976, 1979) together with a detailed examination of the subsample of children who had received traumatic, accurately localisable open head injuries (Shaffer, Chadwick, and Rutter, 1975; Chadwick, Rutter, Thompson, and Shaffer, 1981) has added to what is known of the cognitive and psychiatric consequences of such cortical injuries. Thompson (1976) reported on 282 subjects who had sustained a focal cortical injury in childhood from infancy to 16 years of age. When the entire sample of 282 subjects was categorized by age at injury, then an effect was revealed which is not apparent if only smaller groups with more limited ranges of ages at injury are studied. Full scale IQ rises from 97.05 in those injured when younger than 5 years of age to 106.5 in those older than 15 at injury, a difference which is significant at the 1% level, and which holds for both verbal and performance intelligence scales. All the subtests show this effect, but in the case of Vocabulary, Similarities, and Coding the differences are not significant. Digit Span and Arithmetic, with their demands on attention, both show substantial and significant effects on a one-way analysis of variance. The child's age at injury has been reasonably well established as an important factor in determining the extent of recovery, and in the case of encephalitis, meningitis, and therapeutic irradiation of the brain early injury is the more damaging.

Eiser (1981) reported on 47 patients who had been treated for brain tumours in childhood, and found that those treated before 5 years of age had a mean IQ of 76.5, those in the 5–10 range 91.9, and those older than 10 had IQs of 99.9, a significant difference.

More intensive study was made of a group of 98 children who had received cortical lesions as a result of unilateral compound depressed fractures of the skull with associated dural tear and who had sustained gross damage to the underlying brain substance, which had been confirmed at operation (Thompson, 1976). Standard tests of intelligence and scholastic ability were used to compare these children with normals, and a selection of unstandardised special tests were added to look for potential deficits associated with lesions at particular sites in the brain, in the expectation that the neurosurgical reports would afford the most accurate localisation of injury. A comparison was made between the mean intelligence scores of this sample with traumatic lesions, average age at injury 5 years, and the standardisation sample, and no significant differences were found. The full scale IQ was 97.31, verbal IQ 99.02, and performance IQ 97.11. Only three Wechsler subtests were below the expected value of 10 scaled points: Arithmetic 8.02 ($p < .001$). Picture Arrangement 9.06 ($p < .05$), and Coding 8.98 ($p < .01$).

A major effect on intelligence, however, was revealed when children were

TABLE 2
The Effects of Loss of Consciousness on Intelligence

	Loss of consciousness		
Wechsler IQ	<3 days (N = 75)	3–7 days (N = 13)	7+ days (N = 10)
Full scale	99.2	92.8	88.0
Verbal	100.8	92.8	93.3
Performance	98.8	95.5	85.4

categorised by their posttraumatic loss of consciousness. When subjects were categorised in this way (Table 2), it can be seen that full scale intelligence remained at the average level until the period of unconsciousness suffered exceeded 3 days, and that this drop was further accentuated when subjects had been unconscious for more than 7 days.

When the scores on subtests were categorised by the severity of injury, then Digit Span, a measure of attention, showed a clear gradient of impairment from slight to permanent disability, showing that consciousness as a control process is particularly susceptible to disruption after severe injuries. The locus of the lesion had no effect on the IQ scores, but one subtest, Block Designs, was impaired for those with injuries in the left frontal and the right parieto-occipital lobes.

Tests of learning ability, on the other hand, were able to reveal the true potential of subjects who, on tests of retained knowledge, were able to camouflage their mental deficits. Indeed, the few interlobe differences which occurred were on measures of the learning of new words in which the left hemisphere as a whole, and the left temporal lobe in particular, were impaired and new faces learning, in which right temporals were particularly impaired. These difficulties are in line with adult deficits and suggest the possibility that there were hidden deficits in the sample children which more taxing learning tasks might have revealed. Adults, with less power of restitution, may be demonstrably impaired even on undemanding tasks.

Tachistoscopic dot span, a measure of the span of apprehension of a briefly presented visual display, showed significant impairment with parieto-occipital injuries, a deficit which appeared greater than that which could be accounted for by visual field defects.

Although of normal intelligence, the group shows considerable scholastic retardation, being on an average of 2 years behind their chronological age in both spelling and the accuracy and comprehension of reading. Such backwardness in reading is found in 29% of those unconscious for less than 3 days and in 47% of those comatose for longer periods. There is a clear suggestion that those skills required for successful learning have been disrupted even 2 years after the head injury (and this is not due to amount of absence from school, which is no different from a control group).

The apparent conclusion is that children's brains are plastic enough to take over the functions of the damaged areas. This plasticity holds true within the entire age range studied, in that no age-at-injury effects are found. Functional plasticity is a term which refers to the capacity of cortical areas to take over the functions of damaged zones. Plasticity refers to the degree to which tissue would not normally have specialised. The converse is functional rigidity, in which there is strict division of labour, and cortical areas lack the flexibility to stand in for each other. Only in dealing with the unfamiliar and having to learn on the spot can the children be see to be impaired. The left temporal group not only require more trials to learn the word list, but also take in far less of it on the very first presentation. These same children are capable of learning other, nonverbal, material and so afford us the only example of a material-specific, location-related deficit in the study.

The paucity of lobe effects underlines power of recovery of the young brain, and by implication postpones the age at which functions can be said to be localised. Possibly most cortical areas are potentially capable of taking on any cortical function, although natural preferences exist for unknown structural reasons. At some time, possibly at about age 13, this equipotentiality diminishes, and lobe-related deficits are the result.

A prospective study of children with head injuries is a comparative rarity in this field, but such a study has been done by the time-consuming procedure of contacting subjects immediately after their injuries and testing them repeatedly over the subsequent 2 years. This study (Rutter, Chadwick, Shaffer, and Brown, 1980; Chadwick, Rutter, Brown, Shaffer, and Traub, 1981; Brown, Chadwick, Shaffer, Rutter, and Traub, 1981; Chadwick, Rutter, Shaffer, and Shrout, 1981) compared a group of children with severe injuries resulting in a posttraumatic amnesia of at least 7 days with those whose milder injuries caused a posttraumatic amnesia of less than 7 days, and compared them with a matched control group with only orthpaedic injuries. The children were studied as soon as possible after the accident and then again 4 months, 1 year, and $2\frac{1}{4}$ years after the injury. Parents were given a standardized interview, teachers filled in behavioural questionnaires, and all children were given an extensive neuropsychological assessment.

In order to avoid sampling biases six Regional Neurosurgical Units serving the southeast of England were used to provide unselected consecutive cases meeting the study criteria that they were aged between 5 and 14, and had a posttraumatic amnesia of at least an hour's duration. Inspection of background information revealed that children with severe head injuries, the majority of whom were pedestrians hit by cars, were closely comparable with controls in all crucial respects. Those with mild injuries, who often received their injuries in unsupervised play, were more likely than controls to be boys, to have come from socially disadvantaged backgrounds, and to have had prior adjustment problems at home and at school. These differences had to be taken into account in all analyses, and it is clear that studies which fail to include control groups may often produce misleading results.

The severity of injury measure was the duration of posttraumatic injury up to the point at which the memory for daily events became continuous (Brooks, 1976), which has been found to be a reasonably good predictor of long-term recovery (Russell, 1971; Bond, 1975; and Jennet, 1976). Posttraumatic amnesia was preferred to recovery of consciousness as a measure, because 91% of patients with a coma lasting at least 6 hr have a posttraumatic amnesia of more than a week during which recent events are not remembered reliably.

The overall pattern of intellectual outcome is shown in Fig. 1. The control group shows a slight practise effect. Children with mild injuries show a similar

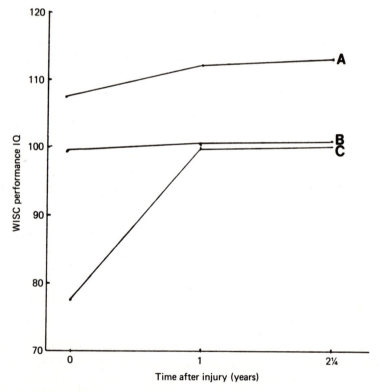

Fig. 1. Head injury and cognitive recovery. (A) Controls; (B) mild head injury; (C) severe head injury.

TABLE 3
Severity of Injury and Cognitive Deficit One Year after Injury

	Posttraumatic amnesia (days)		
Wechsler scales	7–14	15–21	22+
Verbal IQ	+6.6	+2.7	−14.4***a
Similarities	+2.2	+1.0	−3.0***
Vocabulary	+1.1	+0.7	−1.8
Digit Span	−0.2	−0.3	−2.1
Performance IQ	+2.6	−14.7	−25.4***
Block Designs	+2.2*	−1.0	−2.6
Object Assembly	+0.1	−3.0	−4.3***
Coding	−1.1	−2.3	−3.9*

aSignificant differences from matched controls: $*p < .05$, $**p < .025$, and $***p < .01$.

increase, but at a level consistently lower by about 9 IQ points. Children with severe injuries show an initial deficit of 30.2 IQ points, which is equivalent to two standard deviations, and which represents a colossal impairment of intellectual function. However, by 1 year this had reduced to an 11.5-point impairment, remaining at roughly that level thereafter. The severe injury group was less affected in verbal abilities than performance skills, the average deficit being 10.3 points initially, falling to a mere 2 points by 1 year. The subtests of Vocabulary and Digit Span were the least affected by the injury, whilst the Coding performance task was the most impaired. Figures derived from a 4-month follow-up reveal that much of the cognitive recovery had taken place by then.

Turning to the effects of the severity of the injury, it will be seen from Table 3, where the children are compared with matched controls, that the most pronounced impairment is suffered by those children who experienced more than 22 days of posttraumatic amnesia. Once again, the deficits in this group are greater on performance than on verbal items, though both are permanently affected. From the point of view of the pattern of recovery, it can be said that most recovery takes place soon after the injury, that substantial improvement takes place in the following year, and that after that gains are small and largely restricted to those who had most ground to recover in the first place.

How do these injuries affect the child's awareness of himself? In looking at these injured children it is essential to have an assessment of preinjury behaviour, and this was obtained by means of a parental interview and teacher questionnaire given before the consequences of the accident were known. The mild injury group was shown to have had a raised level of behavioural disturbance prior to injury, but this did not get worse after the accident. However, the severe injury children showed a marked increase in psychiatric disorder, remaining roughly double that found in the control group. Despite this finding the "dose response" relationship which had been so clearly revealed in the cognitive sphere was only weakly present, indicating that extrinsic factors are implicated in the presence and nature of the behavioural disturbance. Prior disturbance is a major determinant, such that children without prior abnormality achieve a 29% disorder rate, compared with 55% for those who had prior problems. Similarly, psychosocial adversity, a measure of poor home circumstances, was associated with a 60% disorder rate as compared with 14% for those enjoying more favourable home circumstances.

Is there a pattern to this postinjury disturbance? Most disorders were similar in extent to those found in other disturbed children, but social disinhibition was far more frequent. This involved undue outspokenness without regard to social convention, frequently asking embarrassing questions and making very personal remarks, and getting undressed in social situations. In passing, one should note that the much vaunted link between cerebral injury and hyperkinesis is not supported by this study, and a diagnosis of minimal cerebral dysfunction cannot be sustained on the finding of hyperkinesis alone. Some nonsignificant but suggestive differences are that overtalkativeness, bed-wetting, overeating, general slowness, and stuttering are all more frequent in the head-injury group. Another way of categorising these findings is by extent of posttraumatic amnesia, and those children in whom this extended for more than 22 days have higher rates of speech abnormality, refusal to cooperate, distractibility, and social disinhibition than controls.

Specific cognitive deficits were assessed with special tests, and in general these gave results which were similar to those found on the WISC, such that those who did well on the performance scale showed no deficits. A few children were revealed to have specific deficits despite intact performance intelligence. One year after injury the severe group was impaired on object-naming latency, a continuous performance vigilance task, manual dexterity, finger-tapping speed, and the Stroop test, which assesses susceptibility to distraction. More errors were also made on the Matching Familiar Figures task (Kagan, Rosman, Day, Albert, and Phillips, 1964), which assesses impulsivity, revealing that these children made their decisions slightly more speedily and significantly less accurately. At the final follow-up, $2\frac{1}{4}$ years postinjury, some new tests were introduced, and a simple copying task, similar to the Wechsler Coding subtest, revealed significant impairment for the injured group, but longer and more complex tasks which were intended to simulate school work failed to show significant impairment. The authors speculate that their efforts to motivate the child in the early part of the assessment carried over into the unsupervised complex tasks, and possibly failed to replicate the loose and self-paced context of school work.

11 Conclusions

Recent work on brain-damaged children has identified certain broad findings. Early injuries seem to be most damaging to overall levels of performance, while later damage is more likely to give rise to specific cognitive deficits. Tests in which new material must be learned are more sensitive indicators of potential impairment than well-rehearsed skills, but by no means all special tests show this sensitivity. Loss of consciousness is a crucial severity measure with an overwhelming effect on the postinjury outcome. Children who have received severe head injuries are far more likely than controls to show psychiatric disorders, but these disorders are for the most part like those of uninjured children. Social disinhibition was more frequent in the brain-injured group. Distractibility is a further characteristic of children who have suffered extensive loss of consciousness. In general, loss of consciousness is a sensitive index of the severity of damage, and impairment of apprehension and concentration are significant features of the behaviour of children who have received severe injuries.

References

Bond, M. R. (1975). Assessment of the psychosocial outcome after severe head injury. *In* "Outcome of Severe Damage to the Central Nervous System," (CIBA Foundation Symposium 34, new series). Excerpta Medica, Oxford.

Brooks, D. N. (1976). Wechsler Memory Scale performance and its relationship to brain damage after severe closed head injury. *Journal of Neurology, Neurosurgery and Psychiatry,* **39,** 593–601.

Brown, G., Chadwick, O., Shaffer, D., Rutter, M., and Traub, M. (1981). A prospective study of children with head injuries: III. Psychiatric sequelae. *Psychological Medicine,* **11,** 63–78.

Chadwick, O., Rutter, M., Brown, G., Shaffer, D., and Traub, M. (1981). A prospective study of children with head injuries. II. Cognitive sequelae. *Psychological Medicine,* **11,** 49–61.

Chadwick, O., Rutter, M., Shaffer, D., and Shrout, P. (1981). A prospective study of children with head injuries—IV. Specific cognitive deficits. *Journal of Clinical Neuropsychology,* **3**(2), 101–120.

Chadwick, O., Rutter, M., Thompson, J., and Shaffer, D. (1981). Intellectual performance and reading skills after localised head injury in childhood. *Journal of Child Psychology and Psychiatry,* **22,** 117–139.

Craft, A. W. (1975). Head injury in children. *In* "Handbook of Clinical Neurology" (Eds. P. J. Vinken and B. W. Bruyn), Vol. 23, pp. 445–458. New York, Wiley.

Eiser, C. (1981). Psychological sequelae of brain tumours in childhood: A retrospective study. *British Journal of Clinical Psychology,* **20,** 35–38.

Field, J. C. (1960). Two types of tables for use with Wechsler's intelligence scales. *Journal of Clinical Psychology,* **16,** 3–7.

Fisher, G. M., and Parsons, P. A. (1962). The effect of intellectual level on the rate of false positive diagnoses from the Hewson and Adolescent ratios. *Journal of Clinical Psychology,* **18,** 125–126.

Hebb, D. D. (1942). The effect of early and late brain injury upon test scores, and the nature of normal adult intelligence. *Proceedings American Philosophical Society,* **85,** 175.

Heller, M. D. A. (1963). "A Study of Psychiatric Patients Tested on the Wechsler Intelligence Scales; with Particular Reference to Children with Wide Discrepancies between Verbal and Performance I.Q.s." Unpublished D.P.M. Dissertation, Institute of Psychiatry, University of London.

Herbert, M. (1964). The concept and testing of brain damage in children: A review. *Journal of Child Psychology and Psychiatry,* **5,** 197.

Hewson, L. R. (1949). The Wechsler–Bellevue Scale and the Substitution Test as aids in neuro-psychiatric diagnosis. *Journal of Nervous and Mental Disease,* **109,** 158–183; 246–266.

Holbourn, A. H. S. (1943). Mechanics of head injury. *Lancet,* **2,** 438–441.

Hooper, R. (1969). "Patterns of Acute Head Injury." Arnold, London.

Jackson, J. H. (1874/1932). On the nature of the duality of the brain. *Med. Press,* **1,** 19. (Reprinted in "Selected Writings of John Hughlings Jackson" (Ed. J. Taylor), Vol. II, pp. 129–145. Hodder and Stoughton, London.)

Jennet, B. (1976). Assessment of severity of head injury. *Journal of Neurology, Neurosurgery and Psychiatry,* **39,** 647–655.

Kagan, J., Rosman, B. L., Day, D., Albert, J., and Phillips, W. (1974). Information processing the child: Significance of analytic and reflective attitudes. *Psychology Monograph,* **78,** 1–37.

McFie, J. (1961a). The effects of hemispherectomy on intellectual functioning in cases of infantile hemiplegia. *Journal of Neurology Neurosurgery and Psychiatry,* **24,** 240–249.

McFie, J. (1961b). Intellectual Impairment in children with localized post-infantile cerebral lesions. *Journal of Neurology Neurosurgery and Psychiatry,* **24,** 361–365.

Meyer, V. (1957). Critique of psychological approaches to brain damage. *Journal of Mental Science,* **103,** 80–i09.

Norris, H. (1960). The W.I.S.C. and Diagnosis of Brain Damage. Unpublished dissertation University of London Diploma, Abnormal Psychology.

Ommaya, A. K., and Gennarelli, T. A. (1974). Cerebral concussion and traumatic unconsciousness: Correlation of experimental and clinical observations on blunt head injuries. *Brain,* **97,** 633–654.

Rowley, V. N. (1961). Analysis of the W.I.S.C. performance of brain-damaged and emotionally disturbed children. *Journal Consulting Psychology,* **25,** 553.

Russell, W. R. (1971). "The Traumatic Amnesias" (Oxford Neurological Monographs). Oxford University Press, London.

Rutter, M. L., Chadwick, O., Shaffer, D., and Brown, G. (1980). A prospective study of children with head injuries—I. Design and methods. *Psychological Medicine.*

Rutter, M. L., Graham, P., and Yule, W. (1970). "A Neuropsychiatric Study in Childhood" (Clinics in Developmental Medicine. Nos. 35/36). Heinemann/S.I.M.P., London.

Shaffer, D., Chadwick, O., and Rutter, M. L. (1975). Psychiatric outcome of localised head injury in children. *In* "Outcome of Severe Damage to the Central Nervous System" (Eds. R. Porter and D. W. Fitzsimons), Ciba Foundation Symposium No 34. Elsevier, Amsterdam.

Strich, S. (1969). The pathology of brain damage due to blunt head injuries. *In* "The Late Effects of Head Injury" (Eds. A. E. Walker, W. F. Caveness, and M. Critchley), pp. 501–526. Thomas, Illinois.

Thompson, J. A. (1976). "Cognitive Effects of Cortical Lesions Sustained in Childhood." Unpublished Ph.D. Thesis, University of London.

Thompson, J. A. (1979). Intellectual impairment after childhood cortical injury. *In* "Research in Psychology and Medicine" (Eds. J. Osborne, M. M. Gruneberg, and J. R. Eiser). Academic Press, New York.

Ward, A. A. (1966). The physiology of concussion. *Clinical Neurosurgery,* **12,** 95–111.

3 Causes and Implications of Human Organic Memory Disorders

ANDREW MAYES

*Department of Psychology,
University of Manchester,
Manchester, England*

1 The Varieties of Organic Memory Disorders

Organic memory disorders in humans are usually described and classified in terms of theoretical notions derived from common sense or the experimental study of intact humans. These notions include first, the traditional trichotomy of memory into the stages of registration, storage, and retrieval. Second, they include the more recent view that information is held initially in a short-term store of limited capacity before being transferred into a large-capacity long-term store. Third, they include the idea that different kinds of material and different levels of processing may be mediated by largely independent memory systems.

Reliance on these notions to elucidate the nature of the amnesias faces several problems. First, proper description of some amnesias may be impossible without introducing new theoretical notions. Second, effects of the amnesias on postulated processes may be hard to show. For example, the three memory stages are intimately interdependent. Thus, variations in degree of learning influence both what is registered and how well it is stored, and the effect on memory also depends on the efficiency of later retrieval. These processes are very difficult to tease apart. Third, some of the theoretical ideas are polemical even within the context of studies with intact humans. It has been denied, for example, that both short- and long-term memory stores exist (see Wickelgren, 1974, who argues for a single store) and that semantic and episodic memory are distinct (Anderson and Ross, 1980). Careful study of the pattern of memory breakdown in the amnesias is therefore a useful means of testing, extending, and changing theories based on analysing learning and remembering in intact humans.

Memory disorders can roughly be divided into four groups, using the theoretical ideas enumerated in the first paragraph. *First,* various cortical lesions have been associated with selective short-term memory deficits. The most studied deficit is a disorder of auditory–verbal short-term memory, found in a sub-group of conduction aphasics (see Shallice and Warrington, 1977). These patients, with left parietal lobe lesions, have a disorder characterised by good comprehension and good spontaneous speech but very poor repetition of spoken language. They do badly on short-term memory tests, such as the Digit Span (WAIS) and Peterson tasks, as well as showing a loss of the recency, but not the primacy, component in free recall tasks. These cannot easily be interpreted as output problems because the patients also do badly at verbal short-term tasks, tested by probed recall and recognition, which minimise such problems. The failure is selective, however, since the patients perform within normal limits on short-term memory tests for visually presented verbal material, on auditory non-verbal material, and on long-term memory tests involving paired associates, story recall, and verbal free recall tasks. These claims of normal long-term memory and of a selective deficit in short-term memory have been challenged by Glanzer and Clark (1979). They argue, respectively, that more demanding tests of long-term memory need to be used and that the short-term memory failure may be a subtle output deficit, since Shallice and Warrington's patients performed normally on one matching test of auditory–verbal short-term memory.

Baddeley and Hitch (1974) argued that short-term memory comprises a number of systems which work together to facilitate perception, thinking, and comprehension. The complex was dubbed, appropriately, *working memory*. Shallice (1979) proposed that his subgroup of conduction aphasics had a selective deficit in the short-term verbal input buffer, which stores phonemically coded information. The rarity of paraphasic errors in spontaneous speech in one of the patients suggested that their articulatory loops were normal (Shallice and Butterworth, 1977). In contrast, they did poorly on the harder items in the Token tests, where comprehension of long, complicated, spoken instructions may depend on the ability to maintain phonemic representations over a few seconds. If correct, Shallice's claim that his patients have a selective deficit in their phonemic short-term memories is powerful evidence for the separate existence of an independent, specialized store, because other disorders (to be discussed) affect long-term but not short-term memory, thus creating a double dissociation. It may be, however, that the disorder results from a subtle breakdown in extracting phonemic information under overload conditions, in the face of subsequent normal extraction of semantic information. If so, then slowing the rate of information delivery should disproportionately improve short-term memory in these conduction aphasics. Even if there is a failure in phonemic storage it may not be specific to short-term memory. Storage of meaningless, phonemic inputs may be deficient when tested at long delays although there has been adequate time to process the inputs.

Evidence for other kinds of short-term memory is fragmentary. Thus, Warrington and Rabin (1971) described patients with posterior neocortical lesions, who had normal digit spans but impaired visual "spans of apprehension" for verbal and nonverbal material. Similar modality-specific short-term memory disorders have been reported by others. Thus, Butters *et al.* (1970) and Samuels *et al.* (1972) found that right parietal lesions caused poor recall of visually presented verbal and nonverbal material in the Peterson task, whereas auditorily presented stimuli were recalled normally. Left parietal lesions caused selective short-term memory deficits in both modalities. Finally, De Renzi and Nichelli (1975) have described a group of patients with right posterior lesions, like those of the Butters *et al.* (1970) subjects, who have normal auditory verbal spans but reduced memory spans for spatial locations.

The *second* group of memory disorders comprises cases in which cortical lesions have caused selective long-term memory deficits. It is generally supposed that complex information is stored in widely distributed and interconnected neocortical sites. Information within a particular modality or of a particular material kind may, however, be processed and stored within discrete cortical regions. De Renzi (1982) has argued that focal lesions of association neocortex may cause selective amnesia for faces, colours, or spatial location. Prosopagnosia (inability to recognise even familiar faces), for example, may, he argues, arise from perceptual or memory failure. Although some patients cannot match face photographs of a person taken from different angles or with different illumination or with disguises, others can but still show poor memory for new and old faces. Amnesia for colour in the absence of perceptual or verbal problems has proved harder to isolate; however, De Renzi (1982) believes that the inability to learn a new route or to take one's bearings from familiar surroundings may occur in the absence of global amnesia, and independently of scanning or perceptual problems.

De Renzi's cases display both anterograde and retrograde amnesia, that is, poor learning of new examples of the relevant kind of information and poor memory for such information acquired pretraumatically. If he is correct in proposing that the deficits are not due to perceptual failures and are truly specific, then two interpretations seem plausible. The first is that the specific processing and storage regions in the neocortex have been disconnected from limbic system structures, activity in which is vital for the storage and retrieval of effective memories. These limbic structures are lesioned in global amnesia, which is the fourth kind of memory deficit to be discussed in this chapter. The second interpretation is that the cortical lesions have partially destroyed the specific storage systems. Both interpretations may be true in different cases and to varying degrees.

The first interpretation has been supported by Ross (1980a), who described two cases of selective visual amnesia in patients with bilateral neocortical lesions. One patient had some blind fields, but the sighted fields appeared normal. Despite this he had loss of memory for all recent visual events. He could not draw a plan of the apartment into which he had moved since his stroke although his drawing of his parent's house, where he had lived before his stroke, was very accurate. Unlike De Renzi's cases, those of Ross had severe anterograde amnesia *but* very mild retrograde amnesia. Examination of the lesion suggested that the visual neocortex may have been disconnected from the limbic memory structures within the medial temporal lobe. Ross (1980b) also described three further patients, all with unilateral temporo-occipital cortical lesions, two of whom showed recent memory failure for right-sided tactile stimuli and verbal information, but not auditory nonverbal information, whereas the third had amnesia for left-sided tactile stimuli and auditory nonverbal information. The two cases had left hemisphere lesions and the third one had a right hemisphere lesion. Ross proposed that the sensory inputs were disconnected from their ipsilateral limbic memory structures and that some recovery might occur if these inputs were transferred via the cerebral commissures to the contralateral hemisphere.

Support for the second interpretation has also been claimed by De Renzi (1982) and Warrington (1975). Warrington described three patients with bilateral cortical atrophy who had a form of object agnosia. They appeared to have lost much information about the significance of objects and words. Although their ability to learn most things was severely impaired, Warrington argued that when learning placed minimum demands on semantic interpretation (as in learning abstract pictures) their memory reached normal levels. She proposed that the lesions had degraded the storage of long-established semantic memory. In more recent work Warrington (1981, 1982a) has described other neocortically lesioned patients with syndromes, which suggest that the storage of semantic information may be highly differentiated. One patient had a selective deficit in solving mental arithmetic problems, in which concepts like "quantity" and operations like multiplication were preserved, but problems were still solved slowly, inconsistently, and inaccurately. Warrington (1982a) argued that the patient had lost knowledge of overlearned arithmetical facts like "$2 \times 5 = 10$," access to which facilitates mental calculation. Similarly, Warrington (1981) reported patients who could not identify the meanings of concrete and abstract words, respectively, and suggested that these may be stored separately. It remains disputed, however, to what extent these syndromes are due to degradation of specific semantic stores and to what extent they are due to a failure of certain kinds of input to access a less differentiated store. Such a failure could arise from a high-level perceptual deficit, which is hard to differentiate from a pure memory loss (see Ratcliffe and Newcombe, 1982, for a discussion). This problem bedevils theoretical understanding of all organic problems.

The *third* group of memory problems is caused by prefrontal cortex damage. Although most workers believe that such damage is not associated with a general deficit in recognition and recall, there is evidence for two apparently different kinds of selective memory impairments. First, frontal lesions cause memory problems when good memory depends on elaborative encoding and/or retrieval strategies. This deficit can be related to claims that frontal patients show preservation of cognitive processes if these depend on the performance of routine operations but not if they require the spontaneous initiation and execution of detailed plans (see Shallice, 1982). Thus, Signoret and Lhermitte (1976) found that frontal patients were very poor at learning unrelated paired-associate words, but improved to within normal limits if directed in the use of mediating images. There is also some evidence that frontal lesions cause difficulty in retrieving pretraumatic episodes with no sparing of even the oldest memories. Thus, Albert *et al.* (1981) reported that patients with Huntington's chorea, who have frontal as well as neostriatal atrophy, have a mild retrograde amnesia which affects memory for public events and faces experienced decades before as much as for recently experienced events and faces. In contrast, patients with limbic system lesions showed relative sparing of very old memories. The results suggest that frontal lesions cause a deficit in the elaborative reconstruction of memories.

The second putative memory deficit linked to frontal lesions is specific to temporal or possibly spatiotemporal information. Thus, it has been shown that such patients have a selective difficulty in making memory judgements about item recency and frequency (Milner, 1971; Smith and Milner, 1983). They also tend to show recognition failures only when the task requires them to discriminate which of two items was experienced most recently, rather than simply judge whether an item has been experienced at all (for example, see Prisko, 1963). Whether spatial memory per se is impaired in human frontal patients remains to be properly demonstrated. Spatial memory deficits are frequently claimed in frontally lesioned monkeys, but these deficits are, in fact, usually of spatiotemporal memory, so they can be caused by poor temporal memory. It has been argued that spatiotemporal information is automatically encoded (Hasher and Zacks, 1979). As automatic encoding is supposed to require minimal attentional effort and not to be amenable to intentional modification, it is plausible to argue that the frontal deficit in temporal or spatiotemporal memory is independent of the deficit in memory for information that requires elaborative encoding and retrieval. If so, the two deficits should show a double dissociation with different frontal lesions. On the other hand, it could be that spatiotemporal information is encoded as a consequence of the elaborative encoding of meaning, such that the better the latter is encoded the more accurate will be spatiotemporal memory. If this is so, the two memory disorders will not be dissociable. Evidence of the independence of spatiotemporal memory and memory for target material, however, argues against this second possibility.

The *fourth* type of memory problem is global amnesia (sometimes called the amnesic or, loosely, Korsakoff's syndrome) and is the major theme of the rest of this chapter. It is caused by limbic–diencephalic rather than neocortical damage and is characterised by very poor learning and memory for new information (anterograde amnesia) in association with a variable degree of forgetting of pretraumatic information (retrograde amnesia). These memory failures may be found in conjunction with normal performance on short-term memory tasks, such as digit span, and normal cognitive abilities as assessed by tests such as the WAIS. Although apparently normal short-term memory and cognitive ability is found in "pure" cases of the amnesic syndrome, the memory disorders are usually found in association with unrelated perceptuocognitive failures caused by incidental damage to other brain regions, such as neocortex and brain stem.

Because global amnesics have been reported to learn and retain a variety of simple conditioning and perceptuomotor tasks (see Weiskrantz, 1982b), one might expect to find a fifth variety of human organic memory disorders in which memory for these tasks is poor despite good acquisition and retention of more complex memory. Relevant reports, if they exist, are rare for humans. Recent reports on classical conditioning in rabbits suggest, however, that cerebellar and brain stem lesions may selectively impair memory for simple tasks in humans as well. It has been shown that unilateral lesions of the lateral cerebellum in rabbits prevents learning, retention, and relearning of classical conditioning of the nictitating membrane response of the eye ipsilateral to the lesion, but does not affect the unconditioned response (see Lincoln *et al.*, 1982). Similar effects are found with pontine reticular formation lesions, and neurons in both structures seem to model the learned response (Lavond *et al.*, 1981). Even so, it remains to be shown whether these structures are involved in processing or storage, and whether lesions to them leave memory for more complex tasks unaffected.

The next sections will consider the various etiologies of global amnesia, and then the interrelated issues concerning the locus of the critical lesion in amnesia, whether there is more than one form of amnesia, and the pattern of memory performance seen in amnesia. It will then be possible to relate the brain regions, damage to which is critical in amnesia, to the memory functions probably impaired, and hence to infer what the functions of those regions are in the intact brain. Such speculation is facilitated by anatomical and physiological knowledge, which specifies the informational inputs and outputs of the critical regions. It is, however, impeded by uncertainty about the locus of the critical lesions, and by the methodological problems involved in distinguishing patterns of memory breakdown associated with lesions incidental to amnesia from lesions critical to it. It is also impeded by artifacts which arise from comparisons of poor amnesic memory with good normal memory (see Meudell and Mayes, 1982, for a detailed discussion). For example, amnesics sometimes fail to benefit from semantic cues but do so if their memory is made as good as control subjects by repetition (Wetzel and Squire, 1982).

The form of the syndromes reviewed in this section suggests that sensory information is processed, interpreted, and stored within the association cortex regions, with the frontal cortex playing a key role in integrating and elaborating complex, multimodal inputs. But the stable storage and retrieval of this information somehow depends on further processing, which occurs in one or more limbic–diencephalic system.

2 The Aetiologies of the Global Amnesic Syndrome and Its Diagnosis

Memory problems associated with the amnesic syndrome are relatively common in humans. This is, perhaps, because the critical limbic structures are unusually sensitive to physiological disturbances. Thus, apart from bilateral surgical removal of the medial temporal lobes in the treatment of epilepsy, global amnesia has been associated with chronic alcoholism, thiamine deficiency, nicotinic acid deficiency, anoxia, carbon monoxide poisoning, complications of viral and bacterial diseases such as herpes-induced encephalitis and tuberculous meningitis, strokes affecting, for example, the circulation of the posterior cerebral artery, midline tumours, closed head injury and accidents causing focal lesions, and both normal and abnormal ageing. Multiple electroconvulsive therapy (ECT) courses are also associated with a mild reversible amnesic state, and the transient global amnesic syndrome is believed by some to be caused by a temporary limbic system ischemia. (Fisher [1982], however, described 85 cases of transient global amnesia and noted that 26 cases were triggered by emotional episodes. He argued, therefore, that the syndrome is caused by an electrophysiological disturbance in the hippocampal system, and not by ischemia). Because many of these disturbances disrupt the hippocampal system and its connections, it is interesting to note that recent research suggests that mature rats, whose mothers were malnourished during pregnancy and throughout lactation, show a "hippocampal syndrome," in which they suffer cellular depletion of the hippocampus and learning problems with alternation and spatial-maze tasks (Jordan *et al.*, 1981, 1982).

Although limbic system sensitivity to a variety of physiological insults may explain the frequency of amnesiclike disorders, the detailed mechanisms through which the insults exert their effects are often controversial. It is disputed, for example, whether the critical brain damage in alcoholic amnesia is caused by the direct effects of alcohol ingestion or an associated thiamine deficiency. Research on animal models suggests that learning problems and limbic system damage may be caused by thiamine deficiency and the direct disturbance from ingesting alcohol (see Mayes and Meudell, 1983, for a fuller discussion). Extrapolations from such models to humans can only be made if the pattern of learning disturbance in the animals corresponds to that found in human global amnesics. This assumption has not been fully substantiated. Even so, alcoholic amnesics are behaviourally a heterogeneous group, so that it is likely that their condition has a complex and variable causation. They suffer from differing degrees of frontal cortex atrophy with associated cognitive impairments. This atrophy may be a direct effect of alcohol ingestion (see Thomson, 1982; Ron, 1982). An alcoholic amnesic's precise pattern of cognitive loss may therefore be a function of his sensitivity to thiamine (and other vitamin) deficiency and such factors as his style of drinking (see Mayes and Meudell, 1983).

Just as the amnesic syndrome is usually mixed with other cognitive deficits in alcoholic amnesics, so may the "pure" syndrome be associated with multiple cognitive failures in normal and abnormal ageing. The initial presenting symptom in the dementia known as Alzheimer's disease may be a selective failure of memory, but as the disease progresses this deficit is clouded by disturbances of visuospatial and verbal functions. Such overlap makes it difficult to determine the relationship between the cognitive deficits in both abnormal and normal ageing (where the same problems apply). There is growing evidence that Alzheimer's disease is, at least partially, a consequence of a progressive deterioration of function in basal forebrain cholinergic neurons (see Bartus *et al.*, 1982, for a discussion). Controlled studies suggest that such a deterioration in limbic system cholinergic neurons may cause an amnesic syndrome (see Mayes and Meudell, 1983, for a discussion). Memory failure in normal ageing may be caused by the relatively early deaths of such neurons. In Alzheimer's disease their death is presumably accelerated by an unidentified disease process. It is possible that the dementia may be a viral disease to which genetically predisposed individuals are susceptible. In this connection it is interesting to note that Crow (1982) has proposed that a proportion of schizophrenics, who display mainly negative symptoms (e.g., flattened affect) and respond poorly to drugs, also show a progressive dementia resembling Alzheimer's disease and suffer a progressive loss of limbic system neurons beneath the temporal lobes. Crow argues that this disorder may be virally transmitted.

Diagnosis of the causes of global amnesia depends ultimately on the correct identification of the behavioural syndrome. It might be argued, for example, that the nature of the memory failure in Alzheimer's disease is quite distinct from that in alcoholic amnesia or that following bilateral medial temporal lobe lesions. To resolve such doubts a universally available, sensitive, and discriminating memory test battery would need to be used. The nearest approximation to such a battery is the Wechsler Memory Scale (WMS). Amnesics are required to score appreciably lower on their normalised WMS than on the WAIS. Unfortunately, the WMS is overly sensitive to the short-term component of memory so that amnesics may score well on it and some nonamnesics may score badly (see Meudell and Mayes, 1982). A new battery needs to be standardised which assesses recognition and recall for both verbal and visual material, short-term memory, retrograde amnesia, and learning of a perceptuomotor task (which should be normal in "pure amnesics"). Until such a battery is generally used, and since diagnosis remains based on the WMS or clinical impression, one cannot be confident that the etiologies discussed in this section are all associated with the same kind of memory failure.

3 Location of the Critical Lesion(s) in Amnesia

The minimal lesion(s) critical to amnesia must be sufficient for the symptoms of memory failure to occur, without causing other cognitive deficits. The location of such lesion(s) is polemical for two main reasons. First, there have been hardly any human cases in which the memory deficit has been adequately described in life, which have received postmortem anatomical analysis. Most cases with good postmortem analysis relate to memory failure based on clinical impression. Such cases may possibly not be amnesic or may suffer incidental cognitive damage. When behavioural characterisation has been adequate and the memory failure selective, lesion location has generally been based on relatively insensitive *in vivo* techniques such as computed-axial-tomographic (CT) scanning. Second, although animal models do not face these problems, it has proved difficult to isolate patterns of learning deficits in animals which truly model human global amnesia.

The longest standing view has been that global amnesia arises from lesions of the hippocampus or of serially connected structures, with emphasis placed on the mamillary bodies and the fornical link and less certainly attached to the anterior thalamus and the cingulate cortex. Surgical lesions of the anterior temporal cortex, uncus, and amygdala were not found to cause amnesia unless the hippocampus was invaded. Indeed, with unilateral lesions, severity of amnesia correlated with degree of hippocampal removal (Milner, 1971). Attempts to refine the localisation of the lesion by studying hippocampal lesions in monkeys led, however, to confusion, since the animals did not show the expected learning failures (see Weiskrantz, 1982a). Two additional views of the lesion location subsequently emerged. First, Horel (1978) argued that damage to the temporal stem, linking temporal cortex to amygdala and diencephalic structures, is critical. Second, Mishkin (1978) proposed that combined hippocampal and amygdala lesions are necessary for the appearance of severe permanent amnesia for recognition and associative tasks. Both positions are compatible with the neurosurgical evidence, because amnesia-producing medial temporal operations destroy both temporal stem and the amygdala, as well as the hippocampus.

Criticism of the hippocampal hypothesis was also made by Victor *et al.* (1971). In their study of a large series of alcoholic amnesics, they reported five cases with mamillary body atrophy who did not show amnesia, whereas dorsomedial thalamic atrophy was invariably associated with amnesia. Two interpretations of this finding are plausible. First, destruction of both mamillary bodies and dorsomedial thalamic nucleus is necessary to cause severe, permanent amnesia. Destruction of either structure alone will only cause a mild, probably temporary, amnesia. Second, unless mamillary body destruction is total severe amnesia will only occur if there is extra damage to the dorsomedial thalamus (see Weiskrantz, 1982b). This leaves open the possibility of whether large lesions of the latter nucleus cause severe amnesia. There are reports of amnesia following selective dorsomedial thalamic damage (McEntee *et al.*, 1976; Squire and Moore, 1979; Speedie and Heilman, 1982). Conversely, Mair *et al.* (1979) have described two severe and "pure" amnesics, in whom postmortem analysis revealed no dorsomedial thalamic atrophy. Damage was not, however, confined to the mamillary bodies, because there was also atrophy in the paratenial nucleus. Apropos of Mishkin's (1978) hypothesis this region projects to, and perhaps receives projections from, the amygdala (see Weiskrantz, 1982b). So it remains uncertain whether mamillary body damage alone is sufficient to cause severe amnesia. Similar uncertainty surrounds the role of fornix lesions in amnesia. Squire and Moore (1979) reviewed 50 human cases with fornix lesions and found amnesia in only three cases. In these, damage may have extended into medial thalamus.

Available human data, therefore, do not clearly discriminate between the hippocampal hypothesis, the temporal stem hypothesis, and the view that severe amnesia requires lesions to both the hippocampal circuit and that of the amygdala. In this context, it is worth noting that as well as being bidirectionally linked to frontal neocortex, the dorsomedial thalamus is similarly linked to the amygdala and receives temporal stem projections. To discriminate among the three major hypotheses, recent research has used animal lesion models of amnesia. It was Mishkin (1978) who initially found that monkeys with combined hippocampal and amygdala damage performed much worse on a delayed nonmatching to sample task than did monkeys with either lesion alone. More recently Mishkin (1982) has extended this work with colleagues to show that combined lesions also impair memory for object–reward associations more severely than single lesions. In contrast to Gaffan (1974), no severe recognition impairments were found following fornix lesions. When these lesions were combined with amygdala damage, however, there was very poor performance in the delayed nonmatching to sample task. A similar disturbance was found when hippocampectomy was combined with stria terminalis (a major amygdala–diencephalic pathway) lesions. In an ingenious study, Mishkin disconnected the visual regions of the temporal neocortex (area TE) from underlying hippocampus and amygdala and found an equivalent disturbance of visual delayed nonmatching to sample. He therefore argued that recognition memory involves storage of interpreted inputs in temporal and other association cortices. For such storage to be stable, interpreted sensory information must be processed further in the hippocampal and amygdala circuits. These systems project to the anterior thalamus and dorsomedial thalamus, respectively, and Mishkin has found that a combined lesion of these thalamic nuclei also drastically impaired delayed-nonmatching-to-sample performance. Mishkin postulated two different versions of his hypothesis. In the first, processed information is fed back to association neocortex via reciprocal connections of the hippocampal and amygdala circuits. In the second, both systems feed into the midline thalamic nuclei, which modulate association cortex activity through their diffuse cortical projections. This second postulate is compatible with evidence from single-unit recording studies which have found "familiarity" neurons in the anterior midline nuclei (Perrett *et al.*, in press).

The effects of combined hippocampal–amygdala lesions have also recently been examined by another group and compared with the effects of temporal stem lesions (see Squire and Zola-Morgan, 1983, for an excellent review). It was found that the combined lesion drastically impaired delayed nonmatching to sample performance and minimally affected visual discrimination learning, whereas the reverse pattern of impairment was caused by temporal stem lesions (Zola-Morgan *et al.*, 1982). The experimenters argued that these results disconfirmed the temporal stem hypothesis, since monkeys with lesions of that structure showed effectively normal recognition but were impaired on a task which alcoholic amnesics perform normally (Oscar-Berman and Zola-Morgan, 1980). Their findings and the findings of other studies which they review reveal that monkeys with combined lesions not only perform badly on delayed-nonmatching-to-sample tasks, but also on concurrent learning and delayed-object-discrimination tasks. Although there is some evidence also that the combined lesion is more disruptive of delayed matching and object discrimination than are selective hippocampal lesions, Squire and Zola-Morgan (1983) cast some doubt on the appropriateness of the comparison. They argue that the selective hippocampal lesion often spares the anterior region of the structure, whereas this region is destroyed in the combined lesion. The latter lesion may therefore destroy critical hippocampal structures spared in the selective lesion.

If a lesioned animal is to model human amnesia, it must show good memory for tasks spared in human amnesics and poor memory for tasks that are not. Cohen and Squire (1980) have proposed that human amnesics are normal at procedural learning and memory but poor at declarative learning. The former involves the gradual acquisition of rules, memory for which can only be displayed indirectly in skilled behaviours, whereas the latter involves the often rapid acquisition of memories, the presence of which can be explicitly demonstrated. Squire and Zola-Morgan (1983) argue that delayed matching, concurrent learning, and object discrimination resemble declarative memory in their rapid acquisition and other respects, whereas monkeys' acquisition of visual discriminations is gradual and resembles procedural learning. Unlike Gaffan (1974) they argue that global amnesics may be poor at some kinds of associative memory as well as recognition. Human amnesics may remember procedural skills normally but fail to recognise that they are remembering. Therefore, monkey models of human amnesia should remember many tasks normally but be unable to discriminate whether they are guessing or remembering. Tests of this discrimination have not yet been devised (but see Weiskrantz, 1982a). Nevertheless, on balance, it would seem that hippocampal lesions may cause global amnesia in monkeys, and that the disturbance may be more severe with combined hippocampal and amygdala lesions. Further confirmatory evidence is necessary, however.

4 Is Global Amnesia a Unitary Disorder?

Although Mishkin (1982) believes that the amygdala and hippocampus are functionally equivalent in recognition memory, Squire and Zola-Morgan (1983) question this view, since they found little effect of amygdala lesions on delayed matching tasks (less than with hippocampal lesions). They also cite evidence that selective amygdala lesions do not cause recognition deficits in humans. Even Mishkin (1982) believes that the amygdala circuit may have a special role in forming learned associations. Jurko (1978) has shown, however, that combined left amygdala and center median lesions impair paired-associate learning, although the isolated lesions are ineffective. He suggested that the two structures mediated complementary functions. Even though it remains unresolved whether the amygdala and hippocampus mediate similar or complementary functions in recognition memory, their role in other kinds of learning, such as association learning, is probably distinct. As suggested above, such forms of learning may be impaired in global amnesia.

Apart from the material-specific amnesias caused by unilateral limbic system lesions (see Milner, 1971), the possibility that global amnesia comprises several distinct subforms associated with different lesions has only recently been acknowledged. Two dissociations have been proposed. The first is that medial temporal and diencephalic lesions cause distinct global amnesias. The second is that retrograde and anterograde amnesia may be dissociable. It has been shown with respect to the first putative dissociation, that alcoholic amnesics and patient N.A., who are believed to have diencephalic lesions, learn slowly but then forget at a normal rate (Huppert and Piercy, 1978a; Squire, 1981). In contrast, patient H.M. (who had bilateral medial temporal lobe lesions) and ECT patients (with possible temporal lobe dysfunction) not only learn slowly but also forget more rapidly even when equated for initial degree of learning (Huppert and Piercy, 1979; Squire, 1981). Zola-Morgan and Squire (1982) have reported a similar dissociation in monkeys. Lesioned monkeys were given 10–12 exposures to a sample stimulus in the delayed-nonmatching-to-sample task, so as to equate their performance following a 10-min delay to that of controls. Under these conditions, monkeys with combined amygdala and hippocampal lesions forgot abnormally fast over a day, whereas animals with medial thalamic lesions did not.

Some amnesics, such as case H.M. and ECT patients, show graded retrograde amnesias with abnormal forgetting extending only a few years into the pre-traumatic period (Cohen and Squire, 1981). These patients have putative medial temporal lobe dysfunction. In contrast, diencephalic amnesics with an alcoholic aetiology show retrograde amnesias. which extend back decades (Cohen and Squire, 1981), although this deficit may be a partial result of incidental frontal damage. Thus, Albert *et al.* (1981) have, as mentioned earlier, reported that patients with Huntington's chorea, who have frontal atrophy as well as neo-striatal damage, show a uniform amnesia for pretraumatic events regardless of their age. Temporally ungraded retrograde amnesia for personal episodes has also been reported in functional amnesia (Schacter *et al.*, 1982). As this is a reversible high-level dysfunction of retrieval, it may possibly involve a func-tional distortion of frontal cortex activity. Squire *et al.* (in press) have argued that the rapid forgetting and the graded retrograde amnesia of medial temporal am-nesics are directly linked, that is, disturbance of a prolonged consolidation func-tion underlies both deficits. On the other hand, anterograde and retrograde am-nesia may be dissociable in diencephalic amnesia (L. R. Squire, personal communication). This view is supported by the observations of Winocur *et al.* (1984) of an amnesic with bilateral thalamic lesions, who should not have suf-fered an additional frontal lesion. This patient showed anterograde amnesia in the absence of measurable retrograde amnesia. Speedie and Heilman (1982) have also reported a case in which a patient with a lesion of the left dorsomedial thalamus had an anterograde amnesia for verbal material but did not show mea-surable retrograde amnesia on the Selzer questionnaire. Mair *et al.* (1979) have, however, reported severe and ungraded retrograde amnesia in a diencephalic patient without any frontal atrophy, and the famous selective diencephalic case N.A. apparently has a mild, graded retrograde amnesia (Cohen and Squire, 1981).

It has also been claimed that retrograde amnesia may occur without anter-ograde amnesia. Goldberg *et al.* (1981) described a patient with very dense and extended retrograde amnesia, who did not show any clear signs of residual anterograde amnesia. This case was unusual because of the severity of the retrograde amnesia, which even affected old, much-rehearsed semantic memo-ries. There was, however, no evidence of destruction in the neocortical regions which might constitute the semantic store as the researchers believed that the critical lesion was located in the nonspecific cholinergic and noradrenergic sys-tems in the midbrain. Similar cases, with less severe amnesia, have been re-ported as results of vascular accidents, tuberculous meningitis, and closed head injury (see Wood *et al.*, 1982). Lesion location was not ascertained in these cases, all of which showed an initial anterograde amnesia. Andrews *et al.*, (1982) have, however, recently reported a case with a severe retrograde amnesia, extending back 40 years, without an initial anterograde amnesia. It has been argued that these cases are examples of a new syndrome, associated with a midbrain reticular lesion and an activational failure, which causes particularly severe retrograde amnesia (Goldberg *et al.*, 1982).

According to the view of Squire *et al.* (in press), in temporal lobe amnesia where the graded retrograde amnesia and rapid forgetting of anterograde amnesia are caused by a disturbance of the same mechanism, one would predict that retrograde amnesia will become more severe and prolonged as the duration and severity of anterograde amnesia increases. This is generally the case, and applies whether retrograde amnesia is temporary or permanent. For example, Brazier (1964) reported that electrical stimulation of the hippocampus produced a temporary amnesia, the extent of which was a function of duration of stimulation. Nonetheless, there are exceptions to this rule which have been reported in transient global amnesia. This disorder probably arises from a temporary disturbance of the temporal lobe, recovery is usually associated with a persistent amnesia which includes the entire episode and extends back from half an hour to over 8 hours into the pretraumatic period (Fisher, 1982). Wood *et al.* (1982) have described a case, however, in which retrograde amnesia extending back over years persisted after recovery of the ability to learn new information. The lesion in this case may have affected diencephalic regions. But Penfield and Mathieson (1974) reported that the duration of retrograde amnesia may be a function of the extent to which a lesion extends into the posterior hippocampus. This suggestion receives some corroboration from the work of Fedio and Van Buren (1974). They found that stimulation of the anterior temporal neocortex caused a selective anterograde amnesia in conscious patients, whereas more posterior stimulation caused a selective retrograde amnesia. They were, however, only looking at memory over a few seconds rather than the time scale relevant for Pensfield and Mathieson.

In summary, although Squire *et al.* (in press) may be correct about the association of anterograde and graded retrograde amnesia after damage to some parts of the medial temporal lobe, it remains an open possibility that other temporal and diencephalic (and midbrain) lesions cause selective retrograde and anterograde amnesias. If so, the mechanisms affected are almost certainly distinct from those disrupted in the amnesic syndrome described by Squire *et al.* As human data are likely to remain scanty and inconclusive, the best hope for resolving these issues lies in developing nonhuman primate models of retrograde amnesia.

5 Memory Performance in Amnesia and the Problem of Incidental Frontal Cortex Damage

Attempts to specify the cognitive and memory deficits and hence identify the disturbances responsible for limbic system amnesia are made harder because many amnesics have incidental damage to other structures, including the frontal neocortex. For example, at least 80% of amnesics with an alcoholic etiology have some degree of frontal atrophy (Butters, quoted in Moscovitch, 1982). Fortunately, very severe amnesia can be found without frontal atrophy even in alcoholic amnesias (Mair *et al.,* 1979). It may therefore be possible to distinguish between symptoms essential to amnesia and those incidental to it both by selecting amnesics with damage confined to limbic structures and by examining the effects of frontal lesions.

One influential hypothesis about the functional deficit in amnesia has proposed that the memory deficit of anterograde amnesia arises from a failure to encode spontaneously those features of stimuli the encoding of which, studies of normal subjects suggest, leads to good memory (Butters and Cermak, 1975). In particular, the hypothesis claims that, although amnesics can encode semantic features, they have a habitual tendency not to do so. The hypothesis may be extended to explain prolonged retrograde amnesia if it is supposed that there is also a failure to use semantic features during the retrieval process (although this extension cannot explain graded retrograde amnesia). Butters and Cermak based their hypothesis on observations of amnesics with alcoholic etiologies. For example, such amnesics failed to show release from proactive interference (PI) in the Wickens' paradigm following a semantic shift, although they did show release after an alphanumeric shift. More recently, this group found that their patients' recognition memory for faces approached normal levels when they were encouraged to encode mnemonically effective facial features (Biber *et al.,* 1981).

Similar findings have been reported in patients with frontal lesions. Thus, Moscovitch (1982) found that patients with unilateral frontal lesions failed to show PI release, whereas patients with unilateral temporal lobe lesions did. Consistent with this observation, Squire (1982) has found that alcoholic amnesics' deficit on this task correlates with their performance on "frontal" tests, such as the Wisconsin, and those involving verbal fluency and embedded figures. Furthermore, even when alcoholic amnesics fail to show release on the shift trial, they are usually aware there has been a shift but seem unable, at first, to use this awareness to help their memory (Winocur *et al.,* 1981). This kind of deficit is typical of many frontal patients. The view that alcoholic amnesics' failure to show PI release after semantic shifts arises from incidental frontal damage is also supported by findings of normal release in a patient with a lesion of the left medial thalamus and ECT patients (Squire, 1982), a postencephalitic amnesic (Cermak, 1976), and another amnesic without an alcoholic etiology (see Moscovitch, 1982). Warrington (1982b), however, has reported failure of release in several amnesics, at least one of whom seems not to have had appreciable frontal atrophy, so the issue is not conclusively resolved.

Frontal patients also show very poor learning of weakly associated word pairs, but this deficit largely disappears if the patients are shown how to go about constructing mediating images (Signoret and Lhermitte, 1976). Their memory problem therefore is a secondary consequence of their spontaneous failure to use effective encoding strategies just as has been claimed with alcoholic amnesics. It may be that alcoholic amnesics are only differentially helped by orienting tasks, intended to make them encode semantic and other mnemonically valuable information, if their memory deficit is predominantly caused by frontal cortex atrophy. This possibility is supported by the finding that for both verbal and nonverbal material, memory of a group of alcoholic amnesics was not disproportionately facilitated by orienting tasks, which focussed attention on mnemonically effective semantic features of stimuli (see Meudell and Mayes, 1982, for a review). This series of studies essentially compared memory following spontaneous learning and learning directed toward appropriate or inappropriate strategies in amnesic and control subjects. Although the orienting tasks influenced memory, they did so equally in both groups of subjects.

It is therefore probable that any amnesic problems in the encoding of mnemonically effective features are incidental complications of frontal atrophy. Such atrophy may impair the effortful processes involved in initiating and executing complex plans for learning and remembering. It has also been shown that alcoholic amnesics are disproportionately poor at making recency judgements (Squire, 1982) and that this deficit is related to the finding that alcoholic amnesics confuse recency and frequency judgements (Huppert and Piercy, 1978b; Meudell *et al.*, in preparation). This latter deficit is not a result of comparing poor amnesic with good normal memory, because normal subjects still fail to confuse frequency and recency judgements even when their memories are made as poor as those of amnesics by being tested after a long delay or by being given only brief learning exposures (Meudell *et al.*, in preparation). One might argue that memory failure (not just very poor recency judgements) in all amnesics with limbic system lesions is caused by a deficit in the (probably) automatic encoding of contextual features, particularly temporal ones.

The preceding hypothesis becomes less plausible in the light of Milner's (1971) report that frontal patients are very bad at making recency judgements. Furthermore, Squire (1982) found that the recency judgement deficit in his alcoholic amnesics correlated with performance on other tests impaired by frontal lesions. Squire *et al.* (1981) also found that patient N.A. and ECT patients did significantly better than alcoholic amnesics on recency judgement tests. They were required to judge in which of two lists recognised sentences had been shown, and their performance was compared to that of controls, who were tested at a longer delay so as to reduce their overall level of recognition to that of the amnesics. This was to ensure that poor amnesic recency judgements could not be a mere offshoot of their generally poor memory (the same procedure was used for alcoholic amnesics by Squire). In the event, N.A.'s and the ECT patients' recency judgements were as good as those of the controls.

Once again, therefore, it seems likely that a deficit ascribed to limbic system lesions is a result of incidental frontal damage. The issue is not certain, however, since it still needs to be shown that frontal patients confuse frequency and recency judgements when normal subjects do not. It is also not established convincingly that selective limbic system lesions do not cause a disproportionate problem in making recency judgements. Thus, Hirst (1982) reported that amnesics, with a nonalcoholic etiology, show a recency judgement deficit even when their recognition was matched to that of controls. It was claimed that these patients did not show frontal impairments, and Hirst therefore argued that amnesia is a deficit in automatic encoding of information. Further, it remains possible that N.A. and the ECT patients in the Squire *et al.* (1981) study may have had mild but disproportionate deficits in recency judgements, because the experimental matching procedure made the task harder for controls. Sentence lists were placed 3 min apart and the amnesics began testing 10 sec after list 2, whereas the controls began up to 90 min later. The ratio of list-spacing to the list-testing delay should have been constant to preserve list discriminability at the same level for the controls.

6 Nature of the Functional Deficit(s) in Amnesia

On balance, there is currently no strong evidence that deficits in certain kinds of effortful or automatic encoding processes cause memory failure in either medial temporal or diencephalic amnesics. Encoding problems, when they are found, are probably incidental results of frontal cortex or other nonlimbic system lesions. Although subtler encoding deficits may underlie amnesia it is more plausible to consider the possibility that the deficit is one involving the consolidation and/or maintenance of storage, or of retrieval. It is extremely difficult to tease apart the impaired functions by analyzing the pattern of good and bad memory in amnesics, but this is what has generally been tried. The exercise also depends critically on whether there are several limbic system amnesias and whether retrograde and anterograde amnesias are dissociable. The current status of these issues is not clearly resolved, as has been discussed. There are, however, generalisations about memory in anterograde amnesia, which probably apply to all amnesics, and hence may serve as convenient starting points for identifying the functional deficit(s) in amnesia.

All amnesics are poor at free recall or recognition of any verbal or nonverbal material, which they have recently been shown or given to learn. They do not find such recently presented material to be familiar. In contrast, it is claimed that amnesics learn and retain some tasks normally, although they usually fail to recognise the task they have learned or the materials used in the learning. This dissociation is often called the Claparède effect after the French neurologist who described an instance of it. Normal learning has been claimed for various motor tasks, classical conditioning, identifying degraded perceptual forms, solving jigsaw puzzles and scrambled sentences, learning a numerical rule, the Mc-Culloch illusion, and facilitation of stereoscopic perception of random-dot ster-eograms, as well as other motor–perceptual and cognitive tasks (see Weiskrantz, 1982a; Squire *et al.,* in press). Unfortunately, many of the relevant studies are incompletely reported or fail to include control groups, merely showing that amnesics can learn and retain these tasks. In some cases where controls were included it is apparent that amnesic learning was not completely normal (Brooks and Baddeley, 1976).

The demonstration of complete normality of learning and retention is impor-tant because Meudell and Mayes (1981) have shown that if the testing of control subjects is delayed for over a year, then they also show a Claparède effect, like amnesics, in which they retain the skill of finding shapes embedded in pictures without recognising many of the pictures. Skills may therefore be forgotten more slowly than recognition memory, and amnesics reach an advanced stage of forgetting more quickly. Fortunately, there have been two recent demonstrations of completely normal learning in amnesics. In the first, Cohen and Squire (1980) showed that N.A. and ECT patients and alcoholic amnesics learn and retain normally over 13 weeks the skill of reading mirror reversed words. Although they could read reversed novel words as well as controls, they were not quite as quick at reading previously shown words. This is, perhaps, because normal people can identify familiar reversed words not only by using a perceptual–cognitive skill but also by recognizing an old pattern. Amnesics can only use the acquired skill.

The second demonstration of normal learning and memory in amnesics shows, however, that they can acquire processing skills which apply not only generally to a class of stimuli but also to particular instances of the class. Jacoby and Witherspoon (1982) asked five controls and five alcoholic amnesics visually presented questions involving homophones. For example, "What is an example of a reed instrument?" Later, when asked to spell *read/reed,* subjects tended to give the low-frequency version related to the previous questions. The amnesics did so with a normal or above-normal probability. Even so, they failed to recog-nise the homophones involved in the earlier questions, that is, they showed a Claparède effect. These results not only show that amnesics may acquire both specific and generic information normally, they also suggest that the normal subjects were not using additional strategies dependent on recognition memory. Indeed, Jacoby and Witherspoon found that even in control subjects priming and recognition memory dissociated, in that subjects' priming and recognition were unrelated, that is, whether priming occurred could not be predicted by whether or not a word was recognised. However, it might be argued that the above-normal amnesic tendency reflected the fact that normals' recognition memory inhibited the automatic priming of their spelling.

It is interesting to note that amnesics have been reported to show normal cued recall for recently shown words in the absence of recognition, when cued with the words' first three letters (for example, see Warrington and Weiskrantz, 1974, 1978; Mayes and Meudell, 1981a). Cued recall in normals is typically very poor in these studies, and when their cued recall is better amnesics no longer match them and are not aided differentially by cues (Mayes *et al.,* 1978; Wetzel and Squire, 1982). It is therefore plausible to argue that three-letter cueing often fails to involve recognition and reconstructive abilities and depends more on automatic priming processes, activated by word exposure, which is similar to the kinds of priming shown by Jacoby and Witherspoon (1982). These priming processes are the only ones preserved fully in amnesics' cued recall.

The learning abilities spared in amnesics may form a diverse group although they have been characterised as instances of knowing how rather than knowing that—procedural versus declarative memory (see Squire *et al.,* in press). Such learning may be characterised by its gradual acquisition and by the fact that its presence may only be revealed in action (often skilled action) rather than explicitly declared or displayed. Nevertheless, it probably includes processes as diverse as classical conditioning and cognitive skills, which may be mediated by distinct brain regions. All that is shared may be independence from the limbic memory structures. Contrary to the view of some this independence is not shared by semantic memory, if this is defined as recognisable knowledge, comprising our mental dictionaries and encyclopedias. Amnesics show poor acquisition of new semantic memories and often have some retrograde amnesia for semantic information acquired pretraumatically provided this was not massively overlearned. Their problems, therefore, extend to recall and recognition of both semantic and episodic information. What functions mediate these forms of memory, impairment of which leaves unaffected the kinds of memory spared in amnesics?

One popular suggestion has been that amnesics have selectively poor retrieval because of their excessive sensitivity to interference from competing memories (Warrington and Weiskrantz, 1974; Weiskrantz and Warrington, 1975). On this view, one would predict a retrograde amnesia in which the most distant memories were disturbed as badly as the most recent, but this conflicts with the majority of the evidence, according to which there is sparing of the oldest memories even in the prolonged retrograde amnesias of alcoholic amnesias and some postencephalic amnesias (see Cohen and Squire, 1981). Evidence for this view as it applies to anterograde amnesia came from reports that amnesics may show good cued recall in the face of poor recognition (see Warrington and Weiskrantz, 1974). Amnesics may also show approximately normal learning of strongly related paired-associate words, like "soldier–rifle" (Winocur and Weiskrantz, 1976; Morris *et al.,* in press). Paired-associate learning involves cued recall with semantic cues. It was argued that cues in these tasks were effective because they reduced the number of acceptable competing responses to around 10 words or less and hence massively reduced the degree of interference. This interpretation predicts that the fewer acceptable responses there are, which are associated with each cue, the greater will be the benefit amnesics receive relative to normal subjects. The prediction has not, however, been confirmed (see Warrington and Weiskrantz, 1978). Furthermore, good cued word recall and poor recognition has been found in normal subjects, when their memory is weakened either by testing at long delays or giving them very brief learning exposures (Woods and Piercy, 1974; Squire, Wetzel, and Slater, 1978; Mortensen, 1980; Mayes and Meudell, 1981b). Similarly, retention of highly associated as opposed to moderately associated word pairs has been shown to be differentially preserved over a week (Mayes, Meudell, and Som, 1981). One interpretation of these results is that good cueing is a general feature of poor recognition memory and so may reveal little about the causes of amnesia. The source of amnesics' poor recognition would have to be sought elsewhere.

Even so, the situation in which amnesics show good cued recall has been used to demonstrate their susceptibility to interference in another way. Subjects have learned a first list and then been required to learn a second competing list. For example, with three-letter cues the first list might contain words like "stamp" and the second list words like "station," and with paired-associate learning the first list might contain pairs like "Army–Soldier" and the second list pairs like "Army–Rifle." Several studies have found that although amnesics learn the first list to near normal levels, they (unlike normals) are unable to learn the second list and continue to produce intrusion errors from the first list (Winocur and Weiskrantz, 1976; Warrington and Weiskrantz, 1978; Morris *et al.*, in press). Interpretation of these results is made trickier in light of the criticisms made in the previous paragraph. In terms of the original view that amnesics are excessively susceptible to interference, the findings are corroborative. The view must require, however, that only recognition memory is exposed to high levels of interference and that forms of learning, spared in amnesia, are not. No justification is available for this assumption. Indeed, recognition as distinct from recall (both forms of recognition memory in the above sense) is not very sensitive to interference (see Baddeley, 1976).

There are, however, two other interpretations of the interference results. First, it can be argued that just as good cued recall is a general feature of all poor recognition memory so is high susceptibility to PI. Once again, one could argue that the causes of poor recognition memory in amnesics should be sought elsewhere. The other interpretation iterates what was suggested earlier in this section, namely, good amnesic cued recall for words (and by extension paired-associates) depends on intact automatic priming (a form of spared memory), which is found in the presence of very poor recognition memory. If correct, it would seem that this form of memory is in fact *very* susceptible to PI unless this is moderated by the influence of recognition memory. Amnesics lack this second kind of memory and so do worse than controls in learning the second list. This view actually proposes that priming (and maybe skill learning in general) is very hard to modify unless there is conscious guidance from recognition memory. The sensitivity of priming to PI may be related to the fact that this kind of learning is "context bound." Amnesics have, for example, very poor recall of strongly associated word pairs if they are tested in a different environmental context from that of learning (Winocur and Kinsbourne, 1978). A similar effect is seen in normal subjects tested at a long delay when their recognition memory has weakened (Mayes *et al.,* 1981). The suggestion that priming and skill memory are more susceptible than episodic and semantic memory to contextual shifts requires further testing.

Preliminary support for the above suggestions can be derived from studies of lexical priming, exposure effects on aesthetic judgement, and the priming of spelling, which may be closely related to cued recall in amnesics. Relative to recognition of words, these forms of memory are insensitive to increases of retention interval, decreases in learning exposure, and levels of processing at encoding (see Scarborough, Cortese, and Scarborough 1977; Kurst-Wilson and Zajonc, 1980; Jacoby and Dallas, 1981; Jacoby and Witherspoon, 1982). These observations are consistent with findings in which control subjects, tested after a long delay or after inadequate learning opportunity show, like amnesics, relatively good cued recall and poor recognition. There is also evidence that priming effects are very sensitive to the form of presentation of material at learning and test, which may be related to amnesic susceptibility to contextual shift with paired-associate memory (see Jacoby and Witherspoon, 1982). Sensitivity of these tasks to PI has not yet been studied.

We are, however, currently testing a variant of the view that learning spared in amnesia is very sensitive to PI. One would predict that the cued recall of normal subjects is more susceptible to PI when their recognition memory is attenuated, because they, like amnesics, may only be using priming to achieve cueing. We are currently testing this possibility but have found little evidence of increased PI susceptibility in normals with poor memory. More important, however, neither have we found that amnesics are more susceptible to PI in this paired-associate task (Mayes and Meudell, in preparation). The explanation of these results is unknown, although it probably relates to the conditions which determine whether cued recall is mediated more by priming or recognition memory mechanisms.

Poor learning of second lists by amnesics in cued recall A–B, A–C paradigms only tends to become apparent after a number of trials. The phenomenon should, therefore, perhaps not be interpreted as excessive PI sensitivity but as a species of perseveration. It is well established that hippocampally lesioned animals are slow to extinguish tasks which they acquired normally (see Weiskrantz and Warrington, 1975). Spence (1966) noted that generally humans show much more rapid extinction of classically conditioned responses than animals and argued that this was because their responses were modulated by recognition memory. His argument received support from a study of eye-blink conditioning in which subjects were kept ignorant of the purposes of the experiment. They extinguished the conditioned responses slowly. One would therefore expect that amnesics will acquire classically conditioned responses normally, but extinguish them abnormally slowly, because they lack the modulatory influence of recognition memory (see Weiskrantz, 1982b). Perseveration (rather than PI sensitivity) should therefore be seen as a consequence of amnesics' poor recognition (and poor recognition in general) rather than its cause. Identification of the features of episodic and semantic memory which make them vulnerable to amnesia still needs to be made, therefore.

A recent attempt to do this is the suggestion that amnesia is caused by a disconnection of a semantic memory system in the temporal cortex from a cognitive mediating system in the frontal cortex (Warrington and Weiskrantz, 1982). Episodic memory is dependent on the elaborative and automatic encoding of contextual and other features, for which the frontal cortex is responsible. Semantic memory, except that which has been massively rehearsed, may also depend on the encoding of contextual and other features, which are encoded partly via frontal cortex activities. In amnesics, such encoding should occur, but because the information is not then processed by the lesioned limbic system structures, it is not properly stored and/or properly retrieved (retrieval may require cooperation between frontal and limbic system structures). Simpler kinds of memory which do not lead to recognition (i.e., are not associated with feelings of familiarity) do not depend for their encoding (and perhaps retrieval) on frontal mechanisms. They are therefore spared in amnesia. Weiskrantz (1982b) also proposes that amnesics may also have a disconnection of the frontal mediating system from the midbrain–cerebellar systems, which subserve simple learning (e.g., classical conditioning). This disconnection would not disturb the basic expression of these forms of learning, but rather, their expression in more complex paradigms, such as extinction or latent inhibition.

The strong form of the above view should predict similar effects on memory from frontal lesions and certain limbic system ones. Even assuming that elaborative encoding was made impossible by frontal lesions, which is contrary to the evidence (see Signoret and Lhermitte, 1976), it is generally accepted that frontal patients show good memory for many materials, for example, faces, for which amnesics have very poor memory. The hypothesis also predicts that amnesics should be able to encode elaboratively, but not reliably store the encoded features. This means that they should perform semantic and other high-level orienting tasks normally, but not benefit mnemonically. In fact, high-level orienting tasks have been found not to improve the memory of alcoholic amnesics (Cermak and Reale, 1978; Wetzel and Squire, 1980), to improve it to the same extent as is found for control subjects (Mayes *et al.,* 1978; see Meudell and Mayes 1982 for a review), and to improve it differentially in alcoholic amnesics (Biber *et al.,* 1981). Paradoxically, it seems probable that both the inefficacy of the orienting tasks and their differential efficacy are related to incidental frontal lesions in this group of amnesics (see Mayes and Meudell, 1983). There is, therefore, no strong evidence that limbic system lesions cause special problems with the storage of elaborative encoding. The suggestion is nevertheless bold and original and warrants more rigorous testing.

It is, however, perhaps more plausible to argue that in amnesia information from both temporal and frontal association cortices fails to receive mnemonically essential processing from limbic structures. There is strong evidence, for example, that the hippocampus receives interpreted single-modality and multimodal inputs from temporal association cortex and that there are reciprocal outputs to the projecting cortical sites, probably after further limbic system processing (see Van Hoesen, 1982, for a review). Consistent with this pattern of connections, it is reported that right temporal amnesics can generate visual images and perform well on tests of perceptual encoding, such as the closure test for faces, but are unable to make proper mnemonic use of such encoding (see Milner, 1980). Imagery and perceptual encoding is probably a function of temporal and occipitotemporal neocortex. We need, however, to learn far more about which neocortical regions mediate what kinds of encoding and whether memory for these encoded features is similarly impaired in amnesics. Squire *et al.* (in press) have argued that the interaction between the neocortical regions, where storage probably occurs, and the structures of the medial temporal regions is necessary for the development and maintenance of memory for up to a few years following learning. This medial temporal role in prolonged storage explains why lesions to the structure cause rapid forgetting and a steeply graded retrograde amnesia a few years in extent. Some forms of spared memory may require cortical storage, but will only involve "tuning" or modification of existing representations, rather than the creation of new ones, and this makes them independent of the medial temporal processing system.

Wickelgren (1979) has developed a similar view of medial temporal function which requires memories to continue developing over a period of several years. Squire *et al.,* (in press) main evidence for this process of prolonged consolidation or memory change is based on the pattern of retrograde amnesia in ECT patients. Old memories were tested by examining knowledge of television programmes which had been shown for only 1 year. This test meets the central criterion of equivalence, that is, items were learned to about the same degree and then forgotten at equal rates (Squire and Fox, 1980). ECT patients showed abnormal memory only for items up to 1 or 2 years old—older memories were normally retained. Furthermore, memory for 1- or 2-year-old items was *worse* than for older items (Squire and Cohen, 1979). The disturbance could not, therefore, be only of that subgroup of memories which are remembered only for a short time and which therefore should be disproportionately represented among more recent memories. It must affect all fairly recent memories which are undergoing some prolonged process of change. Although Bartlett (1932) argued that memories change with time so as to become more schematic and less specific, this kind of change does not seem to be involved in the ECT study. Squire and Cohen (1979), in fact, found that ECT disrupted memory for both "schematic" and specific information, if this is recent, but for neither if they were acquired in a distant period. If these results generalise to patients with permanent lesions of the medial temporal regions, then the limbic structures must be associated with different kinds of prolonged consolidatory change.

The nature of the prolonged consolidation and the role of the medial temporal structures remain uncertain. Wickelgren (1979) has proposed that when "free" cortical neurons become part of the storage representation of a new information chunk they gradually become disconnected from arousing hippocampal influences, which would otherwise lead them to be involved in forming new chunks—the gradual disconnection protects them from interference. A more active role is suggested by the Squire *et al.* (in press) view that medial temporal cortex is necessary for a while to maintain the coherence of cortical memories, perhaps by storing the "addresses" of such memories. One might even propose that these "addresses" are temporospatial contexts, partially encoded by frontal cortex, thus creating a rapprochement with Warrington's and Weiskrantz's (1982) hypothesis. Information from associational temporal cortices and frontal cortex may interact in the medial temporal limbic structures, and these structures may temporarily retain a record of part of the interaction—a record which may somehow address the cortically stored memory. It remains to be explained, however, why it ceases to be necessary after a while to maintain memory coherence in this way, particularly if the gradual change is not related to the increasing schematisation of memory as Squire's and Cohen's (1979) study suggests. Because the view that old memories are somehow freed of their contextual origins is so attractive, the generalisability of this study's finding clearly needs to be examined.

Some further discussion of the view that amnesics forget because they cannot use temporospatial and other contextual information is warranted. It is also relevant to consider the implications of this view for semantic and episodic memory. If contextual information does become less important for retrieving semantic and episodic information with the passage of time, this process may not be associated with the loss of *specificity* in information and therefore may be independent of the Bartlettian process in which memories become increasingly schematic. For example, as time passes I may still remember exactly what happened when I fell downstairs on my twenty-first birthday, or remember precise details of French history, but no longer need to use contextual information in retrieving these memories. This would account for the graded retrograde amnesia in medial temporal amnesics if they cannot use contextual information. Acquisition of concepts (a form of semantic memory) probably involves the storage of individual instances, which are context dependent, so both semantic and episodic learning is impaired in amnesics. As time passes memory for the individual instances fails, but the concept remains. Later instances of the concept will have two effects. First, they will produce an episodic memory, but not in amnesics. Second, they will strengthen or ''prime'' the concept, and this process will be spared in amnesics. This second process does not, however, allow semantic representations to change qualitatively and, a fortiori, be created de novo. This account of concept acquisition suggests that concepts are formed slowly by a process impaired in amnesics, and that abstraction occurs because many details of individual instances are eventually forgotten, leaving as a residue what they have in common. Retrieval of the residue and surviving instances will, through rehearsal, become increasingly context free.

What is the evidence that medial temporal amnesics cannot use contextual information? Studies of hippocampally lesioned animals have often been interpreted as showing a contextual processing deficit (see Cormier, 1981). In this chapter, however, it has been argued that human amnesics who display disproportionate problems with recency judgements (and by inference contextual information) do so because of incidental frontal damage. Furthermore, Squire and Cohen (1982) found that amnesic recognition of low-frequency events was not less impaired than that for high-frequency events. If inability to use contextual information underlay the amnesic problem, then low-frequency events should have been better recognised, because retrieval of these events places a minimal strain on use of temporal and spatial features. The apparent conflict of human and animal studies requires resolution.

If, as Squire *et al.* (in press) argue, diencephalic lesions cause a distinct amnesic deficit one must look for other functional failures. The possibility of multiple deficits is consistent with Mishkin's (1982) framework. Not only are there parallel processing pathways through hippocampal and amygdala systems, but there may be feedback loops direct from the medial temporal structures, or later from the medial thalamic structures. It also remains possible that retrograde and anterograde deficits are distinct in diencephalic amnesia. A subtle encoding deficit might underlie the anterograde deficit in diencephalic amnesia although, as already discussed, there is no good evidence for this. Alternatively, the structures may modulate consolidation in the immediate period after learning, either by influencing arousal (perhaps via the nonspecific midline thalamic nuclei) or modulating hormonal activity. Mayes *et al.* (1980) have, indeed, reported that alcoholic amnesics display abnormally low levels of electroencephalographic (EEG) power, but only in the period immediately after word presentation. It remains to be proved that this deficit is related to their poor memories.

Alcoholic amnesics usually show prolonged retrograde amnesias with some sparing of the most distant memories (see Cohen and Squire, 1981). This pattern could be caused by a retrieval deficit arising from incidental frontal damage, which acts in combination with the effects of an anterograde amnesia, getting gradually worse over many years. This prolonged but graded retrograde amnesia may be very different from that caused by selective diencephalic lesions. Such lesions may cause no retrograde amnesia, mild but graded retrograde amnesia, or an ungraded amnesia that may be severe or mild. The cases described by Winocur *et al.* (1984) and Speedie and Heilman (1982) are compatible with there being no impairment. Case N.A. has an impairment compatible with a mild, graded retrograde amnesia, and the two cases described by Mair *et al.* (1979) suggests that there may be a severe, ungraded impairment. Clearly the data are inconclusive and this reinforces the conclusion, made at the end of Section 4, that we need to develop a nonhuman primate model of retrograde amnesia. Even so, some of the inconsistency in the human data may depend on whether lesions involve both mammillary bodies and the dorsomedial nucleus of the thalamus, or only the latter. Whatever the resolution of these issues, diencephalic lesions probably cause processing and/or EEG abnormalities at encoding, and they may also affect aspects of later storage and retrieval as well.

Two final comments will be made before concluding this section. First, several dissociable memory disorders are consequent on specific brain lesions. If, as seems possible, these damaged brain regions mediate the disturbed functions in intact brains, and if the physiological efficiency of these regions emerges selectively through genetic transmission, then one might predict that normal people will show a corresponding set of specific memory abilities. For example, there may be specific memory abilities for colours, faces, and locations, and some people may forget faster than others even when matched for initial degree of learning.

Second, the search for functional deficits in amnesia may be fertilised by, as well fertilise, studies of intact humans. For example, Kunst-Wilson and Zajonc (1980) showed that very brief exposures to polygons changed subjects' aesthetic preferences for the shapes without creating any recognition memory. It might be suggested that any kind of memory, which is minimally impaired by reducing learning exposure in intact subjects, will be spared in amnesics. Another example is Mandler's (1980) research on recognition in normal people, which led him to propose that recognition may depend on two mechanisms: a sense of direct familiarity, which is a function of intraevent integrative processes, and some kind of contextual retrieval, which is a function of interevent elaborative processes. It may be asked whether one or both these processes is impaired in amnesics or, indeed, whether the syndrome and normal memory can be construed in these terms. For example, if the direct sense of familiarity is sufficient for recognition and involves facilitation of the processes of perception—a kind of priming—one should expect it and recognition to be normal in amnesics, but this is clearly not the case.

7 Is Amnesia Caused by a Remediable Biochemical Lesion?

Attempts to alleviate severe global amnesia through the use of better learning strategies and mnemonics are unsuccessful because the patients forget everything, including the mnemonics. Milder amnesics may, however, be more helped by these means, and even severe amnesics may be trained on some skills useful for their rehabilitation. Greater benefits may, in future, be achieved through the use of drug therapy. McEntee and Mair (1978, 1980) showed that a group of alcoholic amnesics had reduced levels of the norepinephrine metabolite 3-methoxy-4-hydroxyphenylglycol (MHPG) in their lumbar spinal fluid. The deficit correlated with the patients' WAIS–WMS discrepancy. Administration of clonidine, a putative α-adrenergic agonist, improved performance on the Peterson task and increased digit span. Although interesting, these findings do not show drug-induced improvements in long-term memory, and it is unlikely that the noradrenergic deficit is responsible for the amnesia (see Mayes and Meudell, 1983, for further discussion).

Weingartner *et al.* (1981) have also reported that administration of vasopressin at the time of learning may improve human memory. The improvement may occur not only in normal subjects but also in ECT patients, and possibly in chronic amnesics (see Mayes, 1983, for a review). It is possible that the hormone is acting centrally on the limbic system neurons responsible for mediating memory, because there is evidence that they contain vasopressin and are modulated by its action (see Mayes, 1983). It should be noted, however, that vasopressin primarily acts as a modulator of norepinephrine activity.

There is growing evidence that Alzheimer's disease, and particularly its associated global amnesia, are related to low levels of the enzymes choline acetyltransferase and acetylcholinesterase, particularly in regions such as the hippocampus (see Bartus *et al.*, 1982, for discussion). The disease may originate in the degeneration of isodendritic neurons of the basal forebrain. These neurons project widely to neocortical and limbic system neurons so that their death may cause widespread dysfunction and later neural death in these latter systems. Whitehouse *et al.* (1982) have, for example, shown that Alzheimer's patients may have a very high degree of neural loss in Meynert's nucleus within the substantia innominata—an isodendritic structure influencing widespread neocortical neurons through its cholinergic projections. Changes in cholinergic markers have also been noted following normal ageing in humans and animals (see Bartus *et al.*, 1982). Drachman (1977) has complemented these observations by modelling dementia in intact subjects who have received the anticholinergic drug scopolamine. The subjects' impaired memory and performance IQ was reversed by physostigmine, but not by the arousing effects of amphetamine. It therefore seems plausible that medial temporal amnesia (and possibly diencephalic as well) is partly caused by a cholinergic lesion. Transient amnesia can also be induced by injections of benzodiazepines (Brown *et al.,* 1982), and it is believed that this group of drugs, like the anticholinergics, may act on medial temporal structures such as the hippocampus. These drug models of global amnesia may then be specifically of medial temporal amnesia. If so, they should be associated with temporally graded retrograde amnesias. This possibility has not been extensively explored, but Brown *et al.* (1982) reported *no* impairment in memory for material learned prior to injection.

Cholinergic agonists and precursors, such as arecoline, physostigmine, choline, and lecithin have been found to improve memory in young humans and animals. Physostigmine and arecoline has also been found to improve memory in aged humans and animals, although the optimal dose seems to vary greatly among individuals (see Bartus *et al.,* 1981, for a review). Although physostigmine and arecoline have been found to improve memory in Alzheimer's disease (see Christie *et al.,* 1981), results with choline and lecithin are more variable. It seems that in the aged and patients with Alzheimer's disease improvements are more consistent the more directly one stimulates appropriate cholinergic receptors. This may be because such subjects suffer from multiple deficits which prevent the conversion of choline to acetylcholine and the release of the latter. This possibility is supported by the finding that memory for passive avoidance is markedly improved in elderly rats by combined treatments with choline and piracetam (a drug which stimulates aspects of neuronal metabolism), although neither drug alone has much effect (Bartus *et al.,* 1981). Encouraging results have also been found in a preliminary study of patients with Alzheimer's disease, and preliminary results with rats suggest that the combined drug treatment may particularly increase hippocampal levels of choline and acetylcholine (see Bartus *et al.,* 1981). It may be found, therefore, that combined drug treatments, which correct several metabolic faults, reliably and significantly improve memory in both medial temporal and diencephalic amnesia. If such treatments can be developed without serious side effects, even severe amnesia may become remediable to some degree.

Coda

Since this chapter was completed in the latter half of 1982, research findings have become available that extend or modify some of its conclusions. Some of these findings will be briefly described here as they relate to the chapter's contents and arguments. First, in connection with possible selective deficits in some forms of procedural memory as considered in Section one, Martone *et al.* (in press) have shown that patients with Huntington's chorea were retarded in learning the skill of reading mirror-reversed words, although their verbal recognition was apparently within normal limits and certainly better than that of patients with Korsakoff's syndrome. Second, although the neuro-anatomical basis of amnesia remains highly controversial, Mishkin's conjoint lesion hypothesis remains a strong contender as it has recently been claimed that separate lesions of the anterior and dorsomedial thalamic nuclei cause only very mild impairments on delayed nonmatching to sample although the combined lesions have a severe effect (Aggleton and Mishkin, 1983). Also, J. P. Aggleton (personal communication) has reported that mamillary body lesions cause an insignificant deficit with this task although others believe the deficit may be greater (S. Zola-Morgan, personal communication). If Mishkin is right and damage to both of two complementary circuits is necessary to produce severe, permanent amnesia, then his view may be compatible with a modified form of the context-memory deficit hypothesis of amnesia. Lesions of the hippocampal–fornix–mammillary body–anterior thalamus circuit may cause spatial memory deficits, whereas lesions of the amygdala–stria terminalis—dorsomedial thalamus circuit may cause deficits in temporal memory and perhaps event-reinforcement associations. In isolation these contextual memory deficits are insufficient to cause severe amnesia, but, if present together, recognition of target material will be very poor. Furthermore, this hypothesis can be extended to encompass possible differences between diencephalic and medial temporal amnesia. These amnesias could represent distinct kinds of failure in memory for the same kinds of contextual information. Similarly, if retrograde and anterograde amnesias are dissociable, a similar argument may be applied to explain them as distinct contextual memory deficits.

Mishkin's hypothesis is, however, not unequivocally proved, and there are serious grounds for doubting the contextual memory deficit hypothesis (for example, frontal lesions seem to cause contextual memory deficits without affecting recognition for target items). It remains a serious possibility that amnesia comprises one or more kinds of functional deficit that affect equally all those forms of information relevant to recognition. Assessment of this nonspecific hypothesis and the context-memory deficit view depends in part on the nature of preserved memory in amnesia. This is a third area in which there have been some important advances. With respect to cued recall and memory for related paired-associates it has been shown that amnesic performance is usually normal only if nonmemory instructions are given (Graf *et al.*, 1984; Shimamura and Squire, submitted for publication). Amnesics performed normally if told to generate the first word that came to mind, beginning with a three-letter cue for a list word or, if told, to free-associate to a word that was a stimulus word in the learning list. When memory instructions were used amnesics did worse than controls. In the experiments concerned, this "priming" memory had disappeared after 2 hours for both amnesics and controls. These findings have several implications for theories of amnesia. They confirm that normal amnesic memory in these tasks does not reflect a form of "propped up" recognition memory but, rather, is a kind of priming similar to that identified by Jacoby and Witherspoon (1982). Therefore, as argued in the chapter, normal amnesic "cued recall" reveals little about the causes of the poor memory of such persons. If memory instructions are given and floor and ceiling effects avoided, then initial letter cueing and memory for paired-associates is usually worse in amnesics. This shows that their recognition memory is probably impaired even when memory cues are given. Therefore, evidence that amnesics have increased sensitivity to proactive interference and contextual shifts in these tasks may be an artifact of their poor recognition. If priming is not modulated by recognition it may be very sensitive to proactive interference and contextual shifts. Finally, the 2-hour delay time for one form of initial letter priming indicates that simulation effects in which normal subjects, tested at long delays, show good cued recall relative to recognition, must be caused by something other than priming. Given that cued recall is determined by recognition memory as well as priming, it may be that different aspects of recognition are lost at different rates. The problem of determining the contribution of priming and recognition to tasks on which amnesics perform around normal levels has not, however, been fully resolved.

Drug trials continue to be run, mainly with cholinergic drugs and on patients with Alzheimer's disease, without very encouraging results. It becomes of increasing interest, therefore, to determine to what extent various drugs model organic amnesias. Little has been done with anticholinergic agents, but Brown *et al.* (1983) have recently shown that lorazepam does not cause retrograde amnesia, nor does it increase rate of forgetting. It would be interesting to see whether anticholinergics accelerate forgetting as these drugs are more likely to mimic the effects of medial temporal lobe damage.

References

Aggleton, J. P., and Mishkin, M. (1983). Memory impairments following restricted medial thalamic lesions in monkeys. Experimental Brain Research, **52**, 199–209.

Albert, M. S., Butters, N., and Brandt, J. (1981). Patterns of remote memory in amnesic and demented patients. *Archives of Neurology,* **38**, 495–500.

Anderson, J. R. and Ross, B. H. (1980). Evidence against a semantic–episodic distinction. *Journal of Experimental Psychology: Human Learning and Memory,* **6**, 441–466.

Andrews, E., Poser, C., and Kessler, M. (1982). Retrograde amnesia for forty years. *Cortex,* **18**, 441–458.

Baddeley, A. D. (1976). "The Psychology of Memory." Harper and Row, New York.

Baddeley, A. D., and Hitch, G. (1974). Working memory. *In* "The Psychology of Learning and Motivation" (Ed. G. H. Bower), Vol. 8, pp. 47–80.

Bartus, R. T., Dean, R. L., III, Beer, B., and Lippa, A. S. (1982). The cholinergic hypothesis of geriatric memory dysfunction. *Science,* **217,** 408– 417.

Biber, C., Butters, N., Rosen, J., Gerstman, L., and Mattis, S. (1981). Encoding strategies and recognition of faces by alcoholic Korsakoff and other brain-damaged patients. *Journal of Clinical Neuropsychology,* **3,** 315–330.

Brazier, M. A. B. (1964). Stimulation of the hippocampus in man using implanted electrodes. *In* "Brain Function: RNA and Brain Function, Memory and Learning" (Ed. M. A. B. Brazier), Vol. 2. University of California Press, Berkeley.

Brooks, D. N., and Baddeley, A. D. (1976). What can amnesic patients learn? *Neuropsychologia,* **14,** 111–122.

Brown, J., Brown, M. W., and Bowes, J. B. (1983). Effects of lorazepam on rate of forgetting, on retrieval from semantic memory and on manual dexterity. *Neuropsychologia,* **21,** 501–512.

Brown, J., Lewis, V., Brown, M., Horn, G., and Bowes, J. B. (1982). A comparison between transient amnesias induced by two drugs (diazepam and lorazepam) and amnesia of organic origin. *Neuropsychologia,* **20,** 55–70.

Butters, N., and Cermak, L. (1975). Some analyses of the amnesic syndromes in brain-damaged patients. *In* "The Hippocampus " (Eds. R. Isaacson and K. Pribram), Vol. 2. Plenum, New York.

Butters, N., Samuels, I., Goodglass, H., and Brody, B. (1970). Short-term visual and auditory memory disorders after parietal and frontal lobe damage. *Cortex,* **6,** 440–459.

Cermak, L. S. (1976). The encoding capacity of a patient with amnesia due to encephalitis. *Neuropsychologia,* **14,** 311–326.

Cermak, L. S., and Reale, L. (1978). Depth of processing and retention of words by alcoholic Korsakoff patients. *Journal of Experimental Psychology: Human Learning and Memory,* **4,** 165–174.

Christie, J. E., Shering, A., Ferguson, J., and Glen, A. I. M. (1981). Physostigmine and arecoline: Effects of intravenous infusions in Alzheimer presenile dementia. *British Journal of Psychiatry,* **138,** 46–50.

Cohen, N. J., and Squire, L. R. (1980). Preserved learning and retention of pattern-analyzing skill in amnesia: Dissociation of knowing how and knowing that. *Science,* **210,** 207–210.

Cohen, N. J., and Squire, L. R. (1981). Retrograde amnesia and remote memory impairment. *Neuropsychologia,* **19,** 337–356.

Cormier, S. M. (1981). A match–mismatch theory of limbic system function. *Physiological Psychology,* **9,** 3–36.

Crow, T. J. (1982). Two syndromes in schizophrenia? *Trends in Neurosciences,* **5,** 351–354.

De Renzi, E. (1982). Memory disorders following focal neocortical damage. *Philosophical Transactions of the Royal Society, London B,* **298,** 73–83.

De Renzi, E., and Nichelli, P. (1975). Verbal and non-verbal short-term memory impairment following hemispheric damage. *Cortex,* **11,** 341–354.

Drachman, D. (1977). Memory and cognitive function in man: Does the cholinergic system have a specific role? *Neurology,* **27,** 783–790.

Fedio, P., and Van Buren, J. M. (1974). Memory deficits during electrical stimulation of the speech cortex in conscious man. *Brain and Language,* **1,** 29–42.

Fisher, C. M. (1982). Transient global amnesia: Precipitating activities and other observations. *Archives of Neurology,* **39,** 605–608.

Gaffan, D. (1974). Recognition impaired and association intact in the memory of monkeys after transection of the fornix. *Journal of Comparative and Physiological Psychology,* **86,** 1100–1109.

Glanzer, M., and Clark, E. O. (1979). Cerebral mechanisms of information storage: The problem of memory. *In* "Handbook of Behavioural Neurobiology" (Ed. M. S. Gazzaniga), Vol. 2. Plenum, New York.

Goldberg, E., Antin, S. P., Bilder, Jr., R. M., Gerstman, L. J., Hughes, J. E. O., and Mattis, S. (1981). Retrograde amnesia: Possible role of mesencephalic reticular activation system in long-term memory. *Science,* **213,** 1392–1394.

Goldberg, E., Hughes, J. E. O., Mattis, S., and Antin, S. P. (1982). Isolated retrograde amnesia: Different etiologies, same mechanisms? *Cortex,* **18,** 459–462.

Graf, P., Squire, L. R., and Mander, G. (1984). The information that amnesic patients do not forget. *Journal of Experimental Psychology: Learning, Memory and Cognition,* **10,** 164–178.

Hasher, L., and Zacks, R. T. (1979). Automatic and effortful processes in memory. *Journal of Experimental Psychology (General),* **108,** 356–388.

Hirst, W. (1982). The amnesic syndrome: Descriptions and explanations. *Psychological Bulletin,* **91,** 435–460.

Horel, J. A. (1978). The neuroanatomy of amnesia: A critique of the hippocampal memory hypothesis. *Brain,* **101,** 403–445.

Huppert, F. A., and Piercy, M. (1978a). Dissociation between learning and remembering in organic amnesia. *Nature (London),* **275,** 317–318.

Huppert, F. A., and Piercy, M. (1978b). The role of trace strength in recency and frequency judgements by amnesic and control subjects. *Quarterly Journal of Experimental Psychology,* **30,** 346–354.

Huppert, F. A., and Piercy, M. (1979). Normal and abnormal forgetting in amnesia: Effect of locus of lesion. *Cortex,* **15,** 385–390.

Jacoby, L. L., and Dallas, M. (1981). On the relationship between autobiographical memory and perceptual learning. *Journal of Experimental Psychology: General,* **3,** 306–340.

Jacoby, L. L., and Witherspoon, D. (1982). Remembering without awareness. *Canadian Journal of Psychology,* **36,** 300–324.

Jordan, T. C., Cane, S. E., and Howells, K. F. (1981). Deficits in spatial memory performance induced by early undernutrition. *Developmental Psychobiology*, **14**, 317–325.

Jordan, T. C., Howells, K. F., McNaughton, N., and Heatlie, P. L. (1982). Effects of early undernutrition on hippocampal development and function. *Research in Experimental Medicine*, **180**, 201–207.

Jurko, M. F. (1978). Center median "alerting" and verbal learning dysfunction. *Brain and Language*, **5**, 98–102.

Kunst-Wilson, W. R., and Zajonc, R. B. (1980). Affective discrimination of stimuli that cannot be recognised. *Science*, **207**, 557–558.

Lavond, D. G., McCormick, D. A., Clark, G. A., Holmes, D. T., and Thompson, R. F. (1981). Effects of ipsilateral rostral pontine reticular lesions on retention of classically conditioned nictitating membrane and eyelid responses. *Physiological Psychology*, **9**, 335–339.

Lincoln, J. S., McCormick, D. A., and Thompson, R. F. (1982). Ipsilateral cerebellar lesions prevent learning of the classically conditioned nictitating membrane/eyelid response. *Brain Research*, **242**, 190–193.

McEntee, W. J., Biber, M. P., Perl, D. P., and Benson, D. F. (1976). Diencephalic amnesia: A reappraisal. *Journal of Neurology, Neurosurgery and Psychiatry*, **39**, 436–441.

McEntee, W. J., and Mair, R. G. (1978). Memory impairment in Korsakoff's psychosis: A correlation with brain noradrenergic activity. *Science*, **202**, 905–907.

McEntee, W. J., and Mair, R. G. (1980). Memory enhancement in Korsakoff's psychosis by clonidine: Further evidence for a noradrenergic deficit. *Annals of Neurology*, **7**, 466–470.

Mair, W. G. P., Warrington, E. K., and Weiskrantz, L. (1979). Memory disorders in Korsakoff's psychosis: A neuropathological and neuropsychological investigation of two cases. *Brain*, **102**, 749–783.

Mandler, G. (1980). Recognizing: The judgement of previous occurrence. *Psychological Review*, **87**, 252–271.

Martone, M., Butters, N., Payne, M., Becker, J. T., and Sax, D. S. (in press). Dissociations between still learning and verbal recognition in amnesia and dementia. *Archives of Neurology*.

Mayes, A. R. (1983). The development and course of long-term memory. *In* "Memory in Animals and Humans" (Ed. A. R. Mayes). Van Nostrand Reinhold, Wokingham.

Mayes, A. R., and Meudell, P. R. (1983). Amnesia in man and other animals. *In* "Memory in Animals and Humans" (Ed. A. R. Mayes). Van Nostrand Reinhold, Wokingham.

Mayes, A. R., Boddy, J., and Meudell, P. R. (1980). Is amnesia caused by an activational deficit? *Neuroscience Letters*, **18**, 347–352.

Mayes, A. R., and Meudell, P. R. (1981a). How similar is immediate memory in amnesic patients to delayed memory in normal subjects? A replication, extension and reassessment of the amnesic cueing effect. *Neuropsychologia,* **19,** 647–654.

Mayes, A. R., and Meudell, P. R. (1981b). How similar is the effect of cueing in amnesics and in normal subjects following forgetting? *Cortex,* **17,** 113–124.

Mayes, A. R., Meudell, P. R., and Neary, D. (1978). Must amnesia be caused by either encoding or retrieval disorders? *In* ''Practical Aspects of Memory'' (Eds. M. M. Gruneberg, P. E. Morris, and R. N. Sykes). Academic Press, London.

Mayes, A. R., Meudell, P. R., and Som, S. (1981). Further similarities between amnesia and normal attenuated memory: Effects with paired-associate learning and contextual shifts. *Neuropsychologia,* **19,** 655–664.

Meudell, P. R., and Mayes, A. R. (1981). The Claparède phenomenon: A further example in amnesics, a demonstration of a similar effect in normal people with attenuated memory and a reinterpretation. *Current Psychological Research,* **1,** 75–88.

Meudell, P. R., and Mayes, A. R. (1982). Normal and abnormal forgetting: Some comments on the human amnesic syndrome. *In* ''Normality and Pathology in Cognitive Functions'' (Ed. A. W. Ellis). Academic Press, London.

Milner, B. (1971). Interhemispheric differences in the localization of psychological processes in man. *British Medical Bulletin,* **27,** 272–277.

Milner, B. (1980). Complementary functional specializations of the human cerebral hemisphere. *In* ''Nerve cells, Transmitters and Behaviour'' (Ed. R. Levi-Montaliani). Pontificia Academia Scientiarum, Vatican City.

Mishkin, M. (1978). Memory in monkeys severely impaired by combined but not separate removal of amygdala and hippocampus. *Nature, London,* **273,** 297–298.

Mishkin, M. (1982). A memory system in the monkey. *Philosophical Transactions of the Royal Society, London B,* **298,** 85–95.

Morris, R. G., Welch, J. L., and Britton, P. G. (in press). The effects of interference on paired associate learning in presenile dementia. *Neuropsychologia.*

Mortensen, E. L. (1980). The effects of partial information in amnesic and normal subjects. *Scandinavian Journal of Psychology,* **21,** 75–82.

Moscovitch, M. (1982). Multiple dissociations of function in amnesia. *In* ''Human Memory and Amnesia'' (Ed. L. S. Cermak). Erlbaum, Hillsdale, New Jersey.

Oscar-Berman, M., and Zola-Morgan, S. (1980). Comparative neuropsychology and Korsakoff's syndrome. II. Two choice visual discrimination learning. *Neuropsychologia,* **18,** 513–528.

Penfield, W., and Mathieson, G. (1974). Memory: Autopsy findings and comments on the role of hippocampus in experimental recall. *Archives of Neurology,* **31,** 145–154.

Perrett, D. I., Caan, W., Rolls, E. T., and Wilson, F. (in press). Thalamic neuronal responses related to visual recognition. II. Memory characteristics.

Prisko, L. (1963). Short-term memory in focal cerebral damage. Ph.D. thesis, McGill University, Montreal, Quebec.

Ratcliff, G., and Newcombe, F. (1982). Object recognition: Some deductions from the clinical evidence. *In* "Normality and Pathology in Cognitive Functions" (Ed. A. W. Ellis). Academic Press, London.

Ron, M. A. (1982). Syndromes of alcohol-related brain damage. *British Medical Bulletin*, **38**, 91–94.

Ross, E. D. (1980a). Sensory-specific and fractional disorders of recent memory in man. I. Isolated loss of visual recent memory. *Archives of Neurology*, **37**, 193–200.

Ross, E. D. (1980b). Sensory-specific and fractional disorders of recent memory in man. II. Unilateral loss of tactile recent memory. *Archives of Neurology*, **37**, 267–272.

Samuels, I., Butters, N., and Redio, P. (1972). Short term memory disorders following temporal lobe removals in humans. *Cortex*, **B**, 283–298.

Scarborough, D., Cortese, C., and Scarborough, H. (1977). Frequency and repetition effects in lexical memory. *Journal of Experimental Psychology: Human Perception and Performance*, **3**, 1–17.

Schacter, D. L., Wang, P. L., Tulving, E., and Freedman, M. (1982). Functional retrograde amnesia: A quantitative case study. *Neuropsychologia*, **20**, 523–532.

Shallice, T. (1979). Neuropsychological research and the fractionation of memory systems. *In* "Perspectives on Memory Research" (Ed. L-G Nilsson). Erlbaum, Hillsdale, New Jersey.

Shallice, T. (1982). Specific impairments of planning. *Philosophical Transactions of the Royal Society, London, B.* **298**, 199–209.

Shallice, T., and Butterworth, E. K. (1977). Short-term memory impairment and spontaneous speech. *Neuropsychologia*, **15**, 729–735.

Shallice, T., and Warrington, E. K. (1977). Auditory–verbal short-term memory impairment and conduction aphasia. *Brain and Language*, **4**, 479–491.

Shimamura, A. P., and Squire, L. R. (1984). Paired-associate learning and priming effects in amnesia: A neuropsychological study. Submitted for publication.

Signoret, J-L., and Lhermitte, F. (1976). The amnesic syndromes and the encoding process. *In* "Neural Mechanisms of Learning and Memory" (Eds. M. R. Rosenzweig and E. L. Bennett). M.I.T. Press, Cambridge, Massachusetts.

Smith, M. L., and Milner, B. (1983). Effects of focal brain lesions on sensitivity to frequency of occurrence. Society for Neuroscience Abstracts, 9.

Speedie, L. J., and Heilman, K. M. (1982). Amnesic disturbance following infarction of the left dorsomedial nucleus of the thalamus. *Neuropsychologia*, **20**, 597–604.

Spence, K. (1966). Cognitive and drive factors in the extinction of the conditioned eye blink in human subjects. *Psychological Review*, **73**, 445–458.

Squire, L. R. (1981). Two forms of human amnesia: An analysis of forgetting. *The Journal of Neuroscience*, **1**, 635–640.

Squire, L. R. (1982). Comparisons among forms of amnesia: Some deficits are unique to Korsakoff syndrome. *Journal of Experimental Psychology: Learning, Memory and Cognition*, **8**, 560–571.

Squire, L. R., and Cohen, N. (1979). Memory and amnesia: Resistance to disruption develops for years after learning. *Behavioral and Neural Biology*, **25**, 115–125.

Squire, L. R., and Cohen, N. J. (1982). Human memory and amnesia. *In* "Handbook of Behavioral Neurobiology" (Eds. J. McGaugh and R. Thompson). Plenum, New York.

Squire, L. R., Cohen, N. J., and Nadel, L. (in press). The medial temporal region and memory consolidation: A new hypothesis. *In* "Memory Consolidation" (Eds. H. Weingartner and E. Parker). Erlbaum, Hillsdale, New Jersey.

Squire, L. R., and Fox, M. M. (1980). Assessment of remote memory. Validation of the television test by repeated testing during a seven-year period. *Behavioural Research Methods and Instrumentation*, **12**, 583–586.

Squire, L. R., and Moore, R. Y. (1979). Dorsal thalamic lesion in a noted case of chronic amnesic dysfunction. *Annals of Neurology*, **6**, 503–506.

Squire, L. R., Nadel, L., and Slater, P. C. (1981). Anterograde amnesia and memory for temporal order. *Neuropsychologia*, **19**, 141–146.

Squire, L. R., Wetzel, C. D., and Slater, P. C. (1978). Anterograde amnesia following ECT: An analysis of the beneficial effects of partial information. *Neuropsychologia*, **16**, 339–348.

Squire, L. R., and Zola-Morgan, S. (1983). The neurology of memory: The case for correspondence between the findings for man and nonhuman primates. *In* "The Physiological Basis of Memory" (Ed. J. A. Deutsch), 2nd edition. Academic Press, New York.

Thomson, A. D. (1982). Alcohol-related structural brain changes. *British Medical Bulletin*, **38**, 87–94.

Van Hoesen, G. W. (1982). The parahippocampal gyrus: New observations regarding its cortical connections in the monkey. *Trends in Neurosciences*, **5**, 345–350.

Victor, M., Adams, R. D., and Collins, G. H. (1971). "The Wernicke–Korsakoff Syndrome. A Clinical and Pathological Study of 245 Patients, 82 with Post-mortem Examinations." Blackwell, Oxford.

Warrington, E. K. (1975). The selective impairment of semantic memory. *Quarterly Journal of Experimental Psychology*, **27**, 635–657.

Warrington, E. K. (1981). Concrete word dyslexia. *British Journal of Psychology,* **72,** 175–196.

Warrington, E. K. (1982a). The fractionation of arithmetical skills: a single case study. *Quarterly Journal of Experimental Psychology,* **34A,** 31–52.

Warrington, E. K. (1982b). The double dissociation of short and long-term memory deficits. *In* "Human Memory and Amnesia" (Ed. L. S. Cermak). Hillsdale, New Jersey.

Warrington, E. K., and Rabin, P. (1971). Visual span of apprehension in patients with unilateral cerebral lesions. *Quarterly Journal of Experimental Psychology,* **23,** 423–431.

Warrington, E. K., and Weiskrantz, L. (1974). The effect of prior learning on subsequent retention in amnesic patients. *Neuropsychologia,* **12,** 419–428.

Warrington, E. K., and Weiskrantz, L. (1978). Further analysis of the prior learning effect in amnesic patients. *Neuropsychologia,* **16,** 169–177.

Warrington, E. K., and Weiskrantz, L. (1982). Amnesia: A disconnection syndrome? *Neuropsychologia,* **20,** 233–248.

Weingartner, H., Gold, P., Ballenger, J. C., Smallberg, S. A., Summers, R., Rubinow, D. R., Post, R. M., and Goodwin, F. K. (1981). Effects of vasopressin on human memory functions. *Science,* **211,** 601–603.

Weiskrantz, L. (1982a). Some aspects of the neuropsychology of memory in animals and humans. *In* "Neuropsychology After Lashley" (Ed. J. Orbach). Erlbaum, Hillsdale, New Jersey.

Weiskrantz, L. (1982b). Comparative aspects of studies of amnesia. *Philosophical Transactions of the Royal Society, London B,* **298,** 97–109.

Weiskrantz, L., and Warrington, E. K. (1975). The problem of the amnesic syndrome in man and animals. *In* "The Hippocampus" (Eds. R. L. Isaacson and K. H. Pribram), Vol. 2. Plenum, New York.

Wetzel, C. D., and Squire, L. R. (1980). Encoding in anterograde amnesia. *Neuropsychologia,* **18,** 177–184.

Wetzel, C. D., and Squire, L. R. (1982). Cued recall in anterograde amnesia. *Brain and Language,* **15,** 70–81.

Whitehouse, P. J., Price, D. L., Struble, R. G., Clark, A. W., Coyle, J. T., and De Long, M. R. (1982). Alzheimer's disease and senile dementia. Loss of neurons in the basal forebrain. *Science,* **215,** 1237–1239.

Wickelgren, W. A. (1974). Single trace fragility theory of memory dynamics. *Memory & Cognition,* **2,** 775–780.

Wickelgren, W. A. (1979). Chunking and consolidation: A theoretical synthesis of semantic networks, configuring in conditioning, S–R versus cognitive learning, normal forgetting, the amnesic syndrome, and the hippocampal arousal system. *Psychological Review,* **86,** 44–60.

Winocur, G., and Kinsbourne, M. (1978). Contextual cueing as an aid to Korsakoff amnesics. *Neuropsychologia,* **16,** 671–682.

Winocur, G., Kinsbourne, M., and Moscovitch, M. (1981). The effects of cueing on release from proactive interference in Korsakoff amnesic patients. *Journal of Experimental Psychology: Human Learning and Memory,* **1,** 56– · 65.

Winocur, G., Oxbury, S., Roberts, R., Agnetti, V., and Davis, C. (1984). Amnesia in a patient with bilateral lesions to the thalamus. *Neuropsychologia,* **22,** 123–143.

Winocur, G., and Weiskrantz, L. (1976). An investigation of paired associate learning in amnesic patients. *Neuropsychologia,* **14,** 97–110.

Wood, F., Ebert, V., and Kinsbourne, M. (1982). The episodic–semantic memory distinction in memory and amnesia: Clinical and experimental observations. *In* "Human Memory and Amnesia" (Ed. L. S. Cermak). Erlbaum, Hillsdale, New Jersey.

Woods, R. T., and Piercy, M. (1974). A similarity between amnesic memory and normal forgetting. *Neuropsychologia,* **12,** 437–445.

Zola-Morgan, S., and Squire, L. R. (1982). Two forms of amnesia in monkeys: Rapid forgetting after medial temporal lesions but not diencephalic lesions. *Society for Neuroscience Abstracts,* **8.**

Zola-Morgan, S., Squire, L. R., and Mishkin, M. (1982). The neuroanatomy of amnesia: Amygdala–hippocampus versus temporal stem. *Science,* **218,** 1337–1339.

4 Neuropsychological Implications of Epilepsy*

CARL B. DODRILL

*Department of Neurological Surgery,
University of Washington School of Medicine,
Seattle, Washington, U.S.A.*

1 Introduction

This chapter deals with a disorder which has significant implications for the study of consciousness. Not only the disorder but also its treatment can produce alterations in consciousness of significance and of practical interest. While the result is often a difficulty in separating the effects of the disorder from its treatment, epilepsy provides a unique setting for studying alterations in consciousness and a basis for hypotheses which may have broader applicability.

In this chapter, the nature of epilepsy will first be discussed along with its etiology and other seizure history variables. A comprehensive method to evaluate changes in neuropsychological functioning will also be described. Attention will then turn to important electroencephalographic (EEG) studies and to the assistance which they offer in providing an index to the degree of consciousness at any moment in time. The implications of antiseizure medications with respect to alterations in consciousness will then be reviewed. Finally, the chapter will close with a section on conclusions and implications.

In this chapter, the term *consciousness* will be used simply to refer to the awareness and integrative responsiveness of the organism to impressions made by the senses. Of particular interest are changes in responsiveness, and epilepsy is a disorder in which many such changes are observed. Such changes may be identifiable by neuropsychological tests. Thus, using results of neuropsychological tests as a basis, this chapter will present data on one particular disorder, with broader implications for an understanding of consciousness. In this way, the

*This project was supported by NIH Grants NS-17277, 17111, and 04053 awarded by the National Institute of Neurological and Communicative Disorders and Stroke, Public Health Service, Department of Health and Human Services, Washington, D.C.

information presented is designed to complement that which is given in other chapters of this volume.

2 Nature of Epilepsy

Epilepsy may be simply defined as a disorder characterized by recurrent seizures. *Seizures* are paroxysmal and episodic events that result from abnormal discharges of cerebral origin and which have a wide variety of manifestations. The best accepted classification is the International Classification of Epileptic Seizures (Gastaut, 1970). In this classification, the majority of seizures are divided according to whether the entire cerebrum is involved from the outset of the seizure or whether only a portion of it is involved. Seizures which involve the entire cerebrum from the outset are called generalized seizures, and seizures which involve only a part of the cerebrum either at the outset of the seizure or throughout the seizure are called partial seizures. Both types of epilepsy are of interest with respect to a study of consciousness, but in different ways. Generalized seizures may take the form of absence attacks (petit mal), myoclonic episodes, infantile spasms, clonic seizures, tonic seizures, atonic seizures, and tonic–clonic seizures (grand mal). Of these types, absence and tonic–clonic are not only the best known but they also have substantial implications for the study of consciousness.

Absence attacks are characterized by lapses in consciousness which typically last a few seconds to a minute. The lapses appear without warning and the person completely ceases voluntary activity during the episode. There is a rapid return to full consciousness with amnesia only for the period during which the attack occurred. In short, this is the type of seizure in which a person is fully conscious and functioning followed by a period wherein momentarily there is partial or complete unresponsiveness, followed by a full return to consciousness. Perhaps nowhere else in nature are such abrupt and complete changes in consciousness evident as with respect to absence seizures. Their EEG manifestations will be discussed in Section 4.

Tonic–clonic seizures represent the second type of generalized attack which will be discussed here. When these seizures represent primarily generalized epilepsy, they involve the entire brain from onset. The body may become rigid (tonic phase) with fully extended extremities and air may be expelled from the lungs, producing a cry. The body may then begin to jerk (clonic phase), and then the jerking tends to slow and stop. After the seizure, the person is typically partially responsive to the environment but is usually obviously confused. Exhaustion may be in evidence as well as a tendency to sleep. Because of the dramatic nature of the attack, many people know about only this one type of seizure and tend to equate all epilepsy with tonic–clonic seizures.

Partial seizures may be divided into two types depending upon whether there is or is not an alteration in consciousness. Elementary partial seizures can arise from any localized portion of the cerebral cortex, and the initial symptoms may be noted in terms of simple movements or sensations. For example, a portion of the body may twitch or may render the impression of having been touched. However, there is no significant alteration in consciousness, and if the seizure does not progress to a generalized attack, the individual is alert throughout the episode. This type of seizure is as clear an example as any that not all forms of epilepsy result in alterations of consciousness.

Partial seizures with complex symptomatology (psychomotor seizures, temporal lobe seizures) are those seizures of focal onset which are typically associated with identifiable alterations in consciousness. Typically, one or the other or both temporal lobes are involved, but closely related parts of the cerebral cortex may be affected as well. Typically also, there are changes in cognition and behavior which may be of a complex nature and which are in some contrast with the relatively simple motor and sensory phenomena associated with elementary partial attacks. Symptoms often found in persons with complex partial seizures take numerous forms and may include feelings of unreality, nausea or abdominal sensations, dizziness, an inability to talk or to hear or both, peculiar tastes or smells, episodes of forced thinking, or déjà vu experiences. The person may also perform a number of nonpurposeful acts during a seizure, including getting up, walking around the room, fingering clothes or objects within the room, and so forth. These phenomena are of considerable interest and seem to be performed irrespective of level of consciousness. For example, actions performed during these episodes do not evidence planning and purpose, but neither are they entirely unreactive to the environment. Thus, if an attempt is made to restrain a person during such an attack, a resistive response may be elicited, but the response is likely to be poorly organized. Is the person conscious or not? Interest in this type of seizure has also been heightened by its prevalence (about 60% of all adults with epilepsy), and by the suggestions that certain behavioral tendencies (e.g., hypergraphia, hyposexuality, hyperreligiosity) may exist with individuals bearing this diagnosis (Bear and Fedio, 1977; Sherwin, 1977; Walker and Blumer, 1977).

From the above, it is apparent that there are various types of epilepsy (including others which are not mentioned here) which are quite different from one to the next. Furthermore, it is apparent that in terms of implications for a study of consciousness, some seizure types are far more relevant than others. These considerations have led a number of investigators to conclude that it is more accurate to speak of ''the epilepsies'' rather than ''epilepsy.''

Before discussing methods of neuropsychological assessment in epilepsy, a few additional points need to be briefly covered concerning seizure disorders themselves. These include etiology of the seizures, age at onset of attacks, and duration of the disorder, seizure frequency, and deterioration in performance over time. Individuals may be identified as having seizure disorders where the cause of seizures is known (symptomatic epilepsy) or where the cause is unknown (essential, idiopathic, or cryptogenic epilepsy). There is a general belief that partial epilepsies are acquired or symptomatic, while the primary generalized epilepsies are idiopathic or cryptogenic. That is, if an individual has a head injury and develops epilepsy, it is commonly believed that the epilepsy will be of focal origin and that even if grand mal seizures are experienced, they will probably be traceable to a focus in one part of the brain. A fairly constant finding is that individuals with acquired seizures perform more poorly on tests of intelligence and on neuropsychological tests than individuals with essential epilepsy (Kløve and Matthews, 1966; Tarter, 1972). Presumably, the decreased intelligence is related to the specific brain insult which caused the epilepsy, but, as will be shown later, intermittent EEG abnormalities may themselves result in decreased alertness, and, furthermore, seizures themselves may in all probability result in additional brain damage.

In general, the literature indicates that the earlier the age of onset of epilepsy and the longer the duration of seizures, the lower the mental abilities (De Haas and Magnus, 1958; Dikmen *et al.,* 1975; Kløve and Matthews, 1969; Lennox and Lennox, 1960). The differences found by the majority of these studies are limited, and it is not entirely clear that other factors such as number of seizures over time may not be equally important. Nevertheless, there is a tendency for individuals who develop epilepsy early in life or who have had seizures for many years to be less alert and less intelligent.

One might conclude that the more frequently one has a seizure, the lower the mental abilities. However, a review of many studies dealing with this topic found no consistent trend (Tarter, 1972). At least part of the difficulty here is that the majority of studies used tests which required alertness to take the test. Furthermore, in most cases persons are not tested at all if they are noted to be postictally confused. Thus, the immediate effects of seizures upon performance have not been adequately measured.

In recent years, more and more attention has been turned to the possibility of deterioration in performance over time with individuals having multiple seizures. It has been shown that there is neural degeneration associated with repeated epileptic attacks in animals, and also that seizures have inhibitory effects upon brain protein synthesis, brain growth, and eventually upon behavioral development (Harris, 1972; Wasterlain and Duffy, 1976). Deterioration in humans over time has also been documented (De Haas and Magnus, 1958; Dodrill and Troupin, 1976; Lennox and Lennox, 1960), although the parameters of such deterioration are as yet poorly described. It appears that generalized seizures other than absence attacks are most likely to be associated with deterioration and especially so if they come without warning, if they result in blows to the head due to falls, and if they are associated with alterations in breathing. Episodes of continuous seizures (status epilepticus) may be particularly destructive to brain tissue (Delgado-Escueta *et al.,* 1983).

3 Neuropsychological Assessment in Epilepsy

Epilepsy may be viewed as a symptom of an underlying brain disorder. At the time of an attack, the individual's brain is clearly not functioning normally. Even between attacks, EEG abnormalities are usually in evidence with persons having seizure disorders. As a consequence, if one examines abilities closely enough even between seizures, one may expect to find some deficits. These deficits may or may not be of practical importance, and they may or may not be associated with specific EEG changes. The complex nature of human mental abilities in the brain is such, however, that if subtle changes in alertness and other skills are to be assessed, some form of equally complex evaluative procedure is required. There are, of course, many ways in which this assessment can be accomplished, and a very large number of neuropsychological tests has been developed. It is beyond the scope of this chapter to review them all. Instead, there will be brief mention of the one comprehensive neuropsychological battery that has been developed specifically with epilepsy in mind and standardized on patients with this disorder. This is the Neuropsychological Battery for Epilepsy (Dodrill, 1978).

In developing the Neuropsychological Battery for Epilepsy, work was begun using as a basis the Halstead–Reitan Neuropsychological Test Battery for Adults (Reitan and Davidson, 1974). To this battery a number of other neuro-psychological test measures were added which cover areas of importance in epilepsy including memory and attention to the task. In adding these test measures, reference was made to the literature for those tests that were demonstrated to be helpful in differentiating among epileptic groups, among various medications, and among other relevant phenomena, such as those pertaining to the EEGs. A total of 100 neuropsychological variables were considered. Through pilot and principal studies these measures were cut to 16, each of which met a series of rigid criteria. These tests cover a broad range of cognitive, perceptual, and motor skills. Included in the battery are tests evaluating attention to the task, memory (verbal and nonverbal), perceptual skills (auditory, tactual, visual), motor abilities (speed, strength, coordination), language-related skills, and visual–spatial functions. The battery has been used in a variety of studies of various EEG phenomena and antiseizure medication side effects, and these studies will be reviewed in subsequent sections of the chapter. In addition, it has been used in clinical contexts to help identify particular brain-related deficits in persons with epilepsy. Some of the tests involve pieces of apparatus, while others are paper and pencil measures. Typically, approximately 4 hours are required for administration of the battery, and usually assessments of general intellectual skills and of personality adjustment are administered in addition.

4 Electroencephalographic Variables

Attention will now be turned to EEG phenomena often seen in epilepsy which have ramifications for alertness and ability to attend to the task. Both epileptiform variables and nonepileptiform variables will be discussed.

EEG epileptiform patterns are those wave forms which are characteristic of seizure disorders. They may be focal or generalized in nature. Focal discharges involve only a portion of the brain. They frequently take the form of spikelike transients which appear intermittently or in clusters. In the vast majority of cases, these discharges have no obvious or clearly discernible effects upon functioning, and even the most sensitive tests of alertness and awareness render findings which are primarily negative (Mirsky *et al.*, 1960; Lansdell and Mirsky, 1964). It is, of course, entirely possible that focal epileptiform discharges produce some limited deficits of a very transient nature, but at least utilizing the technology which currently exists, no discernible effects upon consciousness can be discovered. In contrast, studies of generalized epileptiform discharges almost invariably point to significantly (although temporarily) decreased alertness and functioning (Mirsky, 1969; Goode *et al.*, 1970; Browne *et al.*, 1974).

In addition to the distinction between focal versus generalized epileptiform discharges, the nature of the discharge is also of importance in terms of a study of consciousness. For example, in the studies of the effects of generalized discharges referred to above, it was clear that 3-per-second spike-and-slow-wave patterns were associated with the greatest alterations in alertness. Such patterns are typically found in cases of petit mal epilepsy. Generalized discharges slightly different from this (such as the generalized spike-and-slow-wave discharges which occur at less than $2\frac{1}{2}$ cycles per second) may produce few or no discernible effects. This effect has been illustrated in work done by this author and a colleague (Robert J. Wilkus) (unpublished) with patients having generalized epileptiform discharges. The results on two of these people are presented here. While his/her EEG changes were monitored, the patient played a simple videogame using a standard black and white television. The patient operated a "paddle" and blocked a ball coming across the screen in a simulated table tennis game. The computer operated the paddle on the other side of the screen and unfailingly returned the ball. This is a test which can go on for many minutes without the patient losing interest. Figure 1 shows what typically happened with one of the patients when that individual had a discharge of a generalized nature. The person "missed" the ball. Both before and after the discharge, performance

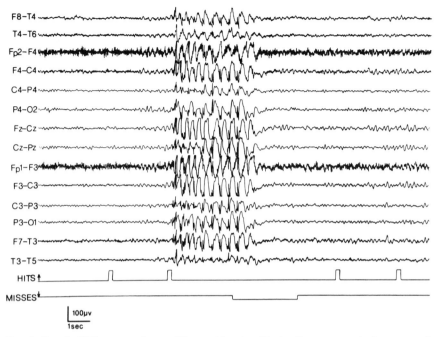

F8–T4

T4–T6

Fp2–F4

F4–C4

C4–P4

P4–O2

Fz–Cz

Cz–Pz

Fp1–F3

F3–C3

C3–P3

P3–O1

F7–T3

T3–T5

HITS

MISSES

100µv
1sec

FIG. 1. Sample EEG segment from a 25-year-old male with simultaneous record of accuracy of responses to an electronic game. The patient performs well before and after the generalized epileptiform discharges but not during it.

was at a normal level. This person has fairly typical diffuse 3-per-second spike-and-wave epileptiform discharges. In the case of the second patient, however, Fig. 2 shows that performances continued unabated before, during, and after the discharges. While these discharges are superficially similar to those in Fig. 1, subtle morphological differences are noted upon close examination. Thus, whereas having a generalized EEG discharge is probably necessary to demonstrate deficits on tasks of this type, it is not a sufficient condition in and of itself.

To make the situation even more intriguing, it should be noted that neither patient suffered a discernible epileptic attack at the time of these recordings. If continuous testing had not been in progress, the momentary loss in performance by the first patient would have been entirely missed. Furthermore, it has been our experience that tests which allow even 1 or 2 seconds of rest between items will permit discharges to appear during these very brief periods so that any losses in functioning are missed. In addition, if the tests are too stimulating, the heightened level of awareness will inhibit discharges, but if they are too dull, the patient will become drowsy and perform poorly. These facts are noted merely to illustrate some of the difficulties encountered in evaluating lapses of attention in these patients.

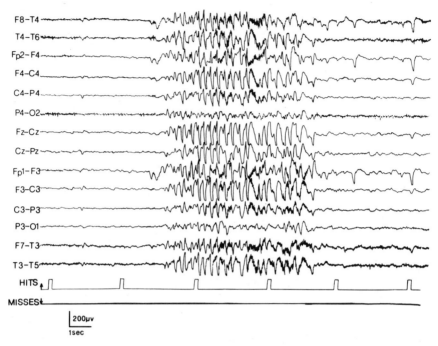

FIG. 2. Sample EEG segment from a 30-year-old female with simultaneous record of accuracy of responses to an electronic game. The patient performs well before, during, and after the generalized epileptiform discharges.

A final word should be offered concerning the general neuropsychological functioning of persons with epilepsy between seizures. Using the Neuropsychological Battery of Epilepsy, it has been discovered that persons whose EEGs typically show no discharges have the best performance, that persons with focal discharges have an intermediate performance, and that persons with generalized discharges have the worst performance (Dodrill and Wilkus, 1976; Wilkus and Dodrill, 1976). In the same studies, it was also discovered that persons with more frequent discharges performed more poorly than persons with few or no discharges. Although EEG records were not simultaneously obtained with the neuropsychological testing, the patients were repeatedly alerted in the performance of the tasks, and it is doubted that the discharges themselves had any significant effects upon performance. Thus, persons with generalized epileptiform discharges appear to be the most impaired, even apart from the immediate effects of their discharges.

We now turn briefly to nonepileptiform EEG abnormalities. In epilepsy, these are typically slow waves for the patient's age and portion of the brain from which they arise. Studies here have tended to focus upon the posterior dominant rhythm ("alpha") frequency (Saunders, 1961; Mulholland, 1969; Dodrill and Wilkus, 1976), but decreased functioning has been related to slowed rhythms from other parts of the brain as well (Vislie and Henriksen, 1958; Lennox and Lennox, 1960; Giannitrapani, 1969; Dodrill and Wilkus, 1978). The general finding from these studies has been that decreased mental abilities accompanies slowed rhythms. As Lennox and Lennox (1960) wrote, "slow waves often match slow wits" (p. 673). Beyond this, nonepileptiform abnormalities in epilepsy do not appear to offer specific implications for a study of consciousness.

5 Antiseizure Medications

The fact that drugs may affect consciousness is well known. In epilepsy, medications given to stop or reduce the rate of seizures represent another opportunity for one to study changes in responsiveness and to at least speculate concerning how these changes occur. Complicating the issue is, of course, the fact that individuals whom we would study for medication effects also have EEG changes, and individuals whose EEG changes we would investigate are receiving antiseizure drugs. An additional problem is that the majority of individuals with epilepsy are receiving more than one medication, and one therefore must consider not only the cumulative effects of the drugs that are taken but also in many cases interaction effects. Moreover, it is a constant observation that individuals with the most frequent seizures also receive the most medications, so that separating the effects of the seizures from the effects of the medications represents an additional problem.

Before discussing the effects of specific drugs, a few comments will be offered concerning how the amount of drug within the person is determined. The simplest form of measurement is to identify how much of the drug is being taken. This method, however, is so crude that it is of almost no value. It is noted, for example, that body size and the amount of blood into which the medication will be diluted varies substantially from one person to the next. A simple formula to help correct for this is to express the drug amount in units administered per unit of weight. Most often, this is done in micrograms of drug giver per kilogram of body weight. Such a formula is a step in the right direction, but it is of limited value because important variables yet remain. The metabolism of the drug varies substantially from one person to the next so that two individuals of the same body mass and receiving the same amount of the same drug cannot necessarily be expected to have the same amount of the drug in their blood serum. Exactly how much is in the serum at any given point in time may be measured by a variety of laboratory techniques having a reasonable degree of accuracy. It is fair to say that this degree of measurement constitutes the standard for the evaluation of the extent of antiseizure medication at the time of this writing. It is also known, however, that only a portion of each drug is able to cross the blood–brain barrier, because usually most of the drug is protein bound. Thus, for example, with phenytoin (Dilantin, diphenylhydantoin) only approximately 10% of the drug serum is not protein bound. There has also been the suggestion that the extent to which a drug is protein bound may vary to some degree from one patient to the next. The extent to which a drug is protein bound may also be related to its effects on functioning, although this area has not yet been well explored. While further discussion of drug measurement will not be included here, it should be clear that the problem of identifying the amount of drug in the individual is a complicated one, which adds substantially to the already difficult task of identifying the effects of the drugs.

The most widely used antiseizure medication in the world today is phenytoin. This drug is effective with a number of types of seizure disorders and does not carry life-threatening risks. With normal therapeutic levels of approximately 10–30 μg of drug per milliliter of serum, patients do not usually report substantial side effects to which they cannot adjust. Nevertheless, low and subtherapeutic serum levels may be associated with decreased performances, at least in normals (Idestrom *et al.*, 1972; Trimble *et al.*, 1980). Within therapeutic ranges, changes from high to low levels have also been associated with improvement on certain tasks of memory, concentration, speed of decision making, and motor performance (Thompson and Trimble, 1982). Perhaps the most consistent finding with the administration of phenytoin is that of decreased motor performance (Booker *et al.*, 1967; Dodrill, 1975).

Carbamazepine (Tegretol) has gained enormous popularity in recent years as an antiseizure medication effective with a number of seizure types but with fewer side effects. A brief review of the literature reveals that it has been associated with relatively fewer side effects than other major drugs such as phenytoin or sodium valporate (e.g., Dodrill and Troupin, 1977; Thompson and Trimble, 1982) and positive psychotropic effects have occasionally been reported (Dalby, 1975). In reviewing large numbers of studies, it is probably fair to say that carbamazepine is associated in many cases with slightly improved alertness and ability to attend to the task in comparison with other antiseizure medications, and that some improvement in mood is also frequently observed.

In at least one study (Dodrill and Troupin, 1977) it was shown that the improvement in alertness with carbamazepine differs depending upon initial level of functioning (persons with lower levels of functioning improved the most with carbamazepine administration). The reason for this is not entirely clear, but it raises the possibility that drugs may differ in their effects from one person to the next.

Phenobarbital (Luminal) administration has frequently been associated with drowsiness or alternatively with restlessness, excitement, and irritability. Phenobarbital has also been related to decreases in ability to attend to the task, in psychomotor performance, and in spontaneous speech. These changes may become more evident as the task is made more difficult and as the degree of external prompting to complete the task decreases (Hutt *et al.*, 1968). These findings are of interest in that they illustrate that both the task and the setting in which it is performed may be of importance in evaluating the effects of drugs upon performance. Stores (1975) cites a series of studies which suggest that learning capabilities in children may be decreased with phenobarbital administration and that there may be negative behavioral consequences as well.

Other studies could be reviewed with respect to the above-mentioned drugs or with respect to other drugs, but it is apparent that detailed evaluations of these medications produce findings which are to a greater or lesser degree suggestive of decreased attentional skills and general alertness. Cognitive abilities may be affected as well. Furthermore, there is evidence that the more medications given to a patient, the lower the performance (Tomlinson *et al.*, 1982). The difficulty, however, is in devising a general model whereby one can with precision predict the side effects of the various drugs with any given patient. No such model exists, and it is not clear that we have the technical knowledge to develop such a model at the present time.

6 Conclusions

We have now looked at several matters pertaining to epilepsy and to their contributions or potential contributions with respect to the study of consciousness. The nature of this disorder is such that it provides a window through which certain aspects of functioning may be studied in a unique way. Of particular value are the abrupt alterations in consciousness often noted in this disorder along with the demonstrable EEG changes. Neuropsychological testing has been shown to be helpful in identifying levels of functioning with relevance to consciousness. There is a sense in which information provided by the study of epilepsy is of great value in the study of consciousness, but, at the same time, it is clear that there are many uncertainties, and this chapter poses more questions than answers. It may be, however, that through the study of epilepsy and related conditions we will ultimately be able to gain insights into the nature of consciousness which would otherwise not have been possible.

References

Bear, D. M., and Fedio, P. (1977). Quantitative analysis of interictal behavior in temporal lobe epilepsy. *Archives of Neurology*, **34**, 454–467.
Booker, H. E., Matthews, C. G., and Slaby, A. (1967). Effects of diphenylhy-

dantoin on selected physiological and psychological measures in normal adults. *Neurology,* **17,** 949–951.

Browne, T. R., Penry, J. K., Porter, R. J., and Dreifuss, F. E. (1974). Responsiveness before, during, and after spike-wave paroxysms. *Neurology,* **24,** 659–665.

Dalby, M. A. (1975). Behavioral effects of carbamazepine. *In* "Advances in Neurology," (Eds. J. K. Penry and D. D. Daly), Vol. 11, pp. 331–344. Raven, New York.

De Haas, A., and Magnus, O. (1958). "Lectures on Epilepsy." Elsevier, New York.

Delgado-Escueta, A. V., Wasterlain, C. G., Treiman, D. M., and Porter, R. J. (Eds.). (1983). Status epilepticus: Mechanisms of brain damage and treatment. *In* "Advances in Neurology," Vol. 34. Raven, New York.

Dikmen, S., Matthews, C. G., and Harley, J. P. (1975). The effect of early versus late onset of major motor epilepsy upon cognitive–intellectual performance. *Epilepsia,* **16,** 73–81.

Dodrill, C. B. (1975). Diphenylhydantoin serum levels, toxicity, and neuropsychological performance in patients with epilepsy. *Epilepsia,* **16,** 593–600.

Dodrill, C. B. (1978). A neuropsychological battery for epilepsy. *Epilepsia,* **19,** 611–623.

Dodrill, C. B., and Troupin, A. S. (1976). Seizures and adaptive abilities: A case of identical twins. *Archives of Neurology,* **33,** 604–607.

Dodrill, C. B., and Troupin, A. S. (1977). Psychotropic effects of carbamazepine and epilepsy: A double-blind comparison with phenytoin. *Neurology,* **27,** 1023–1028.

Dodrill, C. B., and Wilkus, R. J. (1976). Neuropsychological correlates of the electroencephalogram and epileptics: II. The waking posterior rhythm and its interaction with epileptiform activity. *Epilepsia,* **17,** 101–109.

Dodrill, C. B., and Wilkus, R. J. (1978). Neuropsychological correlates of the electroencephalogram in epileptics. III. Generalized non-epileptiform abnormalities. *Epilepsia,* **19,** 453–462.

Gastaut, H. (1970). Clinical and electroencephalographical classification of epileptic seizures. *Epilepsia,* **11,** 102–113.

Giannitrapani, D. (1969). EEG average frequency and intelligence. *Electroencephalography and Clinical Neurophysiology,* **27,** 480–486.

Goode, D. J., Penry, J. K., and Dreifuss, F. E. (1970). Effects of paroxysmal spike-wave on continuous visual-motor performance. *Epilepsia,* **11,** 241–254.

Harris, A. B. (1972). Degeneration in experimental epileptic foci. *Archives of Neurology,* **26,** 434–449.

Hutt, S. J., Jackson, P. M., Belsham, A., and Higgins, G. (1968). Perceptual–motor behaviour in relation to blood phenobarbitone level: A preliminary report. *Development Medicine and Childhood Neurology,* **10,** 626–632.

Idelstrom, C-M., Schalling, D., Carlquist, U., and Sjoqvist, F. (1972). Acute effects of diphenylhydantoin in relation to plasma levels: Behavioural and psychophysiological studies. *Psychological Medicine, 2,* 111–120.

Kløve, H., and Matthews, C. G. (1966). Psychometric and adaptive abilities in epilepsy with differential etiology. *Epilepsia, 7,* 330–338.

Kløve, H., and Matthews, C. G. (1969). Neuropsychological evaluation of the epileptic patient. *Wisconsin Medical Journal, 68,* 296–301.

Lansdell, H., and Mirsky, A. F. (1964). Attention in focal and centrencephalic epilepsy. *Experimental Neurology, 9,* 463–469.

Lennox, W. G., and Lennox, N. A. (1960). "Epilepsy and Related Disorders," 2 vols. Little, Brown, Boston.

Mirsky, A. F. (1969). Studies of paroxysmal EEG phenomena and background EEG in relation to impaired attention. *In* "Attention in Neurophysiology" (Eds. C. R. Evans and T. V. Mulholland), pp. 310–322. Butterworths, London.

Mirsky, A. F., Primac, D. W., Ajmone Marsan, C., Rosvold, H. E., and Stevens, J. R. (1960). Comparison of the psychological test performance of patients with focal and nonfocal epilepsy. *Experimental Neurology, 2,* 75–89.

Mulholland, T. (1969). The concept of attention and the electroencephalographic alpha rhythm. *In* "Attention in Neurophysiology" (Eds. C. R. Evans and T. Mulholland), pp. 100–127. Butterworths, London.

Reitan, R. M., and Davidson, L. A. (Eds.). (1974). "Clinical Neuropsychology: Current Status and Applications." Winston, Washington, D.C.

Saunders, D. R. (1961). Digit span and alpha frequency: A cross-validation. *Journal of Clinical Psychology,* 165–167.

Sherwin, I. (1977). Clinical and EEG aspects of temporal lobe epilepsy with behavior disorder, the role of cerebral dominance. *McLean Hospital Journal* (special issue), 40–50.

Stores, G. (1975). Behavioural effects of anti-epileptic drugs. *Developmental Medicine & Child Neurology, 17,* 647–658.

Tarter, R. E. (1972). Intellectual and adaptive functioning in epilepsy: A review of 50 years of research. *Diseases of the Nervous System, 33,* 763–770.

Thompson, P. J., and Trimble, M. R. (1982). Comparative effects of anticonvulsant drugs on cognitive functioning. *British Journal of Clinical Practice* (Symposium Supplement 18), 154–156.

Tomlinson, L., Andrewes, D., Merrifield, E., and Reynolds, E. H. (1982). The effects of antiepileptic drugs on cognitive and motor functions. *British Journal of Clinical Practice* (Symposium Supplement 18), 177–183.

Trimble, M. R., Thompson, P. J., and Huppert, F. (1980). Anticonvulsant drugs and cognitive abilities. *In* "Advances in Epileptology: The XIth Epilepsy International Symposium" (Eds. R. Canger, F. Angeleri, & J. K. Penry), pp. 199–204. Raven, New York.

Vislie, H., and Henriksen, G. F. (1958). Psychic disturbance in epileptics. *In* "Lectures on Epilepsy" (Ed. A. M. Lorentz De Haas). Elsevier, Amsterdam.

Walker, A. E., and Blumer, D. (1977). Long-term behavioral effects of temporal lobectomy for temporal lobe epilepsy. *McLean Hospital Journal* (special issue), 85–103.

Wasterlain, C. G., and Duffy, T. E. (1976). Status epilepticus in immature rats, *Archives in Neurology,* **33,** 821–827.

Wilkus, R. J., and Dodrill, C. B. (1976). Neuropsychological correlates of the electroencephalogram in epileptics. I. Topographic distribution and average rate of epileptiform activity. *Epilepsia,* **17,** 89–100.

5 Some Problems in the Diagnosis of Schizophrenia and the Concept of Clear Consciousness

MALCOLM P. I. WELLER

Friern Hospital,
Whittington Hospital,
Royal Northern Hospital,
Royal Free Hospital
School of Medicine,
London, England

1 Historical Considerations

The problem of diagnosis permeates psychiatry and is particularly complex in schizophrenia. Early writers, such as Bleuler (1911) and Kraepelin (1919), were impressed by what they saw as a deteriorating condition similar to dementia but which started typically in adolescence and early adulthood. In these cases the onset was often insidious and recovery was either rare or nonexistent, contrasting with episodic disorders in which functioning was restored. The terms *démence précoce* and *dementia praecox,* used by Morel (1860) and Kraepelin (1919), respectively, emphasised irreversible deterioration and chronicity. Bleuler's use of the plural term, the schizophrenias, implied several diseases with common features. Both Bleuler and Kraepelin were impressed by the apathy and indifference shown by many patients with a diminution in emotional force and a seeming disintegration of the personality. This deterioration was not ignored by those whose diagnosis relied on the more easily observed and defined symptoms of delusions and hallucinations, but reliance on these symptoms introduced a checklist approach to diagnosis, based on presenting features, which laid little importance on the recognition of a global deterioration in habits, outlook, and relationships, as well as in thinking.

The growth of interest in biological features has sharpened the desire for an identification of at least a subgroup of unequivocal diagnostic probity. The scheme of Schneider (1957) has enjoyed an ascendancy in defining a core or nuclear group. Interest has shifted once again, however, as biological dif-

Aspects of Consciousness
Volume 4. Clinical Issues

ferences, such as the size of the brain's ventricle, were found in the nonnuclear group. As pointed out by Mackay (1980), autopsy brain studies have been based on chronically hospitalised patients. It is these studies that have added to the evidence for a neurochemical hypothesis that the disease is associated with relative overactivity of central dopamine systems.

The problem of delineating the nature of the nonnuclear group is difficult. A recent survey has shown that most research publications in psychiatry are not written by psychiatrists but by psychologists, biochemists, and other nonmedical scientists (Sadler *et al.*, 1981). These research workers lack clinical expertise and are no doubt anxious to possess a scheme for diagnosis which is acceptable and straightforward to apply. It is unsatisfactory for them to have to rely on the subtle, and sometimes contradictory, judgements of clinicians. This need has intensified the pressure for a greater uniformity in transatlantic diagnostic practise. Research diagnoses focus on the presenting symptoms, while experienced clinicians survey a more comprehensive picture. In his chapter on diagnosis, Bleuler states "We shall always presume that the reader is capable of taking into consideration the accompanying circumstances as well as the total psychic consideration" (1911, p. 295), a position in accord with the later writings of Adolf Meyer (1952).

Diagnostic practices may not coincide in different parts of the world. It was clear from the United States/United Kingdom Diagnostic Project (Cooper *et al.*, 1972) that American psychiatrists had a broader concept of schizophrenia than English psychiatrists. They diagnosed 65% of patients in a consecutive series of 250 admissions to Brooklyn State Hospital as schizophrenic, while only 34% of the patients similarly admitted to Netherne Hospital in South London were so diagnosed. This difference was not sustained when the same population was interviewed by a research team trained in the same institution and using rehearsed interviews and diagnostic approaches. The researchers diagnosed schizophrenia in 32% of the New York and 26% of the London patients. In a second sample from diverse hospitals a similar pattern emerged: 62% of the 192 New York and 34% of the 174 London patients were diagnosed as suffering from schizophrenia. On reexamination by the research team, these figures altered to 29% of New York patients and 25% of London patients. The International Pilot Study in Schizophrenia (IPSS) (World Health Organization, 1973b), a transcultural psychiatric investigation of 1202 patients in nine countries using the Present State Examination (PSE), no doubt contributed to the reappraisal of diagnostic criteria in America. The publication of DSM-III in 1980 has resulted in the American criteria for the diagnosis of schizophrenia becoming more stringent than those of the British. The new American system does not recognise schizophrenia if the patient has an illness which lasts for less than 6 months and/or has significant affective disturbance. This applies also to the Feighner criteria (Feighner *et al.*, 1972) and the Iowa criteria (Morrison *et al.*, 1973).

TABLE 1

Interview Questions from PSE 9th Edition for Symptoms Constituting
the Nuclear Syndrome

Thought echo or commentary	Do you ever seem to hear your own thoughts repeated or echoed? (What is that like? How do you explain it? Where does it come from?)
Third-person auditory hallucinations	Do you hear several voices talking about you? Do they refer to you as "he" (she)? (What do they say) Do they seem to comment on what you are thinking, or reading, or doing?)
Thought broadcast	Are your thoughts broadcast, so that other people know what you are thinking? (How do you explain it?)
Thought insertion	Are thoughts put into your head which you know are not your own? (How do you know they are not your own?) (Where do they come from?)
Thought block	Do you ever experience your thoughts stopping quite unexpectedly so that there are none left in your mind, even when your thoughts were flowing freely before? (What is that like?) (How often does it occur?) (What is it due to?)
Thought withdrawal	Do your thoughts ever seem to be taken out of your head, as though some external person or force were removing them? (Can you give an example?) (How do you explain it?)
Delusions of control	Do you feel under the control of some force or power other than yourself? (As though you were possessed by someone or something else?) (What is that like?) (Does this force make your movements for you without your willing it, or use your voice, or your handwriting? Does it replace your personality? What is the explanation?)

Delusions of alien forces penetrating or controlling the patient's mind or body and primary delusions in which the patient suddenly becomes convinced that a particular set of events has a special inexplicable meaning that is discrepant with the patient's cultural or social group.

Degrees of certainty are recognised. The examiner must be convinced of at least one nuclear symptom. If the delusions are partial, the syndrome is probable but not certain. Two or more firmly held symptoms are unequivocal evidence of a nuclear syndrome.

Delusions of control may be subdivided into made feelings and made impulses.

Nolan Lewis asserted that "even a trace of schizophrenia is schizophrenia" (Lewis and Piotrowski, 1954). This dictum implies a hierarchical diagnostic practice, adopted in the computer programme CATEGO, which incorporates diagnostic rules designed to process data derived from the PSE. On this scheme one of several pathognomonic features obliges a diagnosis of schizophrenia, whatever other psychopathology may coexist (see Table 1). This is discrepant with current American practise and also the position enunciated by Sir Aubrey Lewis (1934) who wrote "The recognition of isolated symptoms as schizophrenic, however, is quite another matter. There are no pathognomic signs, no unequivocal marks of the schizophrenic symptom." In his series of 61 melancholic patients "ideas of reference or of persecution were found in the majority" and he considered that some of the patients had a schizophrenic disorder which was only "slight or subordinate." The CATEGO programme does not assign mood-congruent delusions or first-person auditory hallucinations to schizophrenia and separates off persecutory delusions into a separate category. Nevertheless, Schmid *et al.* (1982), who have evolved their own computer-based diagnostic programme, consider that the CATEGO progamme overdiagnoses schizophrenia. Others as well as Lewis have felt that psychotic symptoms may be secondary phenomena to an affective illness, and terms such as schizoaffective, atypical affective, cycloid psychosis, and schizophreniform psychosis betray an unease in unambiguously assigning some psychotic patients with a strong affective colouring to a schizophrenic category (see Langfeldt, 1939; Holmboe and Astrup, 1957; Achte, 1961; Leonhard, 1961; Procci 1976).

Until recently American training was much influenced by psychoanalytic models in which sufferings in the present are considered expressions of the vicissitudes of early experience. The same underlying psychological mechanisms are considered universal and the same treatment approach is adopted irrespective of the complaint. Diagnosis is unimportant in this procedure. Patients who seemed inappropriate for psychoanalysis included those whose empathetic understanding was low and whose emotional range and responsiveness were restricted. These patients may have included some with schizophrenia as we understand the illness in the United Kingdom, but the group as a whole was designated schizophrenic, leading to a much wider use of the term in North America.

Most of the work of psychiatrists who were training for analytic work in private practice was done in general hospitals where they were separated from the most disturbed patients, who were in the mental hospitals. In his critical paper "Schizophrenia: The Sacred Symbol of Psychiatry," Szasz acknowledged for argumentative purposes that

When Kraepelin, Bleuler and their contemporaries became psychiatrists, psychiatry was already an established form of medical and medico-legal practice. Moreover, the real locus of psychiatric practice was the insane asylum or mental hospital, just as the real locus of surgical practice was the operating room (Szasz, 1976).

British psychiatrists were more likely than their American counterparts to have mental hospital experience and so see the full range of psychiatric morbidity. The terms psychosis and psychotic are used in a different way in psychoanalytic writings and are sometimes equated with schizophrenia. Freud (1894) used the term psychosis to represent successful rejection of an incompatible or intolerable idea. The Freudian usage of the terms psychosis and psychotic is broad and encompasses an aetiological model which, because of equivalence of terms, has contributed to assumed aetiological models of schizophrenia, including those of double bind (Bateson *et al.,* 1956) and pseudomutuality (Wynne *et al.,* 1958). The objection of Laing and his colleagues to recognising schizophrenia at all (Laing and Esterson, 1964) is belied by their pursuit of revolutionary treatments. There is no "right" way to diagnose schizophrenia because there is no criterion by which one can be declared unequivocally right or wrong. This is not so with medical conditions in general, where biochemical or histological techniques can securely establish the diagnosis. In the medical concept of disease, organic pathology is considered the source of the signs and symptoms revealed by the patient (the signs are those features that can be demonstrated and the symptoms those that the patient complains of). Psychopathology is not tissue pathology. In some contexts, such as psychoanalysis, the term psychopathology may be used to indicate the proposed mental mechanisms which produce the signs and symptoms, but generally the term is used for the signs and symptoms themselves.

This point is stressed by Szasz (1960, 1962), who considers that in a philosophical sense mental illness does not exist and that in linking the two terms *mental* and *illness,* we are making what Gilbert Ryle (1949) calls a categorical mistake. Szasz considers that "mental illness" is a metaphor, minds can be "sick" only in the sense that jokes are "sick" or economies are "sick." He is particularly critical of the term schizophrenia, but in Seymour Kety's (1974) sardonic paraphrase, "if schizophrenia is a myth, it is a myth with a strong genetic component" (p. 961). Genetic studies have been dogged by diagnostic difficulties, often being reliant on case records and retrospective proceedings, but, despite criticisms (Paton-Salzberg 1982; Marshall 1984), they repeatedly confirm Kety's assertion (Gottesman and Sheilds, 1982). In any event, the purpose of medical classifications is to group together patients with similar features and to distinguish them from patients with different features.

The recognition of a cluster of characteristic signs and symptoms, or a syndrome, has been the historic route to discovering the underlying cellular pathology. As stated on the first page of a well-known text book of pathology, "the precise aetiology of many diseases is not exactly known." (Thomson and Cotton, 1968). Biological factors have been demonstrated in psychotic disorders. The inconsistency of these biological factors emphasises the probability of distinctive subgroups, as recognised in Bleuler's composite term "the schizophrenias," and the interactions of physical processes with similar consequences following a variety of cellular and biochemical lesions. Paranoid and acute schizophrenia were amongst the best defined syndromes on a cluster analysis of 250 consecutive psychiatric admissions (Everitt *et al.*, 1971). For this author, the arguments of Szasz are stronger for neurotic disorders, particularly for hysteria, a concept that was attacked by Slater (1965) as sometimes masking more sinister conditions, including neurological diseases.

A variety of diagnostic criteria has been applied by Kendall *et al.* (1979) to the same groups of patients, with poor correlation between the various criteria used. This arose in part because of obvious discrepancies, such as the age range, or the chronicity of the disorder necessary for one diagnostic scheme, but not for another. They found that several different schemes based on the presenting features correlated with the eventual diagnosis. Langfeldt's diagnostic scheme was successful, although less clear in defining systems. This scheme seemed to capture some of the more elusive but significant features of the disease. Langfeldt's (1960) guidelines included emotional blunting, low initiative, and altered and often peculiar behaviour as one of a group of symptoms that qualified for a diagnosis of schizophrenia.

Chronicity presents a particular difficulty, since many clinicians are hesitant to diagnose schizophrenia for brief-lived episodes that resolve completely. Various

TABLE 2

Incomplete Recovery from Index Episode[a]

Criteria	N	n	Percentage difference, schizophrenics versus others	χ^2
All patients	134	38	28	
Clinical diagnosis	57	29	51—12	24.8
Carpenter (5)	48	25	52—15	20.7
Langfeldt	37	21	57—18	20.3
Spitzer's research diagnostic criteria	34	19	56—19	17.0
Carpenter (6)	24	15	53—21	16.8
Clinicalt	45	22	49—18	14.1
CATEGO	37	16	43—23	5.6
Schneider	38	16	42—23	4.9
New Haven	48	19	40—22	4.6

[a]Second column shows number of patients exhibiting characteristic in question (incomplete recovery from index episode in this instance). Third column compares frequency of that characteristic in N schizophrenics in $134-N$ other patients. Last column gives χ^2 value of fourfold table expressing this comparison. Critical value of χ^2 for significance at 5% level is 3.6 and at 1% level 6.6, excluding patients with residual schizophrenia. (From Kendell, Brockington, and Leff 1979.)

terms have been applied to these episodes to avoid the use of the term schizophrenia, such as schizophreniform psychosis and acute psychotic reaction. Such terminological distinctions may be appropriate for separating a subgroup of disorder, but if chronicity is a criterion of diagnosis, then in diagnosing this disorder one makes it chronic. "In our view, psychiatric diagnosis must be based on the presenting situation, not on the course taken by the illness" (Schneider, 1957, p. 92). This reasonable viewpoint is being disregarded if a duration of illness of at least 6 months is required as in the DSM-III, the St. Louis (Feighner *et al.*, 1972), or Iowa (Morrison *et al.*, 1972) criteria used in America. The Research Diagnostic Criteria requires only 2 weeks' illness (Spitzer *et al.*, 1977). Recent work (Coryell and Tsuang, 1982) suggests that a period considerably less than 6 months will separate out a group with a very different prognosis.

Schneider identified a series of symptoms which, it is asserted, often occur together (Mellor, 1959) and that are considered pathognomic of schizophrenia in Europe. These are utilised in the table of symptoms comprising the nuclear syndrome (see Table 1). In many ways, this helpful list has come to be seen as exemplifying the key symptoms of the disorder. Because these symptoms have assumed such prominence, they have obscured the original concept of the disease described by Kraepelin (1973) and Bleuler (1911). These pioneers recognised the signs and symptoms emphasised by Schneider, but considered them to be secondary features of a more comprehensive illness. Schneider may have been maligned, and the more global nature of the disease is a theme running through his writings:

This is not to say, however, that we diagnose schizophrenia *only* when first rank symptoms are present. Second rank symptoms and expressive phenomena (Ausdruckserscheinungen) may often justify this diagnosis by virtue of their combination and accumulation.(Schneider,1957)

The difference is really one of emphasis. Some form of primary disturbance, somewhat elusive to specify, was held by Kraepelin and Bleuler to underly a variety of phenomena. By using the term *first-rank symptom*, Schneider appears to ascribe to these a source of the second-rank symptoms, and thus be implying a model contrary to those of Kraepelin and Bleuler.

[T]he weakening of judgement, the mental activity and of creative ability, the dulling of emotional interest and the loss of energy, lastly, the loosening of the inner unity of the psychic life would have to be reckoned among the fundamental disorders of dementia praecox. . . . (Kraepelin, 1919, p. 248)

It has been suggested that undue emphasis has been placed on psychotic experiences, with insufficient attention given to the global deterioration, and that this situation owes much to the writings of Kurt Schneider (Kety, 1980). Clinicians, and especially research workers, may have relied excessively on psychotic

TABLE 3

Frequency of Occurrence of First-rank Symptoms in Selected Published Reports

	Bland and Orn (1980) (38 schizophrenics)	Carpenter et al. (1973) (103 schizophrenics)	Carpenter and Strauss (1974) (466 schizophrenics)	Mellor (1970) (173 schizophrenics)	Lewine et al. (1982) (100 schizophrenics)
Audible thoughts	2%	20%	28%	11.6%	—
Voices arguing	0%	—	22%	13.3%	27%
Voices commenting	24%	—	10%	13.3%	10%
Thought broadcast	24%	33%	26%	21.4%	48%
Thought insertion	47%	20%	23%	19.7%	47%
Thought withdrawal	0%	15%	25%	9.8%	13%
Made affect	29%	11%	16%	6.4%	23%
Made impulse	8%	—	—	2.9%	
Made volition	26%	28%	29%	9.2%	—
Delusional perception[c]	63%	—	—	6.4%	6%
Somatic passivity	—	17%	—	11.6%	—

[a] From Lewine et al. (1982).
[b] The frequency with which particular first rank symptoms occur varies from study to study.
[c] Partial and full delusions combined.

TABLE 4
Correlations of First-rank Symptoms with PSE Items[a]

	PSE item	*r*
Thought insertion	Panic attacks/autonomic	.31
	Obsessional ideas/rumination	.35
	Delusional mood	.34
	Delusions of misinterpretation	.41
	Preoccupation with delusions and hallucinations	.32
Thought broadcast	Restlessness	.36
	Panic attacks/autonomic	.36
	Simple ideas of reference	.41
	Guilty ideas of reference	.40
	Pathological guilt	.35
	Subjective ideomotor pressure	.35
	Grandiose ideas/actions	.30
	Depersonalization	.39
	Delusional mood	.36
	Verbal hallucinations—mood	.42
	True hallucinations	.34
	Visual hallucinations	.35
	Delusional misinterpretation	.34
	Fantastic delusions	.33
	Delusions of catastrophe	.42
	Acting out delusions	.34
	Suspicion	.32
Thought echo	Restlessness	.33
	Morbid jealousy	.39
	Observed anxiety	.43
Thought withdrawal	Morbid jealousy	.36
	Delusions of catastrophe	.43
	Suspicion	.48
Voices discuss patient	Autonomic anxiety, due to delusions	.32
	Hopelessness	.32
	Changed perception	.36
	Voices to subject	.42
	True hallucinations	.48
	Visual hallucinations	.33
	Embarrassing behaviour	.32
Delusions of control	Panic attacks/autonomic	.31
	Changed perception	.32
	Religious delusions	.32
	Fantastic delusions	
Delusions of alien forces	Panic attack/autonomic	.33
	Delayed sleep	.31

(*continued*)

TABLE 4 (*Continued*)

	PSE item	r
Primary delusions	Free-floating anxiety	.31
	Anxious foreboding	.48
	Panic attacks/autonomic	.43
	Situational anxiety	.34
	Specific phobias	.31
	Pathological guilt	.38
	Grandiose ideas/actions	.32
	Depersonalization	.33
	Suspicion	.32

[a]From Lewine *et al.* (1982).

experiences, but this cannot be attributed to Schneider (1957) who throughout his discussion emphasises the "over-all personality change" that occurs in schizophrenia, "without which we should hesitate to assess any hallucinatory experience as a symptom of psychosis" (p. 98). "Psychosis, and in particular schizophrenia, always involves an over-all change. . . . A psychotic phenomenon is not like a defective stone in an otherwise perfect mosaic" (p. 95). The frequency with which particular first-rank symptoms occur varies from study to study. These symptoms tend to cluster together but this can be overemphasised. In many instances the clustering of first-rank symptoms (see Table 4) is seen to be somewhat greater for nonpsychotic symptoms than for other first-rank symptoms. Using clinician's diagnoses based on DSM-III criteria and including patients from a research unit focussed on affective illness, 25% of the affectively ill patients experienced Schneiderian first-rank symptoms (Carpenter and Strauss, 1973).

One study showed that experiences of voices commenting on the patient were associated with a poor outcome (McCabe, 1976). This was confirmed by Bland and Orn (1979) who also found certain other symptoms were associated with a favourable outcome (see Table 5). There was disagreement between the two studies regarding thought broadcasting. McCabe found this associated with poor outcome, in contradiction to Bland and Orn.

In another study delusions and hallucinations in general were associated with a good outcome, whereas disorganisation of thinking was associated with a poor outcome (Tsuang, Woolson, and Simpson, 1981). Vaillant's (1963) findings were largely in accord with this. The various models of schizophrenia have included evidence of left cerebral hemisphere dysfunction (see Davison and Bagley, 1969; Flor-Henry, 1969; Editorial, *Lancet*, 1979; Wexler, 1980; Gruzelier, 1981, for reviews). The symptom of disorganisation of thinking fits this model well and may therefore be indicative of organic pathology.

TABLE 5
Outcome of First-rank Symptoms[a]

Symptoms	Direction of contribution
Thought broadcast	+
Made impulse	+
Delusional perception	+
Made affect	−
Voices commenting	−
Audible thoughts	−
Made volition	+
Thought insertion	+

[a]The outcome is a combination of economic productivity, social adjustment, and psychiatric condition indices. The analysis was by means of stepwise regression and the symptoms are arranged in order of magnitude of effect. (After Bland and Orne, 1980.)

2 Categorical and Dimensional Approaches to Diagnosis

Psychotic experiences are categorically distinct from normal experiences.

If there is a relationship between schizoid personality and psychosis, it is certainly not of the nature of a transition but a sort of leap, as, for example, from the state of chronic alcoholism to delirium tremens. (Jaspers, 1946, p. 654)

The discontinuity between psychosis and normality does not preclude a spectrum between schizophrenia and affective psychotic experiences. Jaspers held such a view: "the major psychoses—schizophrenia, manic-depressive disorder and the epilepsies—have indistinct demarcations" (Jaspers, 1946, p. 518). There is some experimental evidence for this assertion. No separation could be demonstrated between 127 consecutive admissions with functional psychoses and 105 "schizoaffective patients" who fulfilled operational criteria for schizophrenia or paranoid psychosis and for manic or depressive illness (Kendell and Brockington, 1980), who sought unsuccessfully for some discontinuity in either the phenomena or in the outcome of the disorder. Earlier attempts had also failed. (Kendell and Gourlay, 1970, Brockington and Leff, 1979). This accords with the view of Bleuler (1911, p. 304), "All the phenomena of manic-depressive psychosis may also appear in our disease; the only decisive factor is the presence or absence of schizophrenic symptoms," but contradicts the position adopted by the current American diagnostic systems in excluding major affective disturbance from a diagnosis of schizophrenia, even when other schizophrenic features are present. This issue is particularly highlighted when there appears to be a change in diagnosis. Both Cooper (1967) and Sheldrick and her colleagues (1977) were using the CATEGO system of diagnosis. In this hierarchical diagnostic scheme, any single appropriate psychotic symptom dictates a diagnosis of schizophrenia, which might not recur, and apparently did not recur in a subsequent illness. Luxenburger (1939) described similar transitions in diagnosis and anticipated later observations relating epilepsy to psychosis and mood disturbance (Slater *et al.,* 1963; Gibbs, 1951; Donger, 1959; Flor-Henry, 1969; Shukla *et al.,* 1979, Sherwin, 1982). "I even hold the view that one and the same individual can become first an epileptic, then a schizophrenic and finally a manic-depressive" (Luxenburger, 1939). Brief-lived psychotic experiences indistinguishable from schizophrenia occurred in many patients during manic episodes which were rigorously defined (Carlson and Goodwin, 1973). Whether or not schizophrenia is diagnosed in these cases therefore seems reliant on a hierarchical system of diagnosis and frequent scrutiny of a changing state.

When affective illness and schizophrenia coexist, the American diagnostic schemes (DSM-III, Feighner *et al.,* 1973; Morrison *et al.,* 1973) disallow a diagnosis of schizophrenia. The group in whom the two pathologies coexist has a better prognosis than those persons who fulfill the American criteria, but worse than affective illness on measures of marital, residential, occupational, and psychiatric measures (Tsuang and Dempsey, 1974). Weller and Kugler (1979) found that the two-pathologies group was unique in comparison to both schizophrenic and affective patients and to nonpsychiatric controls on a touch localisation task.

Triplets who were indubitably monozygotic on a variety of ontogenetic and biochemical criteria displayed different psychiatric symptoms that could not be adequately explained on the basis of environmental factors. Two had nuclear schizophrenic features, whereas the third was diagnosed as manic-depressive. These original diagnoses were confirmed by two independent doctors unaware of the previous diagnoses. A third independent doctor considered one schizophrenic patient to be manic-depressive, still leaving a diagnostic discordance (McGuffin, Reveley, and Holland, 1982). The triplet who all agreed had manic-depressive illness of the manic type also had an episode of schizoaffective illness of the manic type. The triplets were 28 years old, and with the lapse of time the diagnoses might come to harmonise. In the evolution of a schizophrenic illness affective symptoms may be an early manifestation.

The disintegration of the psychic personality is in general accomplished in dementia praecox in such a way that in the first place the disorders of emotions and of volition dominate the morbid state. (Kraepelin, 1919, p. 283)

Although psychotic experiences are of an either/or variety, apparently normal people can experience them under extreme conditions. One eminent psychiatrist reported a brief psychotic experience during conditions of high arousal, extreme fatigue, and enforced vigilance during the war. Severely sleep-deprived individuals can experience hallucinations and paranoid delusions, and sleep deprivation is used systematically by brutal investigators. Sleep deprivation is common in hypomania and may contribute to hallucinatory experiences in this condition. Psychotic experiences have been reported under experimental conditions of sensory isolation in which the subject is deprived of as much sensation as possible. Prolonged exposure to a homogeneous, perceptual environment has a disrupting effect on perception, thinking, and emotional processes, and is thought by some researchers to generate hallucinations and delusions (Zubek *et al.*, 1963). A similar condition could be imposed functionally on some schizophrenic patients, who apparently lack normal orienting responses to novel stimuli (Gruzelier *et al.*, 1981). Visual hallucinations, which are common in organic psychoses caused by toxic substances, are rare in schizophrenia, which is dominated by auditory hallucinations. A defect in attention would be compatible with the predominance of auditory hallucinations in schizophrenia because the visual stimulus field is, in general, more highly structured than is the auditory stimulus field, and the potential for perceptual errors is less in the visual modality because of the richness of contextual cues. As pointed out by Hebb (1958, p. 198), ''a perception is itself not observable, and it must be regarded as a theoretically-known event; an inference, not a datum.'' The diary of the lone, transatlantic yachtsman, Donald Crowhurst, who developed delusional beliefs before committing suicide (Tomalin and Hall, 1970), exemplifies the effect of total isolation. Russell-Davis (1972) emphasises the need for confirmation of one's perceptions, and considers that social isolation, such as may occur in sensitive people during adolescence, is conducive to the evolution of idiosyncratic perceptions and concepts, which he sees as implicated in the aetiology of schizophrenia. Bannister (1963) predicted a weakening of the integrity of the system of psychological constructs in subjects who experienced repeated invalidation of their responses. Surprisingly, his experimental results showed the reverse effect. On the other hand, Asch (1952) could induce subjects apparently to misjudge length under pressure to conform to false estimates given by ''stooges.'' Even delusional experiences are modified by social factors. A stationary spot of light appears to move when viewed in a darkened room. This compelling experience, the so-called autokinetic movement, becomes concordant for a group of observers communicating with one another (Sherif and Sherif, 1956).

Perceptual abnormalities have been described in schizophrenia patients, including phoneme recognition (Caudrey and Kirk, 1979) and size and distance constancy (Weckowicz, 1960; Weckowicz *et al.*, 1958). They are more affected by the Muller–Lyer illusion (Weckowicz and Witney, 1960). The abnormalities of word associations found in schizophrenic patients (Pavy, 1968) may originate from misperceptions of stimulus words (Moon, 1969), which in turn may arise from phoneme discrimination deficits (Caudrey and Kirk, 1979). Visual and auditory defects have been described in paraphrenia and paranoid psychoses (see Kay *et al.*, 1976, and Cooper *et al.*, 1976) and schizophrenia generally (Burtt and Weller, 1984). All these perceptual abnormalities would be intensified by social isolation, preventing the checking and verification of experience.

3 Personality and Negative Features: The Process-reactive Distinction

There is a group of individuals who seem to display some of the features associated with chronic schizophrenia, such as emotional blunting, poor rapport, and low motivation but to only a slight degree, insufficient for a diagnosis of schizophrenia. Such individuals seem particularly numerous in the families of schizophrenic patients and were considered by Bleuler (1923, p. 432–433) to be suffering from "latent schizophrenia." Kraepelin similarly thought that the relatives of schizophrenic patients sometimes manifested "latent schizophrenia," and Luxenberger (1939) formed the impression that the relatives seemed often to suffer from a milder form of schizophrenia. The concept of latent schizophrenia has affinities with "borderline syndrome" proposed by Grinker *et al.* (1968) and "pseudoneurotic schizophrenia" suggested by Hoch and Polatin (1949).

Romney's initial analysis of the psychological test results of first-degree relatives of schizophrenic probands found more thought disorder in this group. Partialing out intelligence removed this finding (Romney, 1967, 1969a, 1969b). Low intelligence in family members is not normally thought to be associated with schizophrenia. Studies have shown more creativity, superior intelligence, and leadership ability (Hammer and Zubin, 1968; Karlsson, 1968; Jarvick and Chadwick, 1973). Goldberg and Morrison (1963) showed that the clustering of schizophrenia in the lower socioeconomic class is a consequence of illness and not family circumstances as judged by the father's occupation. From Romney's data one must conclude that the relatives of affected probands are either less intelligent than his controls, or that the relatives were indeed more thought-disordered and that this contaminated their performance on the Wechsler Adult Intelligence Scale (WAIS).

In describing the mothers of 100 schizophrenic probands who were interviewed blindly with control groups of 20 neurotic probands and 57 non-psychiatric subjects, Alanen (1958) considered that the experimental group were distinguished by characteristics such as having a "loveless and aggressive attitude towards her child, and at the same time to exhibit a powerful possessiveness." These characteristics are consonant with later evidence that the expression of powerful emotions is perturbing to schizophrenic patients, and relapses are more likely when such patients are restored to highly emotional families (Vaughan and Leff, 1976; Leff and Vaughan, 1980).

Oddities in interactions and behaviour have been observed in uncontrolled American experiments with uncertain diagnostic criteria (Lidz and Lidz, 1949, 1963). In an unbiased sample, Hirsch and Leff (1975) were unable to replicate the evidence of Wynne and Singer (1963; Singer and Wynne, 1966a, 1966b; Wynne 1967, 1968, 1971) who claimed objective evidence for the hypothesis that "the types of thought disorder are functions of the mode of family transactions," although they did find that the fathers of schizophrenic patients were more verbose (Leff and Hirsch, 1972). One has no aetiological indications from these findings. Whilst it is plausible that some of the maternal characteristics might contribute to relapse, it does not follow that they were causative of the disorder. Two alternative possibilities are (1) that both parent and child have a genetic disorder which is expressed in a more muted form in the mother or (2) that the problems of caring for a schizophrenic child induce characteristic parental responses.

The diagnostic criteria were unclear in Alanen's study, although she used patients from the Psychiatric Clinic of Helsinki, where diagnostic practices are close to those of the United Kingdom. Dr. Viitamaki blindly analysed Rorschach findings (a projective inkblot test). The mothers of neurotic patients were indistinguishable from the nonpsychiatric controls, except for showing more reserve and self-criticism. But the mothers of schizophrenic patients showed poverty and coldness of their emotional life, lack of empathy, proneness to unrealistic behaviour and thought patterns, aggressiveness, proneness to domineering patterns of interpersonal relationships, anxiety, inward insecurity, and "schizoid traits."

Luxenberger (1939) would recognise schizoid personality only if there was a positive family history of schizophrenia.

Considered as an individual apart from his family circle the affectionless psychopath is an extreme and inferior variant of the personality with shallow effect. But if I find, for example, that he has a schizophrenic father then there is nothing against my censoring him as a carrier of the schizophrenic disposition and from this point of view calling him a schizoid psychopath. (Luxenberger, quoted in Jaspers, 1959, p. 655)

The concept of a spectrum disorder with a genetic basis was supported by the pioneer adoption study of Heston (1966) who found an excess of sociopaths (antisocial psychopaths) and a variety of distinguishing behavioural indices in his group of adopted probands born to schizophrenic mothers, compared to his control population. The same spectrum was found by Kety *et al.* (1975, 1978) in their Danish adoption studies, but their widely accepted conclusion is open to criticism.

Thirty-three probands were selected out of a possible five hundred seven individuals. The diagnoses were broadly based and included pseudoneurotic schizophrenic and schizoid individuals in the category of definite schizophrenia. One-third of the affected relatives were related to only three of the probands.

According to Paton-Salzberg (1982) there was an arithmetical error in one table that reduced the number of families of the index adoptees containing at least one schizophrenic member from 14 to 8, rendering the difference from the control group insignificant. A review of the genetic evidence convinced Gottesman and Sheilds (1982) that genetic factors have been consistently found in a variety of studies, but they refer to the self-criticism accompanying adoption strategies (Wender *et al.*, 1973, 1974; Kety *et al.*, 1976): only some of the biological parents gave, or were allowed to give, their children for adoption; the children placed within their own families were excluded from analysis; those adoptees who were abnormal before placement were not included in the analysis; those parents who were allowed to adopt children would be biased towards health; a strong correlation was demonstrated between the social class of the adopting parents and the biological parents; those children who were fostered and not adopted were not included in the study; and the fathers were unlike the husbands of schizophrenic women but were more likely to be socially inadequate.

It is customary to specify the criteria for patient selection in a research programme. These stipulative (Moore, 1978) or operational definitions tend to concentrate on psychotic features. Such features are convenient for defining the selection procedure, but exclude a large group in whom only negative features are discernible. From a genetic viewpoint such exclusions may obscure familial factors and reduce the interfamily concordance of illness (Heston, 1966, Kety *et al.*, 1975, 1978). Geneticists are therefore attracted to a wider concept of schizophrenia, which for familial concordance analysis extends to incorporating sociopathy and alcoholism as possible minor expressions of a spectrum disorder. The inclusion of personality deterioration into a widened domain of schizophrenia is emphatically rejected by DSM-III, which disregards entirely the negative features of schizophrenia and relegates these to a category of personality disorder. This is in contrast to Kraepelin's, Bleuler's, and Schneider's position, who all emphasised the global nature of psychosis (see, for example, Kraepelin, 1913, p. 248). The deterioration is poignantly expressed by Holderlin—

> I am here like the shadows, like them,
> I am silent and my shuddering heart
> Has already ceased singing.

In an influential address Kety (1980) stressed the importance of including negative features in patient selection for research. He may have been struck by the computerised axial tomographic (CAT) studies of the Northwick Park group (Johnstone *et al.*, 1976) which found dilated cerebral ventricles in patients with negative symptoms. These patients were designated type II (Crow, 1980) to distinguish them from those with the requisite hallucinations, delusions, and thought disorder, designated type I. Discrepant CAT scan results have been obtained subsequently that possibly reflect patient selection procedures and radiological techniques. Those studies with concordant findings have examined older patients in institutional settings (see Editorial, *Lancet,* 1979, for review). These findings provide support for Kraepelin's concept of a chronic disorder with an organic basis, at least as an important subtype. [On the other hand ventricular dilation has been associated with ECT and chronicity in affective illness, and may contribute to these findings (Calloway *et al.,* 1982; R. Dolan, 1984, personal communication)].

As a geneticist, Kety was arguing from a position of self-interest, but the view he stressed was in accord with Schneider's (1957) assertion that "symptoms of first rank importance do not always have to be present for a diagnosis to be made. . . . We are often forced to base our diagnosis on the symptoms of second rank importance" (p. 135).

Schneider is not exhaustive in defining symptoms of second-rank importance but mentions hallucinations other than those of the first rank, delusional notions, perplexity, depressed and elated moods, and experiences of flattened feeling (p. 134). The mood variation is a troublesome inclusion, and paranoid delusions present a special problem. Schneider stresses the insight necessary for achieving a diagnosis if first-rank symptoms are absent, an insight which must be less in those lacking clinical experience and responsibility, but who may be involved in research (Sadler *et al.,* 1981).

If only symptoms of this order (symptoms of second rank importance) are present, diagnosis will have to depend wholly on the coherence of the total clinical picture. (Schneider, 1957, p. 134)

Kety's genetic findings have been paralleled by psychoneurological and psychophysiological findings in patients lacking positive symptoms, whereas biochemical factors have been found in the contrary florid group (Sandler *et al.,* 1978; van Kammen *et al.,* 1982).

The negative symptoms of schizophrenia are often the first to develop and may be the only manifestation of the disease throughout its course.

The disintegration of the psychic personality is in general accomplished in dementia praecox in such a way that in the first place the disorders of emotion and of volition dominate the morbid state . . . dullness and indifference . . . frequently form the first symptoms. (Kraepelin, 1919, p. 283)

Kraepelin sees the negative symptoms as the core of the illness. In stressing the centrality of these, he contradicts the position adopted by DSM-III of categorising these features as disorders of personality and detaching them from the concept of schizophrenia.

We observe a weakening of those emotional activities which permanently form the mainsprings of volition. . . . It seems to me that the disorders observed in the patients and the complaints to which they give utterance, point exactly to injury to the general scheme of our psychic development as it fixes the substance of our personality. The general trend of volition and also the higher emotions might form the first point of attack. But further the instrument of general conceptions with its regulating influence on the train of thought would then also become worthless, if the will were no longer capable of using it. (Kraepelin, 1919, pp. 74–76)

The group of patients defined by the DSM-III criteria does not correspond to the group described by Kraepelin, Bleuler, or Schneider. Gruzelier and Manchanda (1982) correlated features of the electrodermal orienting response with patients' clinical profiles. These profiles were obtained from the PSE (Wing *et al.,* 1974) and the brief psychotic rating scale (Overal and Graham, 1962) supplied by other workers. In this study certain laterality features discriminated between two profile clusters. The post hoc nature of the initial analysis was overcome by a two-stage experiment. The actual clusters have a quality of special pleading, for example, slowness, social unease, irritability, and simple depression are attributed to mainly negative features of schizophrenia, whereas they might plausibly be related to depression. Surprisingly, conceptual disorganisation is grouped with negative features. Nevertheless, the strategy of correlating symptom profile with objective measures could be extended. Cluster analysis of symptoms gives each symptom an equal weight, whereas diagnosis is typically hierarchical. Nevertheless, cluster analysis has the advantage of exploring the traditional categorisation schemes afresh, unaffected by preconception.

CATEGO diagnoses of schizophrenia were highly concordant with the following psychopathological characteristics (see Table 6). It is interesting to note the high frequency with which voices speaking to the patient occurred in those diagnosed as schizophrenic, especially since there is no exclusion of experiences of voices saying things that were congruent with mood, which we would accept as a psychotic experience in an affective illness. Less than 50% of the patients given the reference diagnosis exhibited poor rapport, suggesting that the population under study was weighted with patients with positive symptoms. Delusions of persecution were frequent, exceeding thought alienation, thoughts spoken aloud, and delusions of control which one would have expected to be particularly common experiences in a group of patients with numerous positive symptoms.

Carpenter *et al.* (1973) identified 69 statistically significant symptom discriminators by analysis of variance from the sample of 1121 patients whose symptoms were collected by the International Pilot Study of Schizophrenia. These symptoms were entered into a stepwise discriminant function analysis using 405 patients with a project diagnosis of schizophrenia and 155 with other diagnoses as the comparison group. The nine most discriminating symptoms, which scored positively, were restricted affect, poor insight, thoughts spoken aloud, poor rapport, widespread delusions, incoherent speech, unreliable information, bizarre delusions, and nihilistic delusions. These became the basis of their flexible system of diagnosis.

TABLE 6
Percentage of Patients with Concordant Features
on Cluster Analysis and CATEGO Diagnoses
of Schizophrenia[a]

Feature	Percentage
Lack of insight	97
Auditory hallucinations	74
Verbal hallucinations	70
Ideas of reference	70
Delusions of reference	67
Flatness of affect	66
Suspiciousness	66
Voices speaking to the patient	65
Delusional mood	64
Inadequate description	64
Thought alienation	52
Thoughts spoken aloud	50
Delusions of control	48
Hearing voices speak full sentences	44
Poor rapport	43

[a]The International Pilot Study in Schizophrenia, Vol. 1, WHO
(1973).

The absence of auditory hallucinations is striking and the final item would commonly be attributed to depression. What is also striking, however, is how well this list corresponds with the classical descriptions of Kraepelin and Bleuler. The evaluation of many of these items, particularly restricted affect, poor rapport, and unreliable information, places difficult demands on raters and introduces subtleties of judgement that researchers attempting to identify an unequivocal group would be anxious to avoid. A comparison of different studies shows that first-rank symptoms are inconsistent in their presence and frequency. Although it is asserted that they cluster together (Mellor, 1970), they have an even closer association with nonpsychotic symptoms (see Table 4).

4 The Paranoid–Nonparanoid Distinction

Certain delusions are described as paranoid. The term is not sharply restricted to delusions of persecution but is commonly extended to include grandiose delusions [e.g., *International Classification of Diseases* (ICD), 9th ed.]. The former commonly accompanies other schizophrenic delusions and may occur in affective illness. Grandiose delusions are characteristic of elated mood disturbance of either mania or hypomania. Paranoid delusions often occur with schizophrenic symptoms and may originate as interpretations of these. If patients have experiences of having thoughts put in their heads, or having their will or body controlled, it is no surprise that they may secondarily develop paranoid interpretations. Many patients who have experienced first-rank symptoms have entertained such interpretations. Paranoid symptoms also occur in affective illness, and, when they do, British psychiatrists accept them as constituting part of a constellation of features consistent with the mood disturbance. Ideas of reference or of persecution were found in most of 61 "depressive state" patients. "They ranged from a mere impression of contempt, jeering, avoidance or hostility on the part of others to a conviction of being poisoned, followed about, shot at, tormented, etc." (Lewis, 1934). Schneider (1957) views the symptoms as merely a subgrouping "unmistakable paraphrenia . . . or paranoia . . . [constitutes] only one type of schizophrenic psychosis."

Separation of paranoid psychoses from schizophrenia would not seem to have been widely practised by the psychiatrists in the IPSS. As pointed out by Roth and McClelland (1979), when the two CATEGO diagnoses were merged the 20% discrepancy rate recorded in seven of the centres declined to 6%, and the 40% figure in Washington was halved to 20%. In Parkes's (1963) diagnostic scheme for schizophrenia commended by Granville-Grossman (1971), delusions of persecution are afforded equal weight with passivity and telepathic experiences, disorders of speech, and thinking. Of the 12 cases that Sheldrick and her colleagues (1977) found whose diagnosis changed from schizophrenia to affective illness, all had paranoid symptoms and some disturbance of mood and sleep. Paranoid symptoms occurring in isolation of other psychotic or affective symptoms may be regarded as constituting a separate disorder (Kahlbaum, 1873; Kraepelin, 1919; DSM-III—Wing *et al., 1974*). Paranoid states, defined according to the *Glossary of Mental Disorders* (1968), were included by Kendell and Gourlay (1970) in the diagnosis of schizophrenia. Paranoia is one of these, and the definition includes sytemised grandiose delusions, which can occur in mania. The definition of involutional paraphrenia states that "Affective symptoms, especially depression, may be present." They were unable to separate affective psychoses and schizophrenia. The separation may have been possible if paranoid states had been omitted or even if they had been assigned to affective psychoses. The same question arises in the literature on schizoaffective disorder when Kendell's criteria of the disorder are adopted (e.g., Brockington and Leff, 1979). A substantial proportion of patients begin their illness with exclusive paranoid symptoms but go on to develop a range of schizophrenic phenomena. In a prolonged follow-up study Tsuang *et al.* (1981) found the paranoid–nonparanoid distinction unstable.

The DSM-III isolates paranoid disorders if certain psychotic symptoms listed

TABLE 7
Final Diagnosis of Paranoid and Nonparanoid Schizophrenia[a]

Final diagnosis	Original diagnostic group	
	Paranoid N = 54	Nonparanoid N = 120
Paranoid schizophrenia	29 (53.7)	12 (10.0)
Nonparanoid schizophrenia	22 (40.7)	101 (84.2)
Bipolar disorder	1 (1.9)	3 (2.5)
Unipolar disorder	0 (0)	2 (1.7)
Undiagnosed psychoses	0 (0)	1 (0.8)
Organic psychoses	1 (1.9)	1 (0.8)
Alcoholism	1 (1.9)	0 (0)

[a]Based on personal and approximate interviews, percentage of *n* in parentheses. (From Tsuang *et al.*, 1981, p. 35.)

in the criteria of psychosis are absent. Although the CATEGO programme separates paranoid disorders, some research workers include this group in their schizophrenic category. The ICD 9 (WHO, 1977) similarly isolates paranoia (codified as 297.1) but is ambiguous in the process and defines it as

A rare chronic psychosis in which logically constructed systematized delusions have developed gradually without concomitant hallucinations or the schizophrenic type of disordered thinking. The delusions are mostly of grandeur (the paranoic prophet or inventor), persecution or somatic abnormality. (295.3)

The confusion arises in differentiating this disorder from schizophrenia of the paranoid type. The definition of the latter contains many permitted inclusive features, indicated by the word *may*. If these features are ignored as being consistent with the diagnosis, but not necessary for it, one is left with a condition indistinguishable from paranoia (see italicised words):

The form of schizophrenia in which relatively stable delusions which may be accompanied by hallucinations, *dominate the clinical picture. The delusions are frequently of persecution but may take other forms (for example, of jealousy, exalted birth, Messianic mission, or bodily change).* Hallucinations and erratic behaviour may occur; in some cases conduct is seriously disturbed from the outset, thought disorder may be gross, and affective flattening with fragmentary delusions and hallucinations may develop.

It is difficult to distinguish between the views that paraphrenia is a late-onset psychosis with well-preserved personality or merely the outcome of schizophrenia in later life when the personality is already well formed, or that it is a

Malcolm P. I. Weller

distinct disorder. Kraepelin separated paraphrenia and paranoia from dementia praecox in part because they occurred later in life and in part because they did not seem to lead to the deterioration which he considered inevitable in dementia praecox. Moreover, the disturbance of feeling and volition, which he regarded as fundamental to dementia praecox, was usually absent.

[D]estruction and finally disintegration of the personality does not take place as in dementia praecox, that much rather the inner unity of the psychic process remains permanently preserved. (Kraepelin, 1919, p. 276)

Meyer (1921) followed up 78 of Kraepelin's cases and found that 40% showed signs of deterioration, some displaying typical schizophrenic symptoms. There was nothing in the original presentation that would have allowed a distinction regarding outcome.

Using the epidemiological data collected from an examination of deafness in paranoid schizophrenia, Kay (1972) found certain differences in that group. In general they were of a prickly, suspicious, premorbid disposition; they were less frequently married; if married they were more often childless, and if they had children these were more likely to have died from diverse causes. It is difficult to disentangle which, if any, of these factors are causally related to the disorder and which are consequential. Psychological abnormalities have failed to differentiate

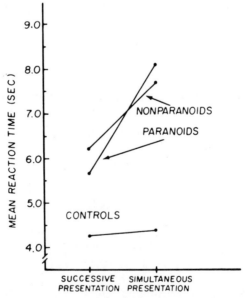

Fig. 1. Reaction time for correct answers on successive presentation mode and simultaneous presentation mode for paranoid and nonparanoid schizophrenics and matched controls.

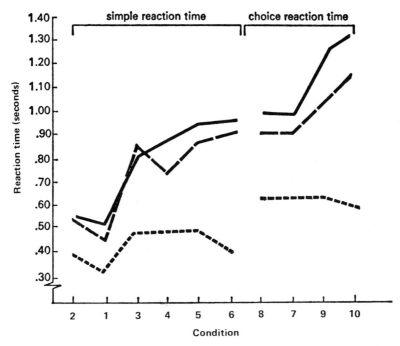

FIG. 2. Comparison of reaction times of paranoid and nonparanoid schizophrenic patients in distracting conditions. 2, 8, No distraction; 1, 7, normal conditions; 3, mild distraction; 4, 9, moderate distraction; 5, severe distraction; 6, 10, mean distraction. (————) Paranoid schizophrenic; (— — —) nonparanoid schizophrenic; (- - - - - - -) nonschizophrenic. (From Payne and Caird, 1967.)

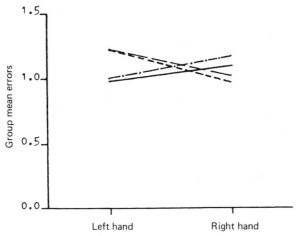

FIG. 3. (————) Normals; (—·—) psychiatric controls; (— — —) paranoids; (——— ——— ———) nonparanoids.

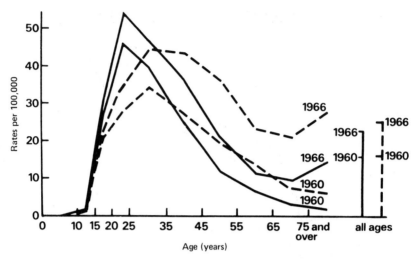

Fɪɢ. 4. Incidence of paranoid states. The 1966 figures include paranoia and paranoid states. They are omitted from 1960 figures. (————) Males; (– – –) females.

the two subgroups (see Fig. 1, 2, and 3) (Payne and Caird, 1967; Gur, 1979; Weller and Ameen, 1982; Burtt and Weller, 1984; Magaro and Chamrad, 1983).

The literature is contradictory, and McGhie (1967) found that hebephrenic patients resembled cases of arteriosclerotic dementia in being unable to screen out irrelevant cues, while paranoid patients were able to do this. Nasrallah *et al.*, (1982) found significantly more left-handedness in their paranoid group, contrasted with the nonparanoid group, suggesting the possibility of greater left hemisphere dysfunction. The same group went on to show greater abnormality of some brain CAT scan indices but no greater degree of neurological soft signs, which were higher in both subgroups than in controls (Nasrallah *et al.*, 1982).

The incidence of paranoia and paranoid states can be estimated from the difference between the 1966 and 1960 statistics. They were included in the former and omitted in the latter (see Fig. 4). Although Kay (1972) suggests that other factors may be operating to affect the age-related incidence of schizophrenia, the change in the accounting procedure between the 1960 and the 1966 figures is obviously important, particularly since it is recognised (Kraepelin, 1919) that paraphrenia has a late onset. Physically and genetically there is a difference in the paranoid subgroup. Conolly (1939), using measurement ratios, found that paranoid schizophrenics had a more pyknic or mesomorphic body build than other types of schizophrenic patients. This finding was confirmed by Verghese (1971) and Verghese *et al.*, (1978).

It has proved possible to differentiate chronic paranoid and nonparanoid schizophrenic patients by the muscle enzyme creatinine phosphokinase

(Melztzer, 1976). Abnormalities have been described of excessive branching of the subterminal motor nerves in psychotic patients (Ross-Stanton and Meltzer, 1981), which also differentiates the two subgroups, but there were only nine paranoid and four nonparanoid patients in the comparison. No significant correlations were found between peak dose of neuroleptic drugs and the morphological features, nor was any relationship found between these features and the duration of illness, or the number of previous psychotic episodes.

Fowler and his colleagues (1975) showed that the risk of relatives of paranoid probands being ill with schizophrenia was only half that of nonparanoid probands (7 versus 14%). The subtype of schizophrenia was not related in probands and relatives, although the age of onset was. Tsuang *et al.* (1974) felt that age of onset may reflect the degree of liability to the illness and account for the difference in the frequency with which relatives were affected in the paranoid and nonparanoid groups. In a later publication and in contradiction to the findings of the Fowler group, 16 schizophrenia cases were subdivided into 4 paranoid and 12 nonparanoid subgroups according to their clinical features at the time of index admission. There was no difference between the rates of schizophrenia in the relatives of the two subgroups, but there was a significant subtype concordance (Tsuang, 1978).

The term paranoid has come to have various meanings. The term delusional disorder was proposed as an alternative by Winokur (1977) to overcome the possibility of confusion and to define a group in whom delusions are not believed to be caused by underlying schizophrenia, affective, or organic conditions. Although Kolle (1931) found an increased risk for schizophrenia in the relatives of probands with delusional disorder, modern familial studies have not supported this finding, or the view that delusional disorder is a subtype of schizophrenia (Winokur, 1977; Kendler *et al.*, 1981). Debray (1975) found that patients with chronic delusions had more relatives with schizophrenia while patients with chronic hallucinations did not, suggesting that paranoia is part of the spectrum of schizophrenia while paraphrenia is not.

5 Phenomenology

Jaspers (1946) separated understandable experiences from those where some putative disease process had placed them outside the range of empathetic understanding. His writings were influential in establishing an approach to diagnosis which relied on detailed descriptions of symptoms, and his disciples included Gruhle, Schneider, and Mayer-Gross. The energetic search for an empathetic understanding of the patient's mental life was an essential characteristic of the approach. It is not part of this procedure to use some form of checklist, possibly with specific probe questions, as in the Present State Examination (Wing *et al.*, 1974), to achieve a diagnosis.

In clinical practice, Jaspers' recommendations are not adhered to since they are difficult to follow and potentially misleading.

Empathy is a very unsure process; it plays an indispensible part in human relations and poetic creations but as a research method it can lead to the greatest self-deception. Since it is so strongly influenced by our prejudices and desires, we accept it as obvious and assured with a considerable degree of certainty. This process is all the more hazardous because we have no yard-stick for measuring the validity of this feeling of certainty. (Kraepelin, 1920, p. 10)

Problems arise even when identical questions are being asked. As in structured interview techniques, such as the PSE, the interview style, verbal emphasis, and examiners' responses may all affect the replies. Further confounding factors are the setting and examiners' expectations, which may produce the same halo effect as has been demonstrated in first impressions, which can be coloured by misleading information deliberately supplied by the investigator (Kelley, 1950). Nevertheless, the clinical scores and categorisation of patients have been found to be reliable (Wing *et al.*, 1967) and the standard interview "introduces a degree of standardization and precision."

When criteria were adopted which excluded acute onset brief-lived episodes or major affective symptoms (Feighner *et al.*, 1972; Morrison *et al.*, 1972), 92.5% of 86 schizophrenic patients were given the same diagnosis over a 30–40 year follow-up period by researchers blind to the original diagnosis. This stability substantially exceeded that obtained for affective illness, where it is often assumed that diagnostic problems are less. The omission of the acute-onset episodic course illness, or those with major affective symptoms, may have removed an important source of variability and provides some justification for viewing the group of patients exhibiting these features as constituting a separate category, a position adopted by DSM-III.

The exclusion of marked affective disturbance finds some justification in the better prognosis when this is present (Vaillant, 1963; Marder *et al.*, 1979) and the instability of diagnosis (M. T. Tsuang, 1983, personal communication). However, this is a departure from historical precedent.

All phenomena of manic-depressive psychosis may also appear in any disease; the only decisive factor is the presence or absence of schizophrenic symptoms. Therefore, neither a state of manic exaltation nor a melancholic depression, nor the alternation of both states has any significance for the diagnosis. Only after careful observation has revealed no schizophrenic features, may we conclude that we are dealing with a manic-depressive psychosis. (Bleuler, 1911, p. 304)

This is the position adopted by Lewis and Piotrowski (1954) in the famous dictum "even a little trace of schizophrenia is schizophrenia" and that of the CATEGO programme.

A potential problem in phenomenology is the possibility of the constellation of features influencing the description of one particular feature. It is imperative that description precedes diagnosis. "We refuse to prejudge when studying our phenomena" (Jaspers, 1959a, p. 56). Inadvertently this obvious precaution may not always be taken. It is difficult to escape pattern recognition, which in essence is the basis of syndromes. But this can make seemingly independent observations dependent on some working hypothesis, which may be culled from other phenomena and the personal and family history.

Frequently we find examples of distinguishing characteristics which fail to stand up to scrutiny. The traditional concepts of thought disorder owe much to the writings of Bleuler:

[T]he peculiar association disturbance is always present, but not each and every aspect of it. Sometimes the anomalies of association may manifest themselves in 'blocking' or in the splitting of ideas. (Bleuler, 1911 p. 13)

In advanced cases, there results a complete word-salad which is entirely unintelligible even though it may be built up, in the main of ordinary words. (p. 155)

Kraepelin (1919) considered defects in language as ranking with equal importance with other schizophrenic symptoms. However, experimentally, there was no correlation between an objective measure of thought disorder, based on sorting photos of individuals into consistent categories (Bannister and Fransella, 1966), and the predictability of schizophrenic speech, measured by deleting words from transcribed speech samples and seeing if these could be correctly substituted (Rutter *et al.*, 1977). Structured interviews were given to 113 patients. Because the interviewers were face to face, additional cues were available and might have been used unwittingly by the researchers. Tangentiality, derailment, incoherence, and illogicality of speech, all of which have been considered pathognomonic of schizophrenia, occurred with nearly equal frequency in both mania and schizophrenia. Blocking was so uncommon that it was thought unlikely to be clinically useful and so were clanging, echolalia, neologisms, and word approximations (Andreasen, 1979).

The CATEGO program does not place language disorder as an isolated finding in the category of schizophrenia, but in a separate category of "other psychosis." In so doing it seems at variance with the recommendations of Bleuler and Kraepelin, but to have anticipated the problems identified by Andreason. There were indications which may have contributed to this prescience. Hawks (1964) was unable to replicate the findings of Payne and Hewlett (1960) and Payne and Friedlander (1962) who, using psychological methods, claimed that schizophrenic patients were overinclusive in their thinking, and McGhie *et al.*, (1964) who had found that hypomanic and obsessional patients had even higher overinclusive scores than did schizophrenic patients. Later, Reed (1968) showed that interobserver reliability was low in assessing concrete thinking on a proverb interpretation test, and Payne and Hewlett (1960) suggested that concrete thinking is a function of low intelligence and not a characteristic of schizophrenia.

The term *pseudomanic* schizophrenia used by Schneider (1957) implies a diametrically opposed position to that adopted in American diagnostic systems, which exclude substantial affective disturbance from the schizophrenic category. A distinction between schizophrenia and mania may not be feasible on clinical ratings of thought disorder.

Claims have been made for a complex but successful distinction based on an objective scoring procedure. Using a technique that lacked theoretical justification, Wykes and Leff (1982) screened acute schizophrenic and manic patients whose speech was particularly difficult to classify clinically. Manics were found to make more links using more pronouns and joining words such as *and, because,* and *so,* although this usage did not necessarily clarify the meaning. Wykes (1981) feels that clinicians' ability to distinguish between the two types of speech can be improved by teaching, but Andreason's study indicates that at the time of writing the distinction cannot be made clinically.

The possibility of fitting observations to diagnosis is illustrated by this issue. The term *flight of ideas* implies a diagnosis of hypomania, whereas "disjointed" or "fragmented" thinking or "inconsequent thought" (Schneider, 1957, p. 99) implies a diagnosis of schizophrenia. If in clinical practice we are actually unable to make the distinction (Andreason, 1979), we may be committing an unwitting error by using different terms to describe clinically indistinguishable phenomena, and fitting our observations to match our diagnoses. The same difficulty is apparent in separating catatonic excitement from overactivity. The former term implies a diagnosis of schizophrenia and the latter of hypomania, but can they be distinguished reliably?

Despite diagnostic differences among psychiatrists (Kreitman, 1961; Kreitman *et al.,* 1961), the consistency of psychiatric observations and inferences was as high as physicians' variability in Fletcher's (1952) study of the physical disorder of pulmonary emphysema (Shepherd *et al.,* 1968). The psychiatrists in this study, however, had received similar training in the same institution.

Psychiatric diagnosis cannot be made entirely by an algorithm. Training and experience cannot be utterly disregarded, and the present findings have to be related to premorbid personality and life history. Checklists are particularly unsuitable when one is dealing with an early or incipient illness when the diagnostic difficulties are greatest. Judgements inevitably have to be made, even in applying apparently clear-cut diagnostic criteria.

According to DSM-III, if the illness has resulted in a deterioration and has been evident for at least 6 months the diagnosis of schizophrenia may be made if there is a "marked loosening of associations." One may be unsure whether associations are, or are not, loosened, and when this point is resolved it is unclear when the loosening is enough to justify the term marked.

Disturbances and inconsistencies in the logical train of thought occur to a subtle degree in normal people under stress (Gottschalk *et al.,* 1972), and depressives as well as schizophrenic patients are less able to abstract than normals (Braff *et al.,* 1974). The presence or absence of a diminished capacity to respond emotionally, known as flattening of affect, is particularly prone to produce differences of diagnosis between trained observers. It is these symptoms, however, that feature prominently in any diagnostic system.

6 Clear Consciousness: Some Conceptual and Identification Problems

Clear consciousness is specified as a requirement for the diagnosis of schizophrenia in the Registrar-General's (1968) *Glossary of Mental Disorders,* and this was implied by Schneider (1957) when he separated somatic factors which lead to clouded consciousness. The object of separating out disorders in which consciousness is not clear is to differentiate organic states, wherein there is a brain dysfunction through known organic causes, from a functional psychosis. Despite this objective, the current 9th edition of the ICD specifies that an acute schizophrenic episode is characterized by a "dream-like state with slight clouding of consciousness and perplexity." An organic basis of schizophrenia was assumed by Kraepelin, and modern findings support such a viewpoint, at least in a subgroup of patients. Such findings create confusion in the nosological system which separates organic disorders from functional disorders. Structural brain changes are implied by the finding of enlarged cerebral ventricles in chronic schizophrenia patients (Johnstone *et al.,*1976; Weinberger *et al.,* 1980), and abnormalities of a variety of brain structures and functions have been described in schizophrenia, including the corpus callosum (Green, Glass, and O'Callaghan, 1979; Bigelow, Nasarallah, and Rauscher, 1983) the cerebellar vermis (Heath, Franklyn, and Shraberg, 1979; Reyes and Gordon, 1981; Coffman *et al.,* 1981), the basal ganglia (see Cumming *et al.,* 1983 for case description and reference to the literature), the mechanism of occulomotor control (Holzman, Proctor, and Hughes, 1973; Latham *et al.,* 1981), the septal nuclei (Heath, 1966; Averbach, 1981a, 1981b), the amygdala (Reynolds, 1983), and the hippocampus (Gruzelier, 1981). The last three are structures that are part of the limbic circuit which subserves emotion and attention and in which various peptide abnormalities have been identified (Roberts *et al.,* 1983).

Cortical damage through strokes, penetrating head injuries, and surgical extirpations seldom has permanent effects on consciousness, although cognitive functions are generally affected. The subcortical structures, however, are of particular interest as their integrity, particularly that of the basal ganglia and midbrain, may be necessary for consciousness (Reichardt, 1929; Jefferson, 1949; Penfield and Jasper, 1947).

Phenomenologically, consciousness often seems disturbed in schizophrenia, but little attention has been directed to this finding, in part, perhaps, because of the conflict with diagnostic requirements. However, clouded consciousness is not always an obvious problem and necessitates careful probing and enquiry. To illustrate the contention that clouding can be demonstrated in schizophrenia, passages from Slater and Roth's celebrated text book (1970) describing clouded consciousness are contrasted with quotations and points from the literature on schizophrenia (see Table 8). It may be seen that many aspects of clouded consciousness seem to be present in schizophrenia if they are sought for. Reservations will immediately spring to mind, which will be more fully dealt with later. Clouding is a fluctuating condition which, like delirium, is a temporary state, in the latter case by definition. Delusions are tenaciously held beliefs, whilst the impressions of delirium are shifting and impermanent, and disorientation is a feature of clouding. On the question of the temporary nature of clouding, this is merely a convention arising perhaps out of a focus on resolving organic conditions, such as febrile illnesses, which leaves us ignorant of the consequences of a prolonged disturbance of consciousness.

In addition to these features and in accord with Lipowski (1980), Slater and Roth mention fluctuations in the intensity of the symptoms, with a tendency for them to become much more prominent at night, and also disturbances of memory and orientation. In order to differentiate "true" schizophrenic phenomena from hypnogogic and hypnopompic experiences, little regard is paid to experiences which occur in bed at night. Nevertheless, patients frequently report such experiences, particularly of being touched, and others describe an intensification of daytime hallucinations. In the words of one author describing a schizophrenic patient, "he continued, however, to suffer from noise in his ears, hearing voices, etc., especially at night " (Rorie, 1862–1863). The abnormal nighttime experiences occurring without any such daytime experiences may represent an incipient phase when psychotic phenomena, like epileptic and delirious phenomena, are highlighted.

Disturbances in memory are revealed in schizophrenia in several different ways. In the World Health Organization's international pilot study of schizophrenia, the test–retest reliability had a mean intraclass correlation coefficient of only .49 (Hays, 1976). Since the patients were describing the same illness episode to trained observers, who used the same structured interview with which the interobserver reliability averaged .83, the memory and reporting of the illness episode must have varied over the few days between the two interviews.

A defect of cumulative memory in schizophrenia has been demonstrated experimentally (Kugler and Weller, 1982). In this study a chain of digits, exceed-

TABLE 8
Clouding in Schizophrenia

Slater and Roth (1978)	Commentary
The patient has difficulty in maintaining attention	It is our contention that many of the behavioural deficits seen in the schizophrenic can be accounted for by a primary attentional disorder (Korntsky and Orzack, 1978)
He tends to be easily distracted	Thinking becomes distracted by external events. It also becomes distracted by irrelevant personal thoughts and emotions which may even become mixed up with the problem (Payne, 1964)
He cannot dismiss from his mind the irrelevant sensory experience or the irrelevant idea	Schizophrenics have difficulty in maintaining a perceptual set and in concentrating on part of the perceptual field to the exclusion of other parts. . . . These patients are less capable of shutting off information which is irrelevant to the task in hand (Weckowicz and Witney, 1960)
Perception is affected so that sense data are misjudged	In early phases of their illness, schizophrenia patients, together with difficulty in thinking, such as an inability to concentrate and to control their thoughts, may experience perceptual difficulty and may even complain of an impairment of vision (Weckowicz, 1960)
	Distance constancy is poorer in schizophrenics than in nonschizophrenics and also . . . related to the poorer size constancy found in these patients. . . . The lack of depth and "flatness" of the visual world of schizophrenics has theoretical implications for the phenomenology of schizophrenia. Together with impaired form constancy it can change, foreshorten and distort the appearance of the perceived objects. Perhaps this change in depth perception would account for the complaint of some schizophrenics that things look different, unfamiliar and strange (Weckowicz, Sommer, and Hall, 1958)
Illusions, especially visual illusions . . . are very much more likely to arise than in the normal state	Schizophrenics are more susceptible to the Muller–Lyer illusion than non-schizophrenics (Weckowicz and Witney, 1960)
There are corresponding difficulties in comprehension	Some investigators [Cameron (1939), Vigotsky (1934), Kasanin *et al.* (1944)] have, on the basis of

(continued)

TABLE 8 (*Continued*)

Slater and Roth (1978)	Commentary
shown at first only at the highest and most abstract level	cognitive testing, concluded that the schizophrenic is unable to form the abstractions necessary for normal thinking in much the same manner in which the patient with organic brain defect is unable to deal with abstractions (Freeman, Cameron, and McGhie, 1958)
Called on to respond to a complex situation, the patient is likely to be slow	Although complete diagnostic specificity is lacking, there seems to be a remarkable correlation between . . . reaction time phenomena and those behaviours that lead diagnosticians at many different times and places to a diagnosis of schizophrenia (Zahn, 1977)
and to show some perseveration in thought and speech	The tendency toward stereotyping, combined with a lack of purposeful goal in their thinking, leads on the one hand to "Klebendenken" (adhesive, sticky type of thinking), to a kind of *perseveration,* and on the other hand to a general impoverishment of thought (Bleuler, 1911, p. 27) We frequently observe written verbrigeration in random repetition of words and sentences, and particularly of single letter and punctuation marks, either in a characteristic pattern or mixed with crosses, circles, triangles and other figures. For many years a hebephrenic always wrote the same row of numbers whose zeros were always continued to the end of each line (Bleuler, 1911, p. 159)
Judgments also will be less balanced and less adequate	The weakening of judgment . . . would have to be reckoned among the fundamental disorders of dementia praecox (Kraepelin, 1913, p. 248)
Gestalts are not sharply circumscribed and finely differentiated; figure–background differentiation is blurred, and is much less open to goal-directed action	Selective perception becomes impossible so that instead of dealing with the essence of the problem irrelevant aspects are perceived and thought about (Payne, 1964) These irrelevant associations to which the normal is also subject but to a much lesser degree would appear to arise from three sources: chance distractors from the environment; irrelevancies from the stimulus situation; and irrelevancies from past experience . . . the mere presence of these irrelevant factors . . . seems to lead the schizophrenic to give them focal rather than ground significance, signal rather than noise import (Shakow, 1962)

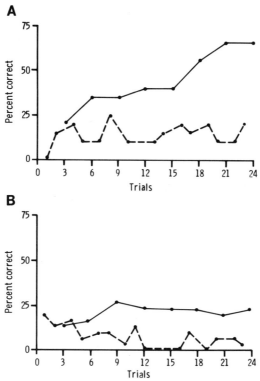

FIG. 5. Performance on the Hebb recurring-digits test. (A) Normal group; (B) schizophrenic group. (————) Recurring digit strings; (— — —) nonrecurring digit strings.

ing the subject's memory capacity, was repeated seven times alternatively with two novel chains. Control subjects, matched for initial digit span, improved their performance steadily and significantly on the repeated chain, while schizophrenic patients did not. (See Figure 5.)

After recovery from an episode of illness, schizophrenic patients often have difficulty in recalling details or even long periods of their illness, and on retesting patients one frequently finds that they have only the haziest recollection of the previous testing procedure (Weller, unpublished; K. Tress, 1983, personal communication). This difficulty has been commented on by early writers. "After acute and agitated phases of the disease we frequently encounter an amnesia varying widely in intensity and extent." (Bleuler, 1911, p. 140).

Stevens *et al.* (1978), supplementing the work of Crow and Mitchell (1975), found that 25% of 357 mental hospital patients with a consistent case-note diagnosis of schizophrenia underestimated their age by more than 5 years; 11% underestimated their age by a mean of 28.9 years. The phenomenon was associated with early onset and a poor prognosis. Six further studies were reviewed with similar findings. (Dahl, 1958; Lanzkron and Wolfson, 1958; Ehrenteil and Jenney, 1960; Michelson, 1968,; Stoffler, 1973; Smith and Oswald, 1976). Crow and Stevens (1978) went on to show what they believed was a "continuum of increasing temporal disorientation" which was associated with age disorientation. Slater and Roth (1970) think the phenomenon of "double orientation," admittedly of person and not of place, is characteristic of schizophrenia and is facilitated by clear consciousness. But elsewhere they state that a "co-existence of two or more totally compatible orientations is a feature of clouding of consciousness" (pp. 601–602).

Lipowski (1980), influenced by the finding of Engel and Ramano (1959), points out that in delirium, slow waves are more prominent in the electroencephalogram. Statistical analysis of the EEG recordings from schizophrenic subjects has shown an excess of slow-wave activity (Coger, Dymond, and Serafetinides, 1979; Weller and Montagu, 1979; Fenton *et al.*, 1980) and an increase in the degree of synchrony between certain brain regions (Flor-Henry, 1969; Weller and Montagu, 1979). Engel and Romano (1959) consider that delirium is "a syndrome of cerebral insufficiency," which takes its origin from changes in the functional metabolism of cerebral neurones. "As with the more familiar concepts of organ insufficiency, this refers to what evolves when the function of the organ as a whole is interfered with, for whatever reason." Regional cerebral blood flow and cerebral metabolism can now be mapped using radioactive isotopes, and Ingvar and Franzen (1974) and Buchsbaum and his colleagues (1982) have shown diminished regional cerebral blood flow activity and cerebral metabolism in schizophrenia, particularly in the frontal area. In an earlier paper, Engel and Romano (1949) stated that "essentially, delirium is a psychotic syndrome in which the basic psychologic symptom is a disturbance in the level of consciousness." As Lipowski (1980) points out in his monograph on delirium, doubt may exist as to whether a patient is suffering from delirium "rather than from one of the functional psychosis. . . . Acute schizophrenic, schizophreniform, or atypical psychoses is particularly likely to give rise to diagnostic difficulties" (p. 210).

Aetiological theories of schizophrenia include autointoxication, biochemical abnormalities, neuroreceptor abnormalities, traumatic brain damage, epilepsy, epileptic kindling, and viral infections. If an organic explanation, such as one of the above, is vindicated at least for some patients, is it likely that consciousness is indeed clear? Is it not equally plausible in such cases that the psychotic experiences are manifestations of disordered brain mechanisms, as postulated by the early writers, and that at least subtle disturbances of consciousness are inevitable and central to the experiences?

When all the instances are assembled, it is difficult to escape the conclusion that at least subtle examples of clouded consciousness can be detected in many schizophrenic patients. This would accord with organic explanations for a certain subgroup of patients and reinforces the arguments of Ferraro (1943) and Roth and McClelland (1979), who challenge Schneider's (1957) view that "the presence of coarse brain disease excludes all other kinds of diagnosis." It is possible that some schizophrenic patients have suffered cerebral damage to regions which will cause both schizophrenic phenomena *and* alterations in the state of consciousness. If an organic explanation is to prevail for even a small subgroup of patients, it would seem unlikely that consciousness is in no way disturbed and a fiction may be being perpetrated in setting forth diagnostic criteria which specify clear consciousness when such a high proportion of patients seem to betray evidence that the sensorium is disturbed.

7 Acknowledgements

Several papers discussed in the chapter were chosen by Dr. A. Mann for Journal Clubs at Friern and the Royal Free Hospitals. I am indebted to the participants for their comments, including Professor A. Wakeling and Professor G. M. Carstairs. Dr. A. Mann and Dr. K. Davison made helpful remarks on the text. Mrs. E. Ames provided help with library facilities. The personal experiments cited in the chapter were supported by grants from the Wellcome Trust and the North East Thames Regional Health Authority.

References

Achte, K. A. (1961). The course of schizophrenic and schizophreniform psychoses. *Acta Psychiatrica et Neurologica Scandinavica Supplement*, **155**, 36.

Alanen, Y. O. (1958). The mothers of schizophrenic patients. *Acta Psychiatrica et Neurologica Scandinavica Supplement*, No. 124.

Albee, G. W. (1977). Silver and golden comments on Dr. Derner. *Clinical Psychologist*, **30**, 7–8.

American Psychiatric Association (1980). "Diagnostic and Statistical Manual of Mental Disorders," 3rd ed. Washington D.C.

Andreason, N. C. (1979). Thought, language and communication disorders. II. Diagnostic significance. *Archives of General Psychiatry*, **36**, 1325–1330.

Averback, P. (1981a). Lesions of the nucleus peduncularis in neuropsychiatric disease. *Archives of Neurology*, **38**, 230–235.

Averback, P. (1981b). Structural lesions of the brain in young schizophrenics. *Canadian Journal of Neurological Science*, **8**, 73–77.

Bannister, D., and Fransella, F. (1966). A grid test of schizophrenic thought disorder. *British Journal of Social and Clinical Psychology*, **5**, 95–102.

Bateson, G., Jackson, D. D., Hailey, J., and Weakland, J. H. (1956). Towards a theory of schizophrenia. *Behavioural Science*, No. 4.

Beaumont, J. G., and Dimond, S. J. (1973). Brain disconnection and schizophrenia. *British Journal of Psychiatry,* **123,** 661–662.

Bland, R. C., and Orn, H. (1979). Schizophrenia: Diagnostic criteria and outcome. *British Journal of Psychiatry,* **134,** 34–38.

Bleuler, E. (1911). "Dementia Praecox or the Group of Schizophrenias." International Universities Press, New York.

Braff, D. L., Aaron, T., and Beck, M. D. (1974). Thinking disorder in depression. *Archives of General Psychiatry,* **31,** 456–459.

Breakey, W. R., and Goodell, H. (1972). Thought disorder in mania and schizophrenia evaluated by Bannister's grid test for schizophrenic thought disorder. *British Journal of Psychiatry,* **120,** 391–395.

Brockington, I. F., and Leff, J. P. (1979). Schizo-affective psychosis: Definitions and incidence. *Pschological Medicine,* **9,** 91–99.

Burtt, C., and Weller, M. P. I. (1984). Diminished auditory acuity in schizophrenia. *Journal of Physiology,* **351,** 208.

Calloway, S. P., Dolan, R. J., Jacoby, R. J., and Levy, R. (1981). ECT and cerebral atrophy; a computed tomographic study. *Acta Psychiatrica Scandanavica,* **64,** 442–445.

Cannon-Spoor, L., and Potkin, S. G. (1980). Poor premorbid adjustment and CT scan abnormalities in chronic schizophrenia. *American Journal of Psychiatry,* **137,** 1410–1413.

Carpenter, J. R., Strauss, J. S., and Bartko, J. J. (1973). Flexible system for the diagnosis of schizophrenia: Report from the WHO international pilot study of schizophrenia. *Science,* **182,** 1275–1277.

Carpenter, W. T., Strauss, J. S., and Muleh, S. (1973). Are there pathogenic symptoms in schizophrenia? *Archives of General Psychiatry,* **28,** 847–852.

Carpenter, W. T., Strauss, J. S., and Muleh, S. (1974). Cross-cultural evaluation of Schneider's first rank symptoms of schizophrenia. *American Journal of Psychiatry,* **131,** 682–687.

Caudrey, D. J., and Kirk, K. (1979). The perception of speech in schizophrenia and affective disorders. In "Hemisphere Assymmetries of Function in Psychopathology" (Ed. P. Flor-Henry). Elsevier, Amsterdam, New York and Oxford.

Chambers, W. R. (1955). Neurological conditions masquerading as psychiatric diseases. *American Journal of Psychiatry,* **112,** 387–389.

Coffman, J. A., Meffero, J., Golden, C. J., Bloch, S., and Graber, B. (1981). Cerebellar atrophy in chronic schizophrenia. *Lancet* **i,** 666.

Coger, R. W., Dymond, A. M., and Serafetinides, E. A. (1979). Electroencephalographic similarities between chronic alcoholics and chronic, non paranoid schizophrenics. *Archives of General Psychiatry,* **36,** 91–94.

Coid, J., and Strang, J. (1982). Mania secondary to procyclidine (kemmadrin) abuse. *British Journal of Psychiatry,* **141,** 81–84.

Conolly, C. J. (1939). Physique in relation to psychology quoted by L. Rees

(1960). Constitutional factors and abnormal behaviour. In "Handbook of Abnormal Psychology" (Ed. H. J. Eysenck). Pitman Medical, London.

Cooper, A. F., Curry, A. R., Kay, D. W. K., Garside, R. F., and Roth, M. (1974). Hearing loss in paranoid and affective psychoses of the elderly. *Lancet* **ii**, 851–854.

Cooper, A. F., Garside, R. F., and Kay, D. W. K. (1976). A comparison of deaf and non-deaf patients with paranoid and affective psychoses. *British Journal of Psychiatry*, **129**, 532–538.

Cooper, J. E. (1967). Diagnostic changes in a longitudinal study of psychiatric patients. *British Journal of Psychiatry*, **113**, 129–142.

Coryell, W., and Tsuang, M. T. (1982). DSM-III schizophreniform disorder. *Archives of General Psychiatry*, **39**, 66–69.

Crow, T. J. (1980). Molecular pathology of schizophrenia: More than one disease process? *British Medical Journal*, **280**, 66–68.

Crow, T. J., and Mitchell, W. S. (1975). Subjective age in chronic schizophrenia: Evidence for a sub-group of patients with defective learning capacity. *British Journal of Psychiatry*, **126**, 360–363.

Crow, T. J., and Stevens, M. (1978). "Age distortion in chronic schizophrenia: The nature of the cognitive deficit. *British Journal of Psychiatry*, **133**, 137–142.

Cumming, S. J. L., Gosenfeld, L. F., Houlihan, J. P., and McCaffrey, T. (1983). Neuropsychiatric disturbances associated with idiopathic calcification of the basal ganglia. *Biological Psychiatry*, **18**, 591–601.

Curran, D., Partridge, M., and Storey, P. (1980). "Psychological Medicine: An Introduction to Psychiatry," 9th ed. Churchill Livingstone, Edinburgh and New York.

Curtis, G. C., and Zuckerman, M. (1968). A psychological reaction precipiated by sensory deprivation. *American Journal of Psychiatry*, **125**, 255–260.

Dahl, M. (1958). A singular distortion of temporal disorientation. *American Journal of Psychiatry*, **115**, 146–149.

Davison, K., and Bagley, C. (1969). Schizophrenia-like psychoses associated with organic disorders on the C.N.S: A review of the literature. *British Journal of Psychiatry* (special publications) **4**, 113.

Debray, Q. (1975). A genetic study of chronic delusions. *Neuropsychobiology*, **1**, 313–321.

Dongier, S. (1959). "Statistical study of clinical and EEG manifestations of 530 psychotic episodes occurring in 516 epileptics between clinical seizures. *Epilepsin*, 117–142.

Editorial. (1979). Psychoses and lateralization of the brain. *Lancet*, **ii**, 1276–1277.

Ehrenteil, O. F., and Jenney, P. B. (1960). Does time stand still for some psychotics? *Archives of General Psychiatry*, **3**, 1–3.

Engel, G. L., and Romano, J. (1944). "Delirium II: Reversibility of the electroencephalogram with experimental procedures. *AMA Archives of Neurological Psychiatry,* **51,** 378–392.

Engel, G. L., and Romano, J. (1959). Delirium, a syndrome of cerebral insufficiency. *Journal of Chronic Diseases,* **9,** 260–277.

Everitt, B. S., Gourlay, A. J., and Kendell, R. E. (1971). An attempt at validation of traditional psychiatric syndromes by cluster analysis. *British Journal of Psychiatry,* **119,** 399–412.

Feighner, J. P., Robins, E., Guze, S. B., Woodruff, R. A., Winokur, G., and Munoz, R. (1972). Diagnostic criteria for use in psychiatric research. *Archives of General Psychiatry,* **26,** 457–463.

Fenton, G. W., Fenwick, P. B. C., Dollimore, J., Dunn, T. L., and Hirsch, S. R. (1980). EEG Spectral analysis in schizophrenia. *British Journal of Psychiatry,* **136,** 445–455.

Ferraro, A. (1943). Pathological changes in the brain of a case clinically diagnosed dementia praecox. *Journal of Neuropathology and Experimental Neurology,* **2,** 84–94.

Finger, S. (1978). "Recovery from Brain Damage: Research and Theory." Plenum, New York.

Fletcher, C. M. (1952). Discussion: The diagnosis of pulmonary emphysemia. *Proceedings of the Royal Society of Medicine,* **45,** 577–584.

Flor-Henry, P. (1969). Psychosis and temporal lobe epilepsy. *Epilepsia,* **10,** 363–395.

Flor-Henry, P., Koles, Z. J., Howarth, B. G., and Burton, L. (1979). Neurophysiology studies of schizophrenia, mania and depression. *In* "Hemisphere Asymmetries of Function in Psychopathology (Ed. P. Flor-Henry), pp. 189–222. Elsevier, North Holland.

Fowler, R. C., Tsuang, M. T., and Cadoret, R. J. (1975). A clinical and family study of paranoid and non-paranoid schizophrenics. *British Journal of Psychiatry,* **124,** 346–359.

Freud, S., Freud, A., Strachey, A., and Tyson, A. (1962). The neuro-psychoses of defence. *In* "Standard Edition of the Complete Psychological Works" (Ed. J. Strachy), Vol. 3, p. 58. The Hogarth Press, London.

Gibbs, F. A. (1951). Ictal and non ictal psychiatric disorders in temporal lobe epilepsy. *Journal of Nervous and Mental Disease,* **313,** 522–528.

Glossary of Mental Disorders (1968). "General Register Office: Studies on Medical and Population Subjects." H. M. S. O., London.

Goldberg, E. M. and Morrison, S. L. (1963). Schizophrenia and social class. *British Journal of Psychiatry,* **109,** 785.

Gottesman, I., and Shields, J. (1982). "Schizophrenia: The Epigenic Puzzle." Cambridge University Press, Cambridge, London.

Gottschalk, L. A., Haer, J. L., and Bates, D. E. (1972). Effect of sensory overload on psychological state. *Archives of General Psychiatry,* **27,** 451–457.

Green, P., Glass, A. and O'Callaghan, M. A. (1979). Some implications of abnormal hemisphere interaction in schizophrenia. *In* "Hemispheric Asymmetries of Function in Psychopathology" (Ed. P. Flor-Henry), pp. 431–448. Elsevier, Amsterdam, New York and Oxford.

Gregory, R. L. (1977). "Eye and Brain: The Psychology of Seeing." Weidenfeld and Nicolson, London.

Grinker, R. R., Werble, B., and Brye, R. (1968). "The Borderline Syndrome." Basic Books, New York.

Grossman, G. (1971). "Recent Advances in Clinical Psychiatry." Churchill, London.

Gruzelier, J., and Manchanda, R. (1982). The syndrome of schizophrenia: Relations between electrodermal response, lateral asymmetries and clinical ratings. *British Journal of Psychiatry,* **141,** 488–495.

Gruzelier, J. H. (1981). Cerebral laterality in psychopathology: fact and fiction. *Editorial in Psychological Medicine,* **11,** 219–227.

Gur, R. E. (1979). Cognitive concomitants of hemispheric dysfunction in schizophrenia. *Archives of General Psychiatry,* **36,** 269–277.

Hammer, M., and Zubin, J. (1968). Evolution, culture and psychopathology. *Journal of General Psychology,* **78,** 154–175.

Hawks, D. V. (1964). The clinical usefulness of some tests of overinclusive thinking in psychiatric patients. *British Journal of Social and Clinical Psychology,* **3,** 186–195.

Hays, W. L. (1976). "Statistics for Psychologists." · Brooks-Cole, New York.

Heath, R. G. (1966). Schizophrenia: Biochemical and physiologic aberrations. *International Journal of Neuropsychiatry,* **2,** 597–610.

Heath, R. G., Franklyn, D. E., and Shraberg, D. (1979). Gross pathology of the cerebellum in patients diagnosed and treated as functional psychiatric disorders. *Journal of Nervous and Mental Disease,* **167,** 585–592.

Hebb, D. O. (1949). "The Organization of Behaviour." Wiley, New York.

Hebb, D. O. (1958). "A Textbook of Psychology. Saunders, Philadelphia and London.

Herbert, M. E., and Jacobson, S. (1967). Late paraphrenia. *British Journal of Psychiatry,* **113,** 461–470.

Heston, L. L. (1966). Psychiatric disorders in foster-home reared children of schizophrenic mothers. *British Journal of Psychiatry,* **112,** 819.

Hill, D. (1963). The EEG in psychiatry. *In* "Electroencephalography (Ed. G. Parr), p. 368. Macdonald, London.

Hoch, P., and Polatin, P. (1949). "Pseudoneurotic forms of schizophrenia," *Psychiatric Quarterly* **23,** pp. 248–276.

Holmboe, R., and Astrup, C. (1957). A follow-up study of 225 patients with acute schizophrenia and schizophrenia psychoses. *Acta Psychiatrica Scandanavica Supplement,* **115.**

Holzman, P. S., Proctor, L. R., and Hughes, D. W. (1973). Eye tracking patterns in schizophrenia. *Science,* **181,** 179–181.

Ingvar, D. H., and Franzen, G. (1974). Abnormalities of cerebral blood flow distribution in patients with chronic schizophrenia. *Acta Psychiatrica Scandanavica,* **50,** 425–462.

Jackson, H. (1931). "Selected Writings." Hodder and Stoughton, London.

Jarvic, L. F., and Chadwick, S. B. (1973). Schizophrenia and survival in psychopathology. *In* "Psychopathology" (Ed. M. Hammer, K. Salzinger, and S. Sutten). Wiley, New York.

Jaspers, K. (1959). "General Psychopathology." University of Chicago Press, Chicago. 4th Impression, 1972.

Jefferson, G. (1949). The nature of concussion. *British Medical Journal,* **i,** 1–5.

Johnstone, E. C., Crow, T. J., Frith, C. D., Husband, J., and Kreel, L. (1976). Cerebral ventricular size and cognitive impairment in schizophrenia. *Lancet,* **ii,** 924–926.

Kahlbaum, K. L. (1873). "Catatonia." Johns Hopkins University Press, Baltimore, Maryland.

Kahlbaum, K. L. (1873). "Catatonia." Johns Hopkins University Press, Baltimore, Maryland.

Karagulla, S., and Robertson, E. E. (1955). Psychical phenomena in temporal lobe epilepsy and the psychoses. *British Medical Journal,* **1,** 748–752.

Karlsson, J. L. (1968). Genealogical studies of schizophrenia. *In* "Transmission of Schizophrenia" (Ed. S. S. Kety). Pergamon, Oxford.

Kay, D. W. K. (1972). Schizophrenia and schizophrenia-like states in the elderly. *British Journal of Hospital Medicine,* **8,** 368–376.

Kay, D. W. K., Cooper, A., Garside, R., and Roth, M. (1976). The differentiation of paranoid from affective psychoses by patients premorbid characteristics. *British Journal of Psychiatry,* **129,** 207–215.

Kay, D. W. K., and Roth, M. (1961). Environmental and hereditary factors in the schizophrenias of old age ('late paraphrenia') and their bearing on the general problem of causation in schizophrenia. *Journal of Mental Science,* **107,** 649–686.

Kelley, H. H. (1950). The warm–cold variable in first impressions of persons. *Journal of Personality,* **18,** 431–439.

Kendell, R. E., and Brockington, I. F. (1980). The identification of disease entities and their relationship between schizophrenia and affective psychoses. *British Journal of Psychiatry,* **137,** 324–331.

Kendell, R. E., Brockington, I. F., and Leff, J. P. (1979). Prognostic implications of six alternative definitions of schizophrenia. *Archives of General Psychiatry,* **36,** 25–31.

Kendler, K. S., Gruenberg, A. M., and Strauss, J. S. (1981). An independent analysis of the Copenhagen sample of the Danish Adoption Society Study of

Schizophrenia III. The relationship between paranoid psychosis (delusional disorder) and the schizophrenia spectrum disorders. *Archives of General Psychiatry,* **38,** 985–987.

Kety, S. (1974). From rationalization to reason. *American Journal of Psychiatry,* **131,** 957–963.

Kety, S., Rosenthal, D., Wender, P. H., and Schulsinger, F. (1976). Studies based on a total sample of adopted individuals and their relatives, why they were necessary, what they demonstrated and failed to demonstrate. *Schizophrenia Bulletin,* **2,** 413–428.

Kolle, K. (1931). "Die Primare Verruckheit" [Primary Paranoia]. Thieme, Leipzig, Germany.

Kornetsky, C., and Orzack, M. H. (1978). Physiological and behavioural correlates of attention dysfunction in schizophrenic patients. *Journal of Psychiatric Research,* **14,** 69–79.

Kraepelin, E. (1919). "Dementia Praecox and Paraphrenia." Livingstone, Edinburgh.

Kraepelin, E. (1920). Patterns of mental disorder. *In* "Themes and Variations in European Psychiatry" (Ed. M. Shepherd). Wright and Sons, Bristol.

Kreitman, N. (1961). The reliability of psychiatric diagnosis. *Journal of Mental Science,* **107,** 876–886.

Kreitman, N. P., Sainsbury, J., Morrissey, J., Towers, J., and Scrivener, J. (1961). The reliability of psychiatric assessment: An analysis. *Journal of Mental Science,* **107,** 887–908.

Kugler, B. T., and Weller, M. P. I. (1983). Hebbs recurring digits in schizophrenic patients, presentation to Second International Conference on Laterality and Psychopathology: Banff, Alberta, Canada. *In* "Laterality and Psychopathology" (Ed. P. Flor-Henry and J. Gruzelier), pp. 493–495. Elsevier, North Holland.

Laing, R. D., and Esterson, A. (1964). "Sanity, Madness and the Family." Tavistock Publications, London.

Langfeldt, G. (1939). "The Schizophreniform States." Munksgaard, Copenhagen.

Lanzkron, J., and Wolfson, W. (1958). Prognostic value of perceptual distortion of temporal orientation in chronic schizophrenics. *American Journal of Psychiatry,* **114,** 744–746.

Latham, C., Holtzman, P. S., and Manschreck, T. C. (1981). Optokinetic nystagmus and pursuit eye movements in schizophrenia. *Archives of General Psychiatry,* **38,** 997–1003.

Leff, J., Kuipers, L., Berkowitz, R., Eberlein-Vries, R., and Sturgeon, D. (1982). A controlled trial of social intervention in the families of schizophrenic patients. *British Journal of Psychiatry,* **141,** 121–134.

Leonhard, K. (1961). Cycloid psychoses: Endogenous psychoses which are neither schizophrenic nor manic depressive. *Journal of Mental Science,* **107,** 633–648.

Lewine, R., Kirchoffer, A., Monsour, M., and Watt, N. (1982). The empirical heterogeneity of first rank symptoms in schizophrenia. *British Journal of Psychiatry,* **140,** 498–502.

Lewis, A. (1934). Melancholia: A clinical survey of depressive states. *Journal of Mental Science,* **80,** 277–238

Lewis, N. D. C., and Piotrowski, Z. A. (1954). Clinical diagnosis of manic-depressive psychosis. *In* "Depression (Ed. J. Zubin), pp. 25–38. Grune and Stratton, New York.

Lidz, R., and Lidz, T. (1952). "Therapeutic Considerations Arising from the Intense Symbiotic Needs of Schizophrenic Patients." International Universities Press, New York.

Lidz, R. W., and Lidz, T. (1949). The family environment of schizophrenic patients. *American Journal of Psychiatry,* **106,** 332–345.

Lipowski, Z. J. (1980). "Delirium, Acute Brain Failure in Man." Thomas, Illinois.

Luxenburger, (1939). Die Vererbung der psychischen Storungen. *In* "Bumke's Handbuch," (Ed. Anonymous).

McCabe, M. S. (1976). Symptom differences in reactive psychoses and schizophrenia with poor prognosis. *Comprehensive Psychiatry,* **17,** 301–307.

McGhie, A. (1967). Studies of cognitive disorder in schizophrenia. *In* "Recent development in schizophrenia. *British Journal of Psychiatry* (Special Publication) No. 1.

McGhie, A., and Lawson, J. S. (1964). Disturbances in selective attention in schizophrenia. *Proceedings of the Royal Society of Medicine,* **57,** 419–422.

McGuffin, P., Reveley, A., and Holland, A. (1982). Identical triplets: Non-identical psychosis? *British Journal of Psychiatry,* **140,** 1–6.

Mackay, A. V. P. (1980). Positive and negative schizophrenic symptoms and the role of dopamine. *British Journal of Psychiatry,* **137,** 379–386.

Magaro, P. A., and Chamrad, D. L. (1983). Information processing and lateralization in schizophrenia. *Biological Psychiatry,* **18,** 29–44.

Marder, S. R., Kammen, D. P. van Doherty, J. P., Rayner, J., and Bunney, W. E. (1979). Predicting drug free improvement in schizophrenic psychosis. *Archives of General Psychiatry,* **36,** 1080–1085.

Mellor, C. S. (1970). First rank symptoms of schizophrenia. *British Journal of Psychiatry,* **117,** 15.

Melztzer, H. Y. (1976). Neuromuscular abnormalities in schizophrenia. *Schizophrenia Bulletin,* **2,** 106–135.

Meyer, A. (1952). "The Collected Papers of Adolf Meyer." Johns Hopkins Press, Baltimore.

Michelson, N. (1968). A note on age confusion in psychosis. *Psychiatry Quarterly,* **42,** 331–338.

Moon, A. F., Messerd, R. B., Wieland, B. A., Pokorny, A. D., and Falconer, G. A. (1968). Perceptual dysfunction as a determinant of schizophrenic word association. *Journal of Nervous and Mental Disease,* **146,** 80–84.

Moore, M. S. (1978). Discussion of the Spitzer-Endicott and Klein proposed definition of mental disorder (illness). *In* "Critical Issues in Psychiatric Diagnosis " (Ed. D. F. Klein). Raven, New York.

Morel, B. A. (1860). "Traites de Maladies Mentales." Mason, Paris.

Morrison, J., Clancy, J., Crow, R., and Winokur, G. (1972). The Iowa 500: I. Diagnostic validity in mania, depression and schizophrenia. *Archives of General Psychiatry,* **27,** 457–461.

Nasrallah, H. A., McCalley-Whitters, M., and Kuperman, S. (1982). "Neurological differences between paranoid and non paranoid schizophrenia. Part I. Sensory-motor lateralization. *Journal of Clinical Psychiatry,* **43,** 305–306.

Nasrallah, H. A., Tippin, J., and McCalley-Whitters, M. (1982). Neurological differences between paranoid and non paranoid schizophrenia. Part III. Neurological soft signs. *Journal Clinical Psychiatry,* **43,** 310–312.

Overall, J. E., and Graham, D. R. (1962). The brief psychiatric rating scale. *Psychological Reports,* **10,** 799–812.

Parkes, C. M. (1963). Interhospital and intrahospital variations in the diagnosis and severity of schizophrenia. *British Journal of Preventative Medicine,* **17,** 85–89.

Paton-Salzberg, R. (1982). Genetic factors in schizophrenia. *Bulletin of the British Psychological Society* **35,** 397–398.

Pavy, D. (1968). Verbal behaviour in schizophrenia: A review of recent studies. *Psychological Bulletin,* **70,** 164–178.

Payne, R. W., and Caird, W. K. (1967). Reactive time, distractability and overinclusive thinking in psychotics. *Journal of Abnormal Psychology,* **72,** 112–121.

Payne, R. W., and Friedlander, D. (1962). A short battery of simple tests for measuring overinclusive thinking. *Journal of Mental Science,* **108,** 362–367.

Payne, R. W., and Hewlett, J. H. G. (1960). Thought disorder in psychotic patients. *In* "Experiments in Personality" (Ed. H. J. Eysenck), Vol. 2. Routledge and Kegan Paul, London.

Penfield, W., and Jasper, H. M. (1947). Highest level seizures. *In* "Association for Research in Nervous and Mental Disease, Proceedings," Vol. 24, pp. 252–271. Williams and Wilkins, Baltimore.

Pool, J. L., and Correll, J. W. (1958). Pschiatric symptoms masking brain tumour. *Journal of Medicine and Sociology,* **55,** 4–9.

Post, F. (1966). "Persistent Persecutory States of the Elderly." Pergamon, London.

Procci, W. R. (1976). Schizoaffective psychosis: Fact or fiction. *Archives of General Psychiatry,* **33,** 1167.

Reed, J. L. (1968). The proverbs test in schizophrenia. *British Journal of Psychiatry,* **114,** 317–321.

Reichardt, M. (1929). Brain and psyche. *Journal of Nervous and Mental Disease,* **70,** 390.

Reyes, M. G., and Gordon, A. (1981). Cerebellum vermis in schizophrenia. *Lancet,* **ii,** 700–701.

Reynolds, G. (1983). Increased concentrations and lateral asymmetry of amygdala dopamine in schizophrenia. *Nature,* **305,** 527–529.

Rizzo, M., and Damasio, H. (1982). Neurological differences between paranoid and non paranoid schizophrenia. Part II. Computerized tomographic findings. *Journal of Clinical Psychiatry,* **43,** 307–309.

Roberts, G. W., Ferrier, I. N., and Lee, Y., *et al.* (1983). Peptides, the limbic lobe and schizophrenia. *Brain Research,* **288,** 199–211.

Robson, J. T., and Suit, B. B. (1962). Space occupying lesions identified following diagnosis of a psychiatric disorder. *Southern Medical Journal,* **55,** 785–791.

Romano, J., and Enger, G. L. (1944). Physiologic and psychologic considerations of delirium. *Medical Clinics of North America,* **28,** 629–638.

Romney, D. (1967). "Aspects of Cognitive Dysfunction in Nuclear Schizophrenics and their Parents and Siblings." Ph.D thesis, University of Newcastle upon Tyne.

Romney, D. (1969a). Psychometrically assessed thought disorder in schizophrenia and control patients, and in their parents and siblings. *British Journal of Psychiatry,* **115,** 999–1002.

Romney, D. (1969b). The validity of certain tests of overinclusion. *British Journal of Psychiatry,* **115,** 591–592.

Rorie, J. (1862–1863). The treatment of hallucinations by electrization. *Journal of Mental Science,* **8,** 363–365.

Ross-Stanton, J., and Meltzer, H. Y. (1981). Motor neurone branching patterns in psychotic patients. *Archives of General Psychiatry,* **38,** 1097–1103.

Roth, M., and McClelland, H. (1979). The relationship of 'nuclear' and 'atypical' psychoses. *Psychiatrica Clinica,* **12,** 23–54.

Russel-Davis, D. (1949). *"Introduction to Psychopathology,"* 3rd ed. Oxford University Press.

Rutter, M., Shaffer, D., and Sturge, C. (1974). "A Guide to Multiaxial Classification Scheme for Psychiatric Disorders in Childhood and Adolescence." Institute of Psychiatry, London.

Rutter, P. R., Draffan, J., and Davies, J. (1977). Thought disorder and the predictability of schizophrenic speech. *British Journal of Psychiatry,* **131,** 67–68.

Ryle, G. (1949). "The Concept of Mind." Penguin, Harmondsworth, England.

Sadler, J., Porter, R., and Evered, D. (1981). Careers of non-medical graduates in British medical research. *Nature,* **293,** 423–426.

Sandler, M., Ruthven, C. R. J., Goodwin, B. L., Tyrer, S. P., Weller, M. P. I., and Hirsch, S. R. (1978). Raised cerebrospinal fluid phenylacetic acid concentration: Preliminary support for the phenylethylamine hypothesis. *Psychopharmacology*, **2**, 199–203.

Schmid, W., Bronisch, T., and Von Zeerson, D. (1982). A comparative study of PSE/CATEGO and Diaska: Two psychiatric computer diagnostic systems. *British Journal of Psychiatry*, **141**, 292–295.

Schneider, K. (1957). Primary and secondary symptoms in schizophrenia. *In* Themes and Variations in European Psychiatry'' (Ed. M. Shepherd). Wright, Bristol.

Schwade, E. D., and Geiger, S. G. (1956). Abnormal EEG findings in severe behaviour disorders. **17**, 307.

Shakow, D. (1962). Segmental set: A theory of the formal psychological deficit in schizophrenia. *Archives of General Psychiatry*, **6**, 1–17.

Sheldrick, C., Jablensky, A., Sartorius, N., and Shepherd, M. (1977). Schizophrenia succeeded by affective illness; catamnestic study and statistical enquiry. *Psychological Medicine*, **7**, 619–624.

Shepherd, M., Brooke, E. M., Cooper, J., and Lin, T. (1968). An experimental approach to psychiatric diagnosis. *Acta Psychiatrica et Neurologica Scandinavica*, **44** (supplement 201).

Sherwin, I. (1982). The effect of the location of an epileptogenic lesion on the occurrence of psychosis in epilepsy. *In* ''Temporal Lobe Epilepsy, Mania and Schizophrenia and the Limbic System'' (Ed. M. R. Timble), pp. 81–97. Karger, Basel, London.

Shukla, G. D., Srivastava, O. N., Katiyar, B. C., Joshi, V., and Mohan, P. K. (1979). Psychiatric manifestations in temporal lobe epilepsy: A controlled study. *British Journal of Psychiatry*, **135**, 411–417.

Simon, W. (1952). The diagnosis of brain tumour masked by mental symptoms. *Mil. Surg.*, **III**, 411–442.

Singer, M. T. (1967). Family transactions and schizophrenia. *In* ''The Origins of Schizophrenia.'' Excerpta Medica International Congress Series, No. 151.

Singer, M. T., and Wynne, L. C. (1963). Differentiating characteristics of parents of childhood schizophrenics, childhood neurotics, and young adult schizophrenics. *American Journal of Psychiatry*, **120**, 234–243.

Singer, M. T., and Wynne, L. C. (1965a). Thought disorder and family relations of schizophrenics. *Archives of General Psychiatry*, **12**, 187–212.

Singer, M. T., and Wynne, L. C. (1965b). ''Stylistic variables in research on schizophrenics and their families.'' Unpublished address presented at Marquette University.

Singer, M. T., and Wynne, L. C. (1966a). Principles for scoring communication defects and deviances in parents of schizophrenics. Rorschach and T.A.T. scoring manuals. *Psychiatry*, **29**, 260–288.

Singer, M. T., and Wynne, L. C. (1966b). Communication styles in parents of normals, neurotics and schizophrenics. *Psychiatric Research Reports,* **20,** 25–38.

Slater, E. (1965). Diagnosis of 'hysteria'. *British Medical Journal,* 1395–1399.

Slater, E., Beard, A. W., and Glitheroe, E. (1963). Schizophrenia-like psychoses of epilepsy. *British Journal of Psychiatry,* **19,** 95–150.

Slater, E., and Roth, M. (1970). "Clinical Psychiatry" 3rd ed. Bailliere, Tindall and Cassell, London.

Smith, J. M., and Oswald, W. T. (1976). Subjective age in chronic schizophrenia. *British Journal of Psychiatry,* **128,** 100, correspondence.

Spitzer, R. L., Endicott, J., and Robins, E. (1977). "Research Diagnostic Criteria for a Selected Group of Functional Disorders, 3rd ed. New York Biometric Research, New York Psychiatric Institute.

Stephens, J. K., Astrup, C., and Mangrum, J. C. (1966). Prognostic factors in recovered and deteriorated schizophrenics. *American Journal of Psychiatry,* **122,** 1116–1121.

Stevens, M., Crow, T. J., Bowman, M., and Coles, E. C. (1978). Age disorientation in chronic schizophrenia: A constant prevelance of 25% in a mental hospital population? *British Journal of Psychiatry,* **133,** 130–136.

Stoffler, F. (1973). Disordered consciousness of time in schizophrenic women. *Münchener Medizinische Wochenschrift,* **115,** 2285–2286.

Symonds, C. P. (1960). Disease of mind and disorder of brain. *British Medical Journal,* **ii,** 1–5.

Szasz, T. (1960). The myth of mental illness. *American Psychologist,* **15,** 113–118.

Szasz, T. S. (1962). "The Myth of Mental Illness." Paladin, London.

Szasz, T. S. (1976). Schizophrenia: The sacred symbol of psychiatry. *British Journal of Psychiatry, Psychiatry,* **129,** 308–316.

Thomson, A. D., and Cotton, R. E. (1968). *Lecture Notes on Pathology,* 2nd ed. Blackwell Scientific, Oxford and Edinburgh.

Tissenbaum, M. J., Harter, H. M., and Friedman, A. P. (1951). Organic neurological disorders. *Journal of American Medical Association,* **147,** 1519–1521.

Tomalin, N., and Hall, R. (1970). "The Strange Last Voyage of Donald Crowhurst." Stein and Day, London.

Toone, B. K., Garralda, M., and Ron, M. A. (1982). The psychoses of epilepsy and the functional psychoses: A clinical and phenomenological comparison. *British Journal of Psychiatry,* **141,** 256–261.

Trimble, M. R., and Perez, M. M. (1982). The phenomenology of the chronic psychoses of epilepsy. *In* "Temporal Lobe Epilepsy, Mania and Schizophrenia and the Limbic System" (Ed. W. P. Koella and M. R. Trimble). Karger, Basel.

Tsuang, G., Fowler, R. C., Cadoret, R. J., and Monnelly, E. (1974). Schizophrenia among first degree relatives of paranoid and non-paranoid schizophrenics. *Comprehensive Psychiatry,* **15,** 295.

Tsuang, M. T. (1978). Familial subtyping of schizophrenia and affective disorders. *In* "Critical Issues in Psychiatric Diagnosis" (Ed. D. F. Klein), pp. 203–211. New York.

Tsuang, M. T., and Dempsey, G. M. (1979). Long term outcome of major psychoses. II. Schizoaffective disorder compared with schizophrenia, affective disorders and a surgical control group. *Archives of General Psychiatry,* **36,** 1302–1304.

Tsuang, M. T., Woolson, R. F., and Fleming, J. A. (1979). Long-term outcome of major psychoses. *Archives of General Psychiatry,* **36,** 1295–1301.

Tsuang, M. T., Woolson, R. F., Winokur, G., and Crowe, R. R. (1981). Stability of psychiatric diagnoses: Schizophrenia and affective disorders followed up over a 30–40 year period. *Archives of General Psychiatry,* **38,** 535–539.

Vaillant, G. E. (1963). The natural history of the remitting schizophrenias. *American Journal of Psychiatry,* **120,** 367–376.

Vaillant, G. E. (1964). Prospective prediction of schizophrenic remission. *Archives of General Psychiatry,* **11,** 509–518.

Van Kammen, D. P. Sternberg, D. E., Hare, T. A., Waters, R. N., and Bunney, W. E. (1982). CSF levels of gamma-amionobutyric acid in schizophrenia. *Archives of General Psychiatry,* **39,** 91–100.

Vaughn, C. E., and Leff, J. P. (1976). The influence of the family and social factors on the cause of psychiatric illness: A comparison of schizophrenia and depressed neurotic patients. *British Journal of Psychiatry,* **129,** 125–137.

Verghese, A. (1971). Body build in mental illness. *Indian Journal of Psychiatry,* **13,** 229.

Verghese, A., Large, P., and Chiu, E. (1978). Relationship between body build and mental illness. *British Journal of Psychiatry,* **132,** 12–15.

Wada, J. A., and Rasmussen, T. (1960). Intracarotid injection of sodium amytal for the lateralization of cerebral speech dominance: Experimental and clinical observations. *Journal of Neurosurgery,* **17,** 266–282.

Waggoner, R. W., and Bagchi, B. K. (1954). Initial masking of organic brain changes by psychic symptoms. *American Journal of Psychiatry,* **110,** 904–9.

Weinberger, D. R., Biglow, L. B., and Kleinman, J. E. (1980). Cerebral ventricular enlargement in chronic schizophrenia: association with poor response to treatment. *Archives of General Psychiatry,* **37,** 11–14.

Weller, M. P. I., and Ameen, M. (1982). Central processing in schizophrenia— Abstracts. *13th C.I.N.P. Congress, Jerusamlem Israel,* p. 756.

Weller, M. P. I., and Kugler, B. T. (1979). Tactile discrimination in schizophrenic and affective psychoses. *In Hemisphere Asymmetries of Function in Psychopathology* (Ed. P. Flor-Henry). Elsevier, North Holland.

Weller, M. P. I., and Montagu, J. D. (1979). Electroencephalographic coherence in schizophrenia: A preliminary study. *In* "Hemisphere Asymmetries of Function in Psychopathology" (Ed. P. Flor-Henry). Elsevier, North Holland.

Wender, P. H., Rosenthal, D., Kety, S. S., Schulsinger, F., and Welner, J. (1973). Social class and psychopathology in adoptees: A natural experimental method for separating the roles of genetic and experimental factors. *Archives of General Psychiatry,* **28,** 318–325.

Wender, P. H., Rosenthal, D., Kety, S. S., Schulsinger, F., and Welner, J. (1974). Cross-fostering: A research strategy for clarifying the role of genetic and experimental factors in the etiology of schizophrenia. *Archives of General Psychiatry,* **30,** 121–128.

Wexler, B. E. (1980). Cerebral laterality and psychiatry: A review of the literature. *American Journal of Psychiatry,* **137,** 279–291.

Wing, J. K., Birley, J. L. T., Cooper, J. E., Graham, P., and Isaacs, A. D. (1967). Reliability of a procedure for measuring and classifying "present psychiatric state." *British Journal of Psychiatry,* **113,** 499–515.

Wing, J. K., Cooper, J. E., and Sartorius, N. (1974). "The Measurement and Classification of Psychiatric Symptoms." Cambridge University Press, London.

Winokur, G. (1977). Delusional disorder (paranoia). *Comprehensive Psychiatry,* **18,** 511–521.

World Health Organization (1973a). "The Pilot Study of Schizophrenia, Vol. 1. WHO, Geneva.

World Health Organization (1973b). "The International Pilot Study of Schizophrenia," Vol. 1. WHO, Geneva.

World Health Organization (1977). International Classification of Diseases. *Vol. I.* Manual of the International Statistical Classification of Diseases, injuries and causes of death. WHO, Geneva.

World Health Organization (1979). "An International Follow-up Study of Schizophrenia." Wiley, Chicester.

Wykes, T. (1981). Can the psychiatrist learn from the psychologist? Detecting coherence in the disordered speech of manics and schizophrenics. *Psychological Medicine,* **II,** 641–642.

Wykes, T., and Leff, J. (1982). Disordered speech: Differences between manics and schizophrenics. *Brain and Language,* **15,** 117–124.

Wynne, L. C. (1967). Family transactions and schizophrenia. II. Conceptual considerations for a research strategy. *In* "The Origins of Schizophrenia." Excerpta Medica International Congress Series.

Wynne, L. C. (1968). Methodologic and conceptual issues in the study of schizophrenics and their families. *In* "The Transmission of Schizophrenia" (Ed. S. Kety). Oxford.

Wynne, L. C. (1971). Family research on the pathogenesis of schizophrenia. *In "Problems of Psychosis, International Colloquium on Psychosis"* (Ed. C. Laurin). Excerpta Medica International Congress Series.

Wynne, L. C. (in press). "Schizophrenics and their families. I. Research redirections." Presented in a condensed version at the Mental Health Research Fund Lecture, London.

Wynne, L. C., Ryckoff, I., Day, J., and Hirsch, S. (1958). Pseudo-mutuality in the family relations of schizophrenics. *Psychiatry,* **21,** 205–220.

Wynne, L. C., and Singer, M. T. (1963). Thought disorder and family relations of schizophrenics. *Archives of General Psychiatry,* **9,** 191–206.

Zahn, T. P. (1977). Comments on reaction time and attention in schizophrenia. *Schizophrenia Bulletin,* **3,** 452–456.

Zubek, J. P., Welch, G., and Saunders, M. G. (1963). Electroencephalographic changes during and after 14 days of perceptual deprivation. *Science,* **139,** 490–492.

6 Anorexia Nervosa: An Enigmatic Disorder

ROBIN STEVENS

*Department of Psychology,
Nottingham University,
Nottingham, England*

1 Introduction

There is a puzzling sex difference in the incidence of obesity and anorexia nervosa. These disorders are at opposite ends of a body-weight continuum so it is unexpected that women are more prone to both. Given that women are more likely to develop one disorder, then men should suffer from the "opposite" disorder. However, women are more likely to be obese than men (see review by Hoyenga and Hoyenga, 1982), and the female-to-male ratio in the incidence of anorexia nervosa is about 19:1. Furthermore, a third eating disorder in which the sufferer vomits or purges after gorging a huge meal—named bulimia nervosa by Russell (1979) or the "dietary chaos syndrome" by Palmer (1979)—is more common in women than in men.

Although these eating disorders are dissimilar, is there a common factor that predisposes women to all three conditions? This cannot be the greater social pressure on women regarding appearance and slimness, since it can apply only to the disorders of anorexia nervosa and bulimia nervosa. An alternative could be a disorder in female hormonal processes that disturbs body-weight regulation. However, as the evidence on anorexia nervosa shows, no simple disruption of the hypothalamic–pituitary–gonadal axis will suffice either. Thus, other factors need to be considered in determining the aetiology of these body-weight disorders, as well as social and endocrinological factors.

It might seem surprising that a book on consciousness should include a discussion on body-weight disorders. However, an important aspect of consciousness is awareness of self, not just in the Cartesian sense of being self-aware, but as an individual with physical characteristics extending in space and time. The terms body image or body schema are used in discussing this attribute of self-awareness. Its evolution can be traced from observations of aberrant self-percep-

Aspects of Consciousness
Volume 4. Clinical Issues

tion in patients with neurological impairments or limb amputations; instances of the latter were chronicled as early as the seventeenth century (see Kolb, 1959). Phantom limbs are the classic example of distorted body image; the basic body schema persists despite surgical or traumatic loss of a body part. Cases of paralysis and paraplegias provide less dramatic instances.

Information about one's shape, size, and extent, as well as those internal cues and stimuli that provide information about needs and emotions, contribute to the body image. Often such information is not immediately available to conscious reflection since dwelling on not being hungry, thirsty, in discomfort, or in pain, is of little psychological or biological value. This is remarked on by Slater and Roth (1969) who propose

> The normal individual, as he himself may discover by introspection, is subject at all times to somatic sensations slightly below the level required to claim the attention of consciousness—feelings of tingling, hotness or coldness in the limbs, even slight pains of a dull or sharp quality, feelings of fullness in the stomach, of distension in bladder or rectum, headaches or sensations of tightness of pressure on the head, etc. . . . The *constant stream of sensation* reaching the central nervous system forms the background from which special perceptions stand out and receive their locations as if from a grid; this is probably the physiological basis of the body scheme or body image.'' (p. 141)

How we reflect on ourselves, how we consider other people see us, and our use of internal and external cues to determine states of need and satiety are important, but often neglected, features of many psychiatric and psychosomatic problems including anorexia nervosa.

2 Phenomenology of Anorexia Nervosa

Sir William Gull (1874) coined the name anorexia nervosa for the emaciated condition that follows self-starvation. At the same time Lasègue (1873) proposed it as a distinct illness, but he called it "hysterical anorexia." However, the current name is a misnomer, since most anorexic patients experience hunger and are obsessed about food. Diagnostic criteria for the disorder have been agreed (see Russell, 1970; Feighner *et al.*, 1972; DSM-III classification, American Psychiatric Association, 1980; see Tables 1 and 2), but differential diagnosis of anorexia nervosa can be difficult since psychiatrically disturbed patients are often anorectic.

The syndrome occurs primarily in adolescent girls from middle-class families, and, in the United States, it is found mainly amongst those with European ancestry. In contrast, proportionately more nonwhite and economically disadvantaged patients suffer from other paediatric disorders (Schwabe *et al.*, 1981). There may be socioeconomic reasons for these differences, that is, differential

TABLE 1
Feighner Criteria for Anorexia Nervosa[a]

For a diagnosis of anorexia nervosa, A through E are required

A Age of onset prior to 25

B Anorexia with accompanying weight loss of at least 25% of original body weight

C A distorted, implacable attitude toward eating, food, or weight that overrides hunger, admonitions, reassurance, and threats; e.g., (1) denial of illness with a failure to recognise nutritional needs; (2) apparent enjoyment in losing weight with overt manifestation that food refusal is a pleasurable indulgence; (3) a desired body image of extreme thinness with overt evidence that it is rewarding to the patient to achieve and maintain this state; and (4) unusual hoarding or handling of food

D No known medical illness that could account for the anorexia and weight loss

E No other known psychiatric disorder, with particular reference to primary affective disorders, schizophrenia, obsessive–compulsive, or phobic neurosis (The assumption is made that even though it may appear phobic or obsessional, food refusal alone is not sufficient to qualify for obsessive–compulsive or phobic disease)

F At least two of the following manifestations: (1) amenorrhoea, (2) lanugo, (3) bradycardia (persistent resting pulse rate of 60 or less), (4) periods of overactivity, (5) episodes of bulimia, (6) vomiting (may be self-induced)

[a]Feighner *et al.*, 1972.

selection according to social class of persons seeking health care. Because racial factors are confounded by class effects in economically developed countries, little can be said about them; however, there are reports of several cases of anorexia nervosa in Japan (Miyai *et al.*, 1975; Yoshikatsu *et al.*, 1978). In contrast, it is a rare condition in Malaysia (Buhrich, 1981), but even there it occurs more in Chinese and Indians than in Malays. Eating customs, cultural

TABLE 2
DSM III Diagnostic Criteria for Anorexia Nervosa

A Intense fear of becoming obese, which does not diminish as weight loss progresses

B Disturbance of body image, e.g., claiming to "feel fat" even when emaciated

C Weight loss of at least 25% of original body weight or, if under 18 years of age, weight loss from original body weight plus projected weight gain expected from growth charts may be combined to make the 25%

D Refusal to maintain body weight over a minimal normal weight for age and height

E No known physical illness that would account for the weight loss attitudes to slimness, and urbanization may all contribute to the difference in incidence.

The sex difference in incidence (19:1 in favour of girls, Halmi, 1974) may reflect the importance that young women place on appearance and thinness. Recent reports show that the prevalence of anorexia nervosa may be higher than once realised. Thus, Crisp *et al.* (1976) found the incidence to be 1 in 100 amongst English schoolgirls aged 16–18 years, and Pope *et al.* (1984) discovered that just under 1% of American suburban women shoppers, aged 13–40 years, met the DSM-III criteria for anorexia. The prevalence may be higher in selected groups: Garner and Garfinkel (1980) diagnosed anorexia nervosa, using rigorous criteria, in 6.5% of a sample of Canadian professional dance students, and Lowenkopf and Vincent (see Lowenkopf, 1982) found 14.5% of women ballet students fulfilled the DSM-III criteria for the disorder. Even nonanorectic students in the second study were abnormally light and had irregular eating habits, so those whose chosen careers place an emphasis on slimness are at considerable risk of developing the disorder. This could reflect the pressures placed by career choice on people who otherwise would not develop anorexia nervosa, or women predisposed to the disorder might select these careers.

Is anorexia nervosa a consequence of societal norms and prejudices about slimness and body weight? The increase in incidence of anorexia in recent years (Willi and Grossman, 1983), which correlates with changing attitudes toward slimness, supports this thesis. Garner and Garfinkel (1980) think that data from *Playboy* centrefolds and "Miss America Pageant" beauty contests reveal a significant trend towards a "thinner ideal shape", while over the last 20 years there has been an increase in average weight for height in women below 30 years according to the American Society of Actuaries. Thus, for example, the "Playmate" of the late 1950s was about 91% of average weight, whereas in the late 1970s she weighed only about 83% of average. Also, winners of "Miss America Pageants" since 1970 have been significantly lighter, at 83% of average weight, than the other contestants.

Button and Whitehouse (1981) found that 6.3% of a randomly selected sample of girls in a tertiary education college in England scored in the "anorexic" range on the Eating Attitude Test (EAT: Garner and Garfinkel, 1979), a self-report questionnaire that assesses the symptoms of anorexia nervosa. Interviews showed that the symptoms of anorexia nervosa were common in high scorers but virtually absent in the others. They concluded that about 5% of postpubertal girls develop a subclinical form of anorexia. Dieting for cosmetic reasons may lead to anorexic behaviour or even to complete anorexia nervosa according to Fries (1974), but then why are so few dieters clinically anorectic? There must be additional aetiological factors. To help delineate these factors we need prospective studies. The retrospective studies that are usual in this area can provide useful insights but are not definitive.

3 Personality Characteristics of Anorexia Nervosa Patients

Patients with anorexia nervosa have various symptoms reflecting a psycho-pathology, but, as is true for other aspects of this disorder, there are problems of cause and effect. Is the illness preceded by a recognised pathology such as depression, anxiety neurosis, or a phobia, or are the symptoms of such disorders, when present in the anorexic, nonaetiological correlates of anorexia nervosa or consequences of it? Since clinical reports on the psychopathological symptoms of anorexics are affected by the biases of the clinician, psychometric studies of anorectic patients are of importance because of their objectivity.

Anorectics respond in an abnormal fashion on various psychometric tests. They are, for example, introverted and neurotic on the Eysenck Personality Inventory (EPI) compared with "normal" control groups (Stonehill and Crisp, 1977; Gomez and Dally, 1980). Also, their L scores are high, which is consistent with the clinical finding that these patients often conceal aspects of their behaviour and feelings from others as well as themselves. Anorectics are no more neurotic than patients with depression or with personality or conduct disturbances but are less extraverted than the latter (Strober, 1980). Beumont (1977) used the EPI to compare anorectics who control weight by restricting intake only with those who also use vomiting or purging. Both groups were more neurotic than normal weight controls, and the "dieters" had lower extraversion scores. Also, "dieters" were more anxious and independent and less extraverted than controls on Cattell's 16PF Inventory, whereas "vomiters and purgers" were indistinguishable from normal people.

According to Eysenck's personality theory (Eysenck and Rachman, 1965), introverted neurotics suffer from dysthymic disorders such as phobias, anxiety neurosis, and depression. Consistent with this is the suggestion by Crisp (1970) that anorexia nervosa is a form of weight phobia, and Cantwell *et al.*(1977) think that depression is an aetiological factor in the disorder. However, Gomez and Dally found that a subgroup of late-onset anorectics, who develop the disorder after the age of 19 had higher neuroticism scores and were more extraverted than controls; this is a profile that is comparable to Eysenck's class of hysterics. Recovery of weight is related to increased extraversion and reduced neuroticism scores.

Other psychometric evidence from Stonehill and Crisp (1977), who used the Middlesex Hospital Questionnaire (MHQ, also called the Crown-Crisp Experiential Index), and Gomez and Dally (1980), using the similar Symptom-Sign Inventory (SSI), supports the view that anorectics suffer from anxiety, depression, and are obsessional. However, there is disagreement on the incidence of hysterical symptoms; on the MHQ they are comparable to "normal" controls, whereas on the SSI some late-onset anorectics score high on the hysteria scale.

After weight restoration the patients show nonsignificant improvements on all the MHQ scales (except for the reported level of somatic complaints which were low); at follow-up, 4-7 years later, most patients had recovered from their anorexia and weight phobia, although they were instead more "phobic in a social sense." A more recent report (Hsu and Crisp, 1980) on these patients and others generally confirmed these findings regarding recovery 4-8 years after treatment. It also showed that the improvements in the MHQ scales measuring anxiety, depression, and somatic symptoms arose primarily from about half the patients who, on independent criteria, had improved most satisfactorily. The remainder were similar in MHQ scores on initial and follow-up testing. Also, lower anxiety, phobia, obsessional, and somatic scores at presentation were predictive of good outcome for weight and menstrual function 4-8 years later.

Beumont (1977), using the Leyton Obsessional Inventory, supported the clinical impression that anorectics are obsessional. His groups of "vomiters and purgers" and "dieters" scored higher than normals on all measures, but "dieters" were presistently more extreme. Strober (1980), using the same inventory, confirmed this finding in young, nonchronic anorectics. Although following weight recovery obsessional symptoms were significantly lower, obsessional traits were unchanged. There is no evidence, however, that anorectics are as obsessional as psychoneurotic patients diagnosed primarily as such (see Crisp *et al.*, 1978).

A comparison, using the Minnesota Multiphasic Personality Inventory (MMPI), of anorectics and patients with schizophrenia by Small *et al.* (1981) showed no significant differences on any of the clinical or validity scales. A product-moment correlation between the two profiles, obtained via a measure of distance between the two groups ($D^2 = .83$). Both scored highest on the same five scales, although not in the same rank order; these were depression, psychopathic deviate, psychasthenia, paranoia, and schizophrenia. These data suggest that anorexics have affective or depressive thoughts and may have more profound thought disorders.

4 Endocrinological Factors

Some symptoms that anorectics suffer from are a consequence of malnutrition, but others are less obviously so caused. Among the latter are depression, obsessions, and amenorrhoea. Since amenorrhoea is an essential symptom in the definition of anorexia nervosa in postpubertal girls under all three currently used diagnostic systems, its importance in understanding the disorder is clear. The loss of menstruation is often dismissed as being akin to "weight loss amenorrhoea" since similar effects are found in externally induced starvation. However, many anorectic women stop menstruating *before* they lose weight. Fries (1977), in a review of 628 cases, found amenorrhoea preceded the onset of symptoms of anorexia in 16%, and in 55% of patients cessation of menstruation was coincident with onset of anorectic behaviour or early weight loss. Similar effects were found by Fairburn (personal communication) in a survey of 500 sufferers of bulimia nervosa; 65% who were previously anorectic reported irregular or absent menses, but, more remarkably, 46% of bulimics who had never been anorectic also were irregular in menstruation. Beumont and Russell (1982) argue that the menstrual disturbance that precedes significant weight loss in some anorectics is secondary to dieting and the consequential small variations in weight. As they point out, amenorrhoea can occur in young women who leave their parental home for a job or to undertake further education. In these girls, altered diets and increased exercise may precede a small weight loss. But they are also subject to many other stressors that could disturb menstruation. Since many patients develop amenorrhoea before notable weight loss there could be a psychogenic origin to the disorder.

Several other symptoms in anorexia nervosa, such as hypothermia, cold intolerance, and peripheral oedema are characteristic of a variety of endocrinological abnormalities. Although there is no incontrovertible evidence for an aetiological role for the hypothalamus or pituitary gland in anorexia nervosa (or bulimia nervosa), this must be a distinct possibility. There will be no attempt to comprehensively discuss the findings of studies on the endocrine status of patients with anorexia since there are many recent reviews (Vigersky, 1977; Halmi, 1978; Drossman *et al.*, 1979; Schwabe *et al.*, 1981; Beumont and Russell, 1982). The evidence outlined below needs to be interpreted with care, since weight loss induced by starvation, in otherwise normal people, can produce similar effects. The deviant hormonal response often can be reversed by nutritional rehabilitation, but on occasions insufficient time is allowed for an abnormal response to potentially recover. Also, because of the low incidence of the disorder, conclusions are drawn from studies with few subjects. Despite these caveats, the evidence for a profound hypothalamic–endocrine disturbance in anorexia nervosa has to be seriously entertained.

5 Hypothalamic–Pituitary–Gonadal Axis

Although the control of menstrual cyclicity is not well understood in women, it is known that the anterior and medial preoptic regions of the hypothalamus are involved, as well as the anterior pituitary gland. The hypothalamus produces, at intervals of about 1 hr, pulses of gonadotrophic releasing hormone (GnRH) that reach the pituitary via a portal plexus of capillaries. Early in the cycle GnRH drives a similar pulsatile production by the pituitary of follicle stimulating hormone (FSH) and luteinizing hormone (LH) that in turn cause the ovaries to produce oestrogen. This has negative and positive feedback effects, the former being a rapid response to low levels of oestrogens and almost certainly a function of the pituitary which can be viewed as becoming less sensitive to stimulation by GnRH. The slower positive feedback effect requires high levels of plasma oestradiol (200–400 pg/ml maintained for at least 36 hr); it results in an LH surge that precedes ovulation.

Anorectics with low body weights have greatly reduced or undetectable urinary and plasma levels of FSH, LH, and oestrogens; nor do they show negative or positive feedback effects when given ethinyl oestradiol. Their pituitary response to exogenous GnRH is variable, abnormal in some, but well preserved in others. Administration of clomiphene, an antioestrogen that blocks the negative feedback effects of oestrogen on the hypothalamus and pituitary in normal women, does not bring about an increased secretion of gonadotrophins in anorectics (Aono *et al.*, 1975; Wakeling *et al.*, 1976). Some of these effects can be explained by the pituitary stores of FSH and LH being depleted (see below).

When anorectic patients regain weight many of these changes are reversed. Urinary and plasma levels of gonadotrophins and gonadal steroids gradually rise without necessarily resuming normal cyclic patterns. Although the negative feedback effects of oestrogen can be elicited by ethinyl oestradiol treatments (Wakeling *et al.*, 1977), or blocked by clomiphene, which causes an inconsistent elevation of LH, the positive feedback effect of oestrogen is delayed until full weight is restored. But even this is not invariable (Wakeling *et al.*, 1976, 1977). In the anorectic patient who is regaining weight, bolus injections of GnRH produce an exaggerated FSH response and a normal or supranormal LH response (Warren *et al.*, 1975). These are reminiscent of the effect seen in normal children entering puberty and therefore add credence to the suggestion that the anorectic has an "immature" hypothalamic–pituitary system.

Continuous infusion of GnRH in normal adults produces a biphasic LH response that Bremner and Paulson (1974) think shows the presence of two functional pools of LH in the pituitary. One pool may be released immediately on stimulation while the other needs prolonged activation. The relative sizes of the pools may be determined by the interaction of GnRH and oestrogen on pituitary gonadotrophins (Yen, 1977). For the patient in an emaciated condition, neither functional pool is available, but with the restoration of weight, endogenous GnRH stimulation reinstates the first pool and probably also the second. Emaciated patients who are continuously infused with GnRH are unable to release LH from either of the depleted pools, but on regaining 80% standard weight they develop a good early LH response, showing that the first pool has been restored. The second LH pool is not functional at this body weight, reflecting either insufficient gonadotrophin or, more probably, a deficient positive feedback effect to oestrogen. Recovery of 95% of standard body weight restores a full biphasic LH response to infused GnRH (Beumont and Abraham, 1981).

Katz *et al.* (1978) proposed that the untreated adult anorexic has an "immature" hypothalamic–pituitary–gonadal system, since her LH secretory patterns are characteristic of prepubertal or early pubertal girls. In early puberty LH is secreted in 15- to 30-min pulses during nocturnal sleep, and later these pulses increase in amplitude and persist into and throughout the day. The untreated anorectic either has no LH bursts or those that occur are associated with sleep. An inactive or abnormal hypothalamic GnRH generation would account for this. Katz *et al.* found that women who had partially or totally recovered ideal weight, but who otherwise remained symptomatic, did not regain adult (mature) patterns of LH secretion. Those who had recovered symptomatically were more likely to have a mature pattern of LH secretion, but even they did not necessarily resume menstruating. Since amenorrhoea frequently persists in "weight-recovered" anorectics (Bell *et al.*, 1966; Wakeling *et al.*, 1976, 1977) it seems the resumption of menses requires more than an adult circadian LH secretory pattern. Frisch and McArthur (1974) claim that each woman must achieve a "critical degree of fatness"—about 17%—before cyclic gonadotrophin secretion and menses can occur. However, the evidence on the normalization of gonadotrophic secretion in weight-recovered anorexics is difficult to reconcile with Frisch's (1977) suggestion that a higher body-fat content of at least 22% is required to reestablish menses that has been lost through dieting. Possibly the recovered anorexia nervosa patient is still eating so abnormally that there are insufficient precursors for critical neurotransmitters or hormones. Alternatively, the hypothalmus and the pituitary, or both, were abnormal before all the symptoms of anorexia nervosa developed, or became so during the period of starvation and weight loss.

6 Hypothalamic–Pituitary–Thyroid Axis

Patients with anorexia nervosa show several symptoms that suggest hypothyroidism, including hypothermia, cold intolerance, bradycardia, low basal metabolic rate, delayed relaxation of the Achilles tendon reflex, raised serum levels of cholesterol and carotene, and constipation. Also, there are abnormalities in the metabolism of testosterone and cortisol, but these may be related to the pituitary–gonadal dysfunction and an adrenal–stress response, respectively. Although the profile of thyroid hormones in anorexia nervosa does not match that seen in true hypothyroidism, in general plasma levels of these hormones are depressed. Basal levels of thyroid stimulating hormone (TSH) are within the normal range, and the increase in TSH after treatment with exogenous thyroid releasing hormone (TRH) is normal in quantity but release is delayed and more prolonged than in control subjects (Miyai *et al.*, 1975; Vigersky *et al.*, 1976; Brown *et al.*, 1977; Casper and Frohman, 1982). These changes are similar to those found in malnourished states other than anorexia nervosa. Wakeling *et al.* (1979) studied levels of TSH and thyroid hormones in anorectics. They started 2 weeks after initiation of a refeeding programme to contral for the reversible changes in levels of thyroid hormones that occur with acute starvation, calorie deprivation, or carbohydrate deprivation. Thyroxine (T_4) levels remained low even after significant weight gains over 4–6 weeks, but triiodothyronine (T_3) concentration rose with weight gain—possibly because a deficit in hepatic monodiodination of T_4 to T_3 in the starvation phase resolved with refeeding.

The aetiological significance of the alterations in thyroid function in anorexia nervosa is contested. Moshang and Utiger (1977), Halmi (1978), and Walsh (1982) argue that the normal levels of TSH, and "essentially normal" response to TRH in anorexia nervosa (but see above) reflect a "hypometabolic" state but not true hypothyroidism. Thus, the changes in the hypothalamic–pituitary–thyroid axis observed in the emaciated anorectic are an adaptive physiological response to severe caloric restriction. However, unlike T_3 levels, T_4 levels do not recover rapidly with refeeding, and TSH responses to TRH stimulation remain abnormal in some weight-recovered anorectics. This evidence persuades Casper and Frohman (1982) to argue for a persistence of disordered neuroendocrine function.

Serum growth hormone (GH) is elevated in one-third to one-half of patients with anorexia nervosa, but refeeding with high-calorie diets corrects this (Brown *et al.*, 1977). Comparable effects are found in cases of protein–calorie malnutrition such as kwashiorkor, but in that disease the abnormality in GH release is related to amino acid deficiency, particularly of alanine, and is normalized after refeeding with proteins.

In normal people L-dopa and apomorphine stimulate GH release, and TRH and GnRH have no effect, whereas in some anorectics dopamine agonists are less effective (Sherman and Halmi, 1977), and, paradoxically, the releasing hormones increase GH output (Macaron *et al.*, 1978; Gold *et al.*, 1980; Brambilla *et al.*, 1981; Casper and Frohman, 1982). In the latter study, Casper and Frohman found an increase in GH after exogenous TRH in patients who had gained weight on the days before treatment. Thus, acute malnutrition is not an explanation for the deranged anterior pituitary response.

7 Abnormalities in Adrenocortical Activity

Levels of cortisol in plasma (Boyar *et al.*, 1977; Brown *et al.*, 1977; Gerner and Gwirtsman, 1981; Gwirtsman and Gerner, 1981), and in cerebrospinal fluid (Gerner and Wilkins, 1983) are elevated in emaciated anorectics, although diurnal variation is normal. This could occur if normal amounts are produced and breakdown is slowed. The daily production of cortisol is about the same in emaciated anorectics as in normal people (Walsh *et al.*, 1978), but in proportion to body size the amount is greater in the anorexia nervosa patient. Boyar *et al.* (1977) found a prolonged half-life of cortisol (from 60 to 78 min) in anorectic patients. Loss of body fat could explain the reduction in the metabolism of cortisol in the emaciated anorectic. Moreover, during recovery from anorexia nervosa there is a fall in the production rate of cortisol, measured by radioactively labelled cortisol and the number of cortisol secretory episodes per 24 hr (Doerr *et al.*, 1980; Walsh *et al.*, 1981). Thus, Walsh (1982) thinks the elevated plasma cortisol levels in the emaciated anorectic results from slower cortisol metabolism and increased adrenocortical activity.

Other evidence for abnormal adrenocortical activity comes from use of the dexamethasone suppression test (DST). Normal individuals treated with a small amount, about 1 mg, of the potent synthetic glucocorticoid dexamethasone suppress adrenal activity for about 24 hr. But patients with anorexia nervosa do not suppress cortisol production as much, nor for as long, when given dexamethasone (Walsh *et al.*, 1978; Gerner and Gwirtsman, 1981; Gwirtsman and Gerner, 1981). This may reflect an increased "drive" to produce cortisol in anorexia nervosa; similar effects are found in patients with depression. Furthermore Walsh (1982) thinks that "the degree of increase in adrenal activity in anorexia nervosa is out of proportion to the malnutrition—perhaps because of a concurrent depression." This issue will be considered later. The DST is thought to be a measure of altered corticotrophin releasing factor (CRF) regulation in the hypothalamus, that in turn affects the secretion of adrenocorticotrophic hormone. Gwirtsman and Gerner (1981) found that most patients still failed to suppress normally after refeeding, thus the DST may be identifying a hypothalamic–pituitary abnormality that is independent of low body weight.

8 Body Image Disturbance—Myth or Reality?

It is claimed that a body image disturbance of delusional proportions is a clinical feature of special importance in the syndrome of anorexia nervosa. Furthermore, Bruch (1973) considers its amelioration to be "a precondition for recovery from anorexia nervosa". Thus, the concept of "body image" is of clinical and theoretical interest. According to Henry Head's (1920) views the body schema is derived from past experiences and current sensations and is organised in the sensory cortex. It is used for localising incoming sensory information on the body surface and makes possible delicate motor actions, since it maintains the relationship of the body to other objects. This extension of the body schema to incorporate relationships between self and the external world has been emphasised in other theoretical contributions. Thus, Schilder (1935) thought that the body image included an individual's perception of her body and its parts, as well as interpersonal, environmental, and temporal factors. Similar notions were proposed by Feldman (1975) who writes

It [The body image] is in a sense the sum of the attitudes, feelings, memories and experiences an individual has towards his own body—both as a more or less integrated whole, and in respect to its component parts. It is not in the ordinary sense an "image" (though visual and kinaesthetic imagery may play a part), and can perhaps more satisfactorily be described as a representation, within the individual's psychological organization or "inner world." (p. 317)

Both Schilder and Feldman treat body image as having characteristics additional to purely perceptual phenomena; for them it takes on attributes of the psychoanalytic concept of ego.

Does the person suffering from anorexia recognise her emaciated condition and the extent of her weight loss? Many anecdotal reports imply that these patients are unaware of their condition and that they persist in claims of being "too fat," even when confronted with other equally thin anorectics whom they recognise as being underweight. Are they truly unaware of their physical condition, or do they recognise it but then deny it for some reason? Studies on body image estimation have not resolved these issues. But other evidence that anorectics show disturbances in a range of perceptual processes makes it likely that aberrations in perception, or cognition, or both, are fundamental in the aetiology of anorexia nervosa.

Glucksman and Hirsh (1969) introduced a technique for measuring body image that requires the subject to judge actual size from their own full-length photographic image projected on a screen. An adjustable anomorphic lens in the optical path allows the image to be changed by 20% in a "fat" or "thin" direction. An alternative method of measuring body image, developed by Reitman and Cleveland (1964), allows several measures of body size to be compared directly with real size. The subject is asked to imagine their body contours projected on a screen a few feet in front of them, and to adjust calipers to correspond to their estimates of different body widths such as their face, shoulders, waist, and hips. A variation of this technique is the image marking method devised by Askevold (1975). The subject stands in front of a large piece of paper mounted on a wall and is asked to imagine herself before a mirror; with a pencil in each hand she marks the places where she "sees" certain points corresponding to widths across specific regions of her body.

Slade and Russell (1973) provided the first systematic examination of body image in anorectics using the movable caliper method. Their 14 hospitalized patients overestimated own body width by 25 to 55%, in contrast to the accurate estimates of normal subjects. These patients accurately estimated their own height and the size of other objects. Accuracy of self-perception improved as weight was gained, and weight loss after discharge from hospital was related to in-hospital overestimation of size. Fries (1977) and Goldberg *et al.* (1977) confirmed a self-overestimation tendency in 21 and 44 anorectic patients, respectively, and accurate estimates in controls. However, Crisp and Kalucy (1974), despite confirming this tendency to overestimate body width in six anorectics, found that normal weight control subjects overestimated body size to a comparable extent. Garner *et al.* (1976) compared 18 patients with anorexia nervosa with normal weight controls, thin controls, and psychiatric patients, and found all groups overestimated body width by 12 to 27%. However, in a replication of Slade's and Russell's study, Button *et al.* (1977) found overestimation of body size in 20 anorectics *and* 16 normal weight controls, but patients who do not vomit were less inaccurate in their judgements and less likely to have an early relapse than those who do. In the largest available study using the adjustable caliper technique, Casper *et al.* (1979) found greater overestimation of body width and depth in 79 female anorexia nervosa patients than in age-matched controls, but both groups were inaccurate. Thus, most evidence from studies using the movable caliper technique shows that overestimation of body size is not unique to anorexia nervosa but is a widespread phenomenon. Casper *et al.* point out that age may be a significant factor in explaining some of the discrepancies; in the original study by Slade and Russell (1973), the patients and controls were not matched for age. Halmi *et al.* (1977) found a learning or maturational factor since older normal weight adolescent girls overestimated body size less than younger ones. Since Slade's and Russell's controls were older than the anorectic patients, the difference in size estimation may be partially explained.

Pierloot and Houbon (1978), Wingate and Christie (1978), and Strober *et al.* (1979) used Askevold's image marking technique on anorectics; all found that age-matched controls were more accurate in estimating body size than were the patients. Also, juvenile anorectics who use restrictive methods of weight control are poorer in estimating body size than those who vomit (Strober, 1981b). An interesting feature of Wingate's and Christie's study was that low ego strength—measured on the *Es* scale of the MMPI, which may be linked with a *general* distortion of perception and judgement—was associated with greater size overestimation.

Using the distorting photograph method of body size estimation, Garner *et al.* (1976) found that anorectic patients overestimated their size but controls did not. But Garfinkel *et al.* (1978) reported that size estimation varied considerably in anorectics and controls. Although generally the anorectic group overestimated their size, a few patients underestimated size by more than 10%, while none of the controls did. Body size estimations were reliable from week to week.

Strober (1981a) examined the relationship between MMPI scores and two separate measures of body image. One was an estimation of body size using the distorting photograph technique, the other was from the Fisher body distortion questionnaire that requires yes–no answers to questions on a range of distorted body experiences such as loss of body boundaries, blockage of orifices, and unusual sensations. A multivariate analysis showed there were two orthogonal dimensions defining the relationships between body image and personality scores. On one dimension, size overestimation and subjective body image distortion were associated with MMPI scales measuring somatization, anxiety, and atypical thinking. These relationships are to be expected, since anorectics display neurotic symptoms and are deluded about their body schemata. However, there was an interesting divergence on the second dimension. Some anorectics were depressed and introverted and their body image deviance was expressed mainly in size overestimation. But others had personality scores characteristic of psychosomatic tendencies and ideational disorders, and their body schema disturbances were in the realm of peculiar phenomenological experiences such as depersonaliztion, ambiguous sensations, fragmented boundaries, and so on.

Clearly there are discrepancies in the studies on body image in patients with anorexia nervosa and normal weight individuals.

If body image estimation is inaccurate in normal people, why are clinicians such as Bruch convinced that body image distortion is so important in the disorder? At an operational level the importance of body schema disturbance in anorectic patients is well founded. Those who overestimate size most have lower pretreatment weight, gain less weight during treatment, are more likely to deny the seriousness of their illness, have greater loss of appetite, are more sexually immature, are more dissatisfied with their body, are more depressed and anxious, experience greater physical anhedonia, and have a poorer prognosis (see Casper *et al.*, 1979; Garner, 1981).

One explanation for the discrepancy between objective measures and claims about body image in anorectics is that denial plays a substantial role in their overt disturbed self-perception. Patients with anorexia nervosa readily deny the seriousness of their illness despite the concern of their family and medical staff regarding their cachetic condition, and severity of illness is related to this tendency. However, anorectics can be "persuaded" to estimate their size more accurately. Pierloot and Houbon (1978) confronted patients with their mirror image and gave them instructions to produce more accurate estimations than in the initial tests. A similar procedure of repeating the size estimations was used by Crisp and Kalucy (1974), but before the second measure they undermined the patient's denial with statements such as "Drop your guard for a moment and tell me again how wide you really judge yourself to be." Denial may be part of a defense mechanism that alleviates conflict and anxiety arising from acknowledgement of true appearance (and hunger sensations).

Bruch (1973) argues that normalisation of body image is necessary for recovery in anorexia nervosa, so procedures that hasten this should be beneficial. Although coercive means for breaking down the patients' denials of their true appearance can produce short-term reductions in the overestimation of body size, there is no evidence for long-term benefits. Just confronting the anorectic with her image in a mirror (Pierloot and Houbon, 1978; Garfinkel *el al.*, 1978) does not have even immediate effects on size perception. But Biggs *et al.* (1980)

found that patients with anorexia nervosa had lower self-esteem after seeing themselves on a TV recording. No attempt was made to obtain estimates of body size, so no conclusions can be drawn about the effectiveness of video feedback on a direct measure of body image. However, Biggs *et al.* claim that the poorer self-evaluation that follows video feedback is beneficial for the anorectic, since it arises from the undermining of the patient's strategies for maintaining self-esteem. This could reduce the tendency toward denial in these patients and thus aid recovery.

Less direct attempts at investigating body image have been pursued. Crisp and Fransella (1972), Feldman (1975), and Fransella and Crisp (1979) explored cognitive constructs related to body image in patients with anorexia nervosa using repertory grid techniques. The first of these studies provided repertory grid data confirming a pervasive concern with body weight in some anorectic patients, but idealized body weight can fluctuate considerably (see Fransella and Crisp, 1979). They cite the case of a woman who maintained her restored weight only after showing, in her constructs, that she no longer attached such importance to normal body weight. A surprising finding by Fransella and Crisp (1979) was a positive correlation between the constructs "*self at normal weight*" and "*ideal weight*" instead of the negative correlation that would be expected from clinical experience. They also found that anorectics were different in construct patterning from normal weight controls and a group with various neurotic disorders. However, all three groups thought being an ideal weight was an important component of sexual attractiveness, while neither the neurotic group, nor the anorectics, saw themselves at present as being sexually attractive. Also, the anorectics, unlike the other groups, consider being fatter (than their present condition) to mean being sexually attractive and to be closer to their ideal self.

Two explanations proposed by Fransella and Crisp for the positive correlation between "*self at normal weight*" and "*ideal weight*" in the anorectic group are worth noting. The patients could be conforming—to what other people wanted of them—to get out of hospital, thus they construe at two levels: one concerned with what they really think, the other with what is expedient. Alternatively, the patients could be behaving like several other groups with long standing disorders like alcoholism, smoking, and obesity in showing the "as if" syndrome. " 'If only' I were not an anorectic I would be physically attractive, successful, and in full control of my life." But like these other disorders, anorexia nervosa is resistant to treatment; possibly the implication of being "normal" makes that condition impossible to consider so the status quo is maintained. The anorectic shows a classic approach–avoidance conflict; a normal weight is an ideal condition that can be achieved only with difficulty, and moreover, is a condition she fears greatly. Further studies using the contruct technique are clearly desirable.

Bruch (1973) and Palazzoli (1978) suggest that defects in ego structure underpin the body image disturbance, disordered perception, and the problems of "establishing a sense of control and identity" in the anorectic. Furthermore, they argue, anorexics have ego boundary disturbances and thus find difficulty in differentiating between self and nonself, between inner experience and external perception, and between independent objects. This is exemplified in the anorectics' experience of gastric fullness on seeing others eat or when thinking about food, and in their fear of close contact with those perceived as "fat". The only empirical support of an ego boundary disturbance in anorectics is that on the Rorschach test they score higher than depressed patients on scales that measure internal–external boundaries (Strober and Goldenberg, 1981). But on penetration, which is purported to measure substantiality of boundaries, their scores were lower. Since normal controls were not used, their conclusion that anorectics have a hazy differentiation of inter–external boundaries must be treated with caution. Moreover, a study on Rorschach patterning in anorexia nervosa by Wagner and Wagner (1978) reported no boundary disturbances but did find responses similar to those seen in conversion hysteria.

9 Perceptual Defects

Could the anorectic have faulty perception of the cues that signal need and satiety? They may be insensitive to the former and oversensitive to the latter, whereas bulimics (and obese people) could be insensitive to satiation cues. However, there are few studies of interoceptive cue perception in anorexia nervosa, and none as yet on bulimia nervosa. Anorectics have normal hunger awareness but are oversensitive to satiation cues, reporting feelings of bloatedness after eating small amounts of food. Although gastric motility is poorly related to hunger, on this measure there is no difference between controls and anorectics (Silverstone and Russell, 1967). Some anorectics fail to interpret stomach contractions as signals for hunger, but this is common even in normal weight individuals.

Despite frequent complaints by anorectics of early satiety, epigastric discomfort, and spontaneous vomiting, there are few studies of gastrointestinal function in the condition. Acute gastric dilation has been reported in patients with anorexia nervosa (Russell, 1966; Jennings and Klidjian,, 1977), and in emaciated prisoners of war. Also, nonobstructive dilation of the proximal duodenal loop or jejunal loop, but with normal gastric emptying of a barium meal, was found by Scobie (1973). Recently, however, Dubois *et al.* (1979) showed slower gastric emptying rates and a reduction in gastric acid output in anorectic patients. Holt *et al.* (1981), using a noninvasive scintiscanning procedure, confirmed that anorectics had slower gastric emptying for the liquid and solid components of a meal compared with normal controls. Emptying rates improved with weight gain but were still significantly slower than in controls (Dubois *et al.,* 1979). Abnormal gastric emptying may be further proof of a primary hypothalamic disorder in anorexia nervosa, since gastrointestinal function is controlled in part by a hypothalamic–parasympathetic mechanism.

Metoclopramide, a potent antiemetic that hastens gastric emptying as well as relaxing the duodenal cap, may restore gastric functioning in anorectic patients. Moldofsky *et al.* (1977) had partial success with the drug, and Saleh and Lebwohl (1979) found it normalised gastric emptying in some patients who initially had delayed emptying. Such treatment may be a useful adjuvant in the overall management of selected patients with anorexia nervosa.

Normal people find the taste of sucrose more pleasant before they ingest glucose than after a load, whereas obese individuals rate it equally pleasant on both occasions (Cabanac and Duclaux, 1970). Obese people may be less sensitive or responsive to cues related to food requirements than are the nonobese. Garfinkel *et al.* (1978) showed that anorectics failed to develop an aversion to sucrose after eating either of two isocaloric meals whose contents denoted "high" or "low" calories. This failure to develop a "satiety" aversion was related to body size overestimation. They suggest that abnormal responsiveness to internal cues related to food requirements, particularly for carbohydrates, may be related to the development of bulimia. It is not clear whether the lack of satiety–aversion to sucrose in anorexia nervosa is a facet of a more general perceptual disturbance or is of special significance.

Lacey *et al.* (1977) reported heightened taste sensitivity to sucrose because of carbohydrate avoidance, and this may be linked to hypoglycaemia and delayed blood glucose clearance in anorectic patients (Casper *et al.*, 1977; Silverman, 1977). When refed with a normal diet, these patients became less sensitive to the taste of sucrose. Thus, altered sensitivity to sucrose may be another example of a compensatory physiological process by means of which the body attempts to reestablish a normal nutritional condition.

10 Is Anorexia Nervosa an Affective Disorder?

Severe depressive illness can be accompanied by a profound anorexia, enough to create serious malnutrition. But is anorexia nervosa a variety of primary affective disorder? According to the Feighner *et al.* (1972) criteria for anorexia nervosa, patients with other known psychiatric illnesses are specifically excluded. But Cantwell *et al.* (1977) think that anorexia nervosa is an atypical affective disorder that develops in an adolescent girl at a time in her life when body image issues are important.

Many anorectics have symptoms of depression during the acute stage of the illness; the reported incidence varies from less than 40% (Hsu *et al.*, 1979) to 93% (Piazza *et al.*, 1980). In the latter study, onset of anorexia was associated in

78% of individuals with loss, through death, separation, or, symbolically, of someone important to the patient—classic "triggers" of reactive depression. A significant proportion of patients are depressed premorbidly or after recovery of body weight (Cantwell *et al.*, 1977; Crisp *et al.*, 1980). Anorectics show less severe symptoms than comparably aged females suffering from endogenous or neurotic depressions, but are more depressed than normal controls (Stonehill and Crisp, 1977; Ben-Tovim *et al.*, 1979; Eckert *et al.*, 1982). Also, according to Eckert *et al.* they are as depressed as anxious neurotics.

Many close relatives of anorectics have affective disorders (Crisp *et al.*, 1974; Morgan and Russell, 1975; Cantwell *et al.*, 1977; Winokur *et al.*, 1980; Gwirtsman and Gerner, 1981). Although Cantwell *et al.* emphasise this factor, the incidence of affective disorders in the families of their anorectics cannot be calculated, since total of probands is not specified, nor had they any control data. However, the Winokur *et al.* well-designed study shows that the incidence (22%) of primary affective disorders in relatives of anorectics was significantly greater than in families of matched controls (10%), and is similar to that reported in families of primary affective disorder patients.

Patients with primary affective disorders can be detected from biological markers such as high plasma cortisol levels, failure to show cortisol suppression to dexamethasone (see Walsh, 1982), and low urinary levels of 3-methoxy-4-hydroxyphenylglycol (MHPG) (Schildkraut *et al.*, 1973)—a major metabolite of brain norepinephrine. Similar changes are found in patients suffering from anorexia nervosa, and some of these were reviewed previously. In addition, MHPG levels are abnormally low during the acute phase of anorexia (Halmi *et al.*, 1978; Abraham *et al.*, 1981; Gerner and Gwirtsman, 1981; Gwirtsman and Gerner, 1981). Increases in MHPG concentration after weight gain treatment correlate with decreases in symptoms of depression according to Halmi *el al.* but Abraham *et al.* contend this was not true in their patients and that increases in MHPG correlated only with weight gain. Since some of the patients in the former study were taking cyproheptadine, whereas bed rest and refeeding was the only treatment in the latter, the studies are not fully comparable. However, Halmi *et al.* found no evidence that cyproheptadine affected depression ratings or MHPG levels.

Maas (1976) suggested that depression is related to abnormalities in catecholamine transmitter mechanisms, and Halmi *et al.* (1978) and Walsh *et al.* (1978) think that anorexia nervosa is a disorder involving noradrenergic pathways. Thus, it is significant that failure to suppress cortisol and low levels of MHPG were found in anorectics who were below 80% of ideal body weight (Gerner and Gwirtsman, 1981; Gwirtsman and Gerner, 1981); this was true regardless of mood. The linking of MHPG and abnormal cortisol suppression in the same patients is consistent with a common mediation through low norepinephrine levels in the hypothalamus. Norepinephrine in the hypothalamus has a tonic inhibitory effect on CRF and thus helps regulation of adreocoricotrophic hormone. Moreover, noradrenergic systems are implicated in the regulation of feeding behaviour; an α-noradrenergic system in the ventromedial hypothalamus excited feeding and a β-noradrenergic system in the ventrolateral hypothalamus suppresses it (Morley, 1980). To be consistent with an "anorexia–depression" model, depletion of norepinephrine should lead to depressive symptoms and to decreased eating. Evidence on the former is indirect and tenuous, but in monkeys depletion of central norepinephine interferes with satiety (Redmond *et al.,* 1977), and the α-noradrenergic agonist clonidine causes hyperphagia and weight gain (Schlemmer *et al.,* 1979). Depletion of norepinephrine may be a factor in producing some of the symptoms of anorexia, especially of depression, and may be involved in the eating disturbance.

Recent attempts to delineate subcategories of anorexia nervosa have focussed on those who resort to vomiting in comparison to the "restricters". According to Strober (1981b), the former are more prone to affective symptoms, and their parents have a higher incidence of affective disorders. Nonanorexic bulimics are particularly likely to exhibit mood disturbances, with some (a reported 70%) even contemplating suicide following bulimic episodes (Abraham and Beumont, 1982; Johnson and Larson, 1982). The possibility that only some types of anorexia are causally linked with affective disorders deserves further investigation.

11 Other Causal Models of Anorexia Nervosa

Several current theories on the aetiology of anorexia nervosa implicate family pathologies in the disorder. But early investigators of anorexia nervosa also considered the families of anorectic patients to have an adverse effect on their charges. Lasègue (1873) believed there was a dynamic pathological interaction in the patient–parent relationship, Gull (1874) thought the relatives to be the "worst attendants", while Charcot (1889) considered separation from the family to be essential for recovery. More recently Bruch (1973) suggested the anorectic is struggling to obtain a separate identity from her parents, and uses starvation as a means of stating her independence and of demonstrating that she can control at least some aspect of her life.

According to the "Family Pathology Theory" proposed by Minuchin *et al.* (1975, 1978), there are typical anorectic families who interact in a pathological fashion. They suggest that particular family characteristics are related to the development and maintenance of childhood psychosomatic symptoms, and anorexia nervosa is a form of psychosomatic illness used to maintain family homeostasis. Families of anorectics are considered to be over protective, enmeshing, rigid, and lacking in strategies for resolving conflicts. Open family conflict is avoided, and a semblance of unity maintained, by the parents protect-ing or blaming the anorectic child who is wrongly considered to be the only family problem. However, attempts to identify typical anorectic parents have been inconclusive (Kalucy *et al.,* 1977; Crisp *et al.,* 1980; see review by Yager, 1982). There is no evidence that specific pathological family interactions exist *before* anorexia nervosa develops or that such pathologies are causal in nature. Retrospective studies fail to distinguish such specific pathologies and family difficulties arising as stress reactions to this exasperating illness (Yager, 1982). Surprisingly, Branch and Eurman (1980) found that the friends and relatives of anorectics admire their slimness, specialness, and self-control; this may help explain the recidivistic tendency of anorectics.

Another model that has similarities to the family pathology view is the "weight-phobia" theory of Crisp (1970, 1977). He thinks that anorexia nervosa centers around the phobic avoidance of normal adult weight, and consequently the disorder arises during the biological and psychological maturational changes of puberty. The adolescent anorectic tries to delay the changes associated with adulthood by preventing weight gain. This behaviour is reinforced because the anorectic continues to experience childhood (biologically and psychologically), and the parents are not confronted by the threat of a child's desiring the freedom that comes with maturity. Crisp thinks the parents of some anorectics have buried or denied conflicts as well as psychiatric and behavioural pathologies. Although anorectics will agree to eat provided they do not gain weight, this is insufficient evidence for a weight-phobia. Salkind *et al*'s (1980) empirical test of the weight-phobia hypothesis proved negative, since anorectics did not show appropriate psychophysiological responses when asked to imagine a series of food and weight-related stimuli; two patients who had other phobias responded when imagining the feared stimuli. Thus, support for the theory is circumstantial: anorectics are amenorrheic and their pattern of gonadotrophin release is imma-ture, and pubertal changes necessary for normal menstrual cyclicity are depen-dent on the attainment of critical increases in white fat (Frisch, 1972, 1977).

Clearly, anorectics have dysfunctional hypothalamic processes. Russell (1970, 1977), amongst others, argued that such abnormalities are only partially dependent on weight loss or psychopathology, but the form and aetiology of the malfunction is unknown. Although hypothalamic tumours can produce symp-toms that are indistinguishable from true anorexia nervosa (Weller and Weller, 1982), there is no evidence that anorectics have a *disease* of the hypothalamus. A good reason for implicating the hypothalamus aetiologically in anorexia is its postulated involvement in feeding. But recent theories of hunger are less hypo-thalamocentric (Friedman and Stricker, 1976); extrahypothalamic structures, such as the amygdala, can control aspects of feeding behaviour such as satiety (Donohoe and Stevens, 1981). Moreover, the lateral hypothalamic syndrome (extreme aphagia and emaciation) is not an equivalent condition to anorexia nervosa, although it is superficially similar. For instance, aphagia in the former condition arises partly from lack of appetite, whereas anorectics have normal and even strong appetites.

Some evidence does support a persistent hypothalamic dysfunction in anorexia nervosa. Thus, recovery of normal or near normal body weight is often insufficient to restore menstruation. Frisch (1977) has argued that a critical threshold of body weight, that may be higher than ideal or premorbid weight, has to be attained for recovery of cyclicity. Knuth *et al.* (1977) encouraged a group of amenorrheic women to increase weight. Those who gained weight (about 3.7 kg) resumed menstruation, and those who remained acyclic gained little weight (mean of 0.7 kg). Normal cyclicity may fail to resume in anorectics because too little time is allowed for total recovery of hypothalamic functioning (Wakeling *et al.*, 1977), or because their eating remains chaotic (starving, bingeing, and purging), or to selective avoidance of carbohydrates (Kalucy *et al.*, 1977; Hsu *et al.*, 1979).

Anorectics have a central thermoregulatory disorder that might reflect a generalised hypothalamic dysfunction (Mecklengerg *et al.*, 1974). Their body temperature is low because of malnutrition, but their thermal distress is out of proportion to the degree of hypothermia. Some anorectics fail to shiver in the cold and also respond abnormally to heat stress (Vigersky and Loriaux, 1977). Luck and Wakeling (1982) showed that anorectics prefer abnormally high temperatures even when their core temperatures are similar to those of controls. They ruled out an abnormal thyroid status in these patients—serum-free thyroxin levels were comparable in the two groups—and the unusual preferences persisted after substantial weight gains, showing that malnutrition was not a direct agent. An abnormally high set point for behavioural temperature regulation, because of a hypothalamic malfunction, is one explanation of these findings. Alternatively, anorectics may be disturbed in perception of cutaneous pain, and the findings are another example of disordered perception in anorexia nervosa. The preferred temperature for skin stimulation was about 45°C, which would feel painful to healthy people and which indicates disruption in endogenous opioid mechanisms.

The importance of opioid (or peptidergic) mechanisms in various processes, including feeding, has been commented on recently, and anorexia nervosa may be causally linked to such compounds. Trygstad *et al.* (1978) isolated and identified an anorexigenic tripeptide from the urine of 10 patients with anorexia nervosa; a total dose of 12 nmol over 20 days of the peptide induced food refusal and weight reduction in mice. It took 6 months for the mice to recover normal weight and apetite. However, this interesting finding needs corroboration, and it has to be shown that this peptide is of aetiological importance in anorexia nervosa.

Endogenous opiate-type peptides, such as β-endorphin and met-enkephalin, can initiate feeding in sated animals, and conversely opioid antagonist drugs suppress appetite in a dose-related fashion (see Morley, 1980). Naltrexone, an opiate antagonist, produces anorexia in people to cause a weight loss of up to 5 kg in 3 weeks (Sternbach *et al.*, 1982), and these effects occur in persons not dependent on opiates (Hollister *et al.*, 1981). Thus, a subtype of anorexia nervosa may be caused by an underactive endogenous opioid system; either too little is produced or there are deficiencies in receptor binding. However, this view is contradicted by the finding of higher than normal levels of opioids in the cerebrospinal fluid of severely underweight anorectics; these levels revert to normal with weight gain (Kaye *et al.*, 1982). Furthermore, continuous infusion of naloxone (an opiate antagonist) facilitated weight gain in anorectic patients (Moore *et al.*, 1981), although the reason for this is in dispute. Gillman and Lichtigfeld (1981) contend that naloxone blocks opiate receptors in the chemoreceptor trigger zone, thereby reducing vomiting. But Moore *et al.* think that the weight gain followed a reduction in lipolysis. A more plausible explanation is that increased levels of endogenous opiates are consequences of malnutrition. This view is similar to that of Margules (1979), who thinks the endorphinergic system aids survival in famine by conserving nutrients and water, and decreasing energy-expending activities. Elevated endorphin levels in emaciated anorectics may reflect a mechanism for stimulating appetite, as well as conserving energy. High levels of endogenous opiates may inhibit GnRH release, since naloxone, an opioid antagonist, increases LH in normal women (Moult *et al.*, 1981) and raises LH levels in cases of amenorrhoea (Blankenstein *et al.*, 1981). Whether opioid antagonist drugs should be used in treating anorexics is not clear. Normalisation of gonadotrophins may be gained at the expense of reduction in appetite.

Indirect evidence for the involvement of endogenous opioids in appetite regulation is that food deprivation produces analgesia which is diminished by naloxone, an opioid antagonist drug (Bodner *et al.*, 1978). This may explain why anorectics prefer a temperature for skin stimulation in the range found to be painfully aversive in healthy individuals. (Luck and Wakeling, 1982).

An interesting comparison has been made between anorexia nervosa and running (Yates *et al.*, 1983). "Obligatory runners" show the same type of obsession as anorectics except that fitness is the goal of one and attractiveness of the other. Their personality profiles are similar—introvert—and many runners are depressed before they begin to run as a pastime. Like anorectics, about 20% of women athletes cease menstruating *before* they start running. The two conditions may be linked by endogenous opioids. Yates *et al.* think that excessive exercise to states of fatigue could increase opioid levels and thereby create the subjective "high" that many runners report—a floating sensation accompanied by a loss of feelings of fatigue. Similarly, anorectic women often seem elated and in constant motion, and they report feeling no tiredness. Increased levels of circulating endorphins could account for the altered states of consciousness in both running and anorexia; the rewarding properties of this state makes both conditions exceptionally resistant to change.

The endocrinological and other physiological evidence on anorexia nervosa is consistent with it being a variety of stress disorder (Walsh, 1982; Donohoe, 1984). Psychological stress alone cannot create anorexia nervosa. But in a predisposed person—one with a particular personality profile, who has difficult family and interpersonal problems, and with a biological predisposition [the "setting conditions" of Slade's (1982) model]—additional stress arising from the problems of adolescence, for example, might produce disturbed eating behaviour. In some girls the consequence of stress could be bulimia alone; this is consistent with animal studies that show that some stressors, like pain, increase feeding behaviour (see Morley *et al.*, 1983). But why, alternatively, should stress create anorexia? We recently confirmed that "confinement stress" in female rats reduces appetite and body weight (Hayward *et al.*, 1984), and that this effect is compounded by oestrogenic stimulation which is known to reduce food intake (Donohoe and Stevens, 1983). The effects of stress on feeding was not reversed by naloxone, but we have evidence that it can be blocked by cyproheptadine, an antiserotonergic drug.

Activation of the hypothalamic–pituitary–adrenal axis in states of stress is effected by CRF. When injected intracerebrally, CRF produces stress-type responses on catecholamine levels, heart rate, and metabolism, and *suppresses* feeding (Levine *et al.*, 1983). This may contribute to, if not totally account for, the excessive restriction in food intake in anorexics.

In summary, there is no entirely convincing explanation for anorexia nervosa. Particular theories emphasise specific facets of the baffling variety of symptoms or environmental conditions of the patients, but the important aetiological factors are not obvious. Most probably, several variables determine whether a person will develop anorexia, and there may be subtypes of the disorder that are linked to particular aetiological factors. Some anorectics may have disturbed hypothalamic functions *before* the disorder develops, others may primarily be depressives, and yet others may have endorphinergic problems.

12 Treatment of Anorexia Nervosa

As would be expected from the variety of theories for anorexia, there is no consensus about its treatment. However, it is generally accepted that restoration of body weight is necessary if treatment is to be successful. For many anorectics a conservative approach to treatment is satisfactory. The patient is admitted to hospital and continuously encouraged to eat a high-energy balanced diet of about 3000 calories a day, but under the supervision of skilled nursing staff, since many will attempt to cheat. If the patient is very undernourished (35–40% below usual weight, or 25–30% if weight loss occurred in fewer than 3 months) weight restoration can be started by enteral or parenteral means, since the anorectic is likely to be at risk (Drossman *et al.*, 1979). Overenthusiastic use of nasogastric feeding is criticised by Browning (1977) because of complications such as acute gastric dilation and aspiration of vomit. In recent years "hyperalimentation," in which all essential nutrients are given intravenously, has been used successfully (Finkelstein, 1972; Maloney and Farrell, 1980; Pertschuk *et al.*, 1981). An advantage with this technique is that the patient recovers body weight without being forced to eat. Pertschuk *et al.* compared patients given "hyperalimentation" with anorectics receiving standard behaviourally oriented inpatient therapy. Weight gain was greater with parenteral nutrition, and most patients were weaned to normal feeding with continued weight gain. Careful management of parenteral treatment is essential to prevent complications such as electrolyte imbalance and infection.

Halmi's group considers that appetite enhancement by cyproheptadine is beneficial in those anorectics with low body weights and a history of previous treatment failures (Goldberg *et al.*, 1979). Cyproheptadine also has antidepressant properties, so it is interesting to compare it with amitriptyline, another antidepressant that has been successfully used in a few open trial (Mills, 1976; Neddleman and Waber, 1977) and single-case studies (Moore, 1977; Kendler, 1978) of anorectics. A recent double-blind study by Halmi *et al.* (1983) showed that patients treated with cyproheptadine (in a high dose of 32 mg/day) gained more weight and were less depressed than the controls; others, given amitriptyline, did not do so well. Both of these antidepressant drugs are serotonergic antagonists (as well as affecting other neurotransmitter systems). Serotonergic mechanisms are implicated in the pathogenesis of depression (Asberg *et al.*, 1976) and in the regulation of feeding, so anorexia nervosa might reflect a dysfunction of this transmitter system.

Various versions of psychotherapy are used as adjuncts in treating anorectics, although psychoanalytic approaches are ineffective (Bemis, 1978). The family therapy approach of Minuchin *et al.* (1978) is also of use, but not as a sole treatment in other hands (see Piazza *et al.*, 1980). Various behaviour therapies have their adherents; of these, operant conditioning techniques are popular for weight restoration since they avoid unpleasant side effects or risks. The basic component of a behaviour therapeutic approach is to make access to privileges (favourite activities or pastimes or social facilities) contingent on weight gain; a variation is to make reinforcement contingent on the amount of food eaten (Bhanji and Thompson, 1974). A review of the research, some 20 papers involving 132 patients, on behaviour modification in anorectics by Garfinkel *et al.* (1977) concludes that it facilitates weight gain but does not prevent recurrence (no other treatment does either), or prove harmful, or result in worse outcomes than other therapies. These findings are corroborated by a study by Eckert *et al.* (1979) on 81 anorectics, half of whom were on a behaviour modification programme, whereas the other half were treated by various traditional techniques.

Bruch (1973) criticises behaviour therapeutic approaches but misinterprets their techniques, aims, and efficacy (see Hauserman and Lavin, 1977; Kellerman, 1977). She argues that "coerced feeding" through an operant regime only reinforces submissive behaviours thereby exacerbating nonassertive tendencies in anorectic patients, and that weight gain per se is not an adequate therapeutic goal, since underlying problems need to be dealt with if therapeutic success is to be achieved. As Wolpe (1975) points out in answer to Bruch, a therapy has to be properly applied before it is condemned as being ineffective. In a well-formulated behaviour therapeutic programme the therapeutic focus is determined by a *behavioural analysis* that elicits information from the patient regarding "the total context of stimulus antecedents". This would be followed by one or several treatment methods. These include extended operant contingency contracting (the patient contracts to consume a specific number of calories a day, or to gain a given weight in a specified time; otherwise a penalty is required), change of maladaptive eating behaviour patterns such as ritualised or secretive eating (Rosen, 1980), building of assertive behaviours (Hauserman and Levin, 1977), shaping independence from an overprotective family, or systematic desensitization to reduce food- or eating-related anxiety. Most clinicians who treat anorectics would agree with such a programme.

13 Prognosis

There are several recent reviews of follow-up studies on anorexia nervosa (Hsu, 1980; Schwartz and Thompson, 1981; Steinhausen and Glanville, 1983) and reports from individual groups on treatment outcome for significant numbers of patients (Halmi *et al.*, 1979; Hsu *et al.*, 1979; Crisp *et al.*, 1980). The following conclusions are drawn from these papers. There are difficulties in determining prognostic indicators and good estimates for treatment outcomes from many follow-up studies on anorectics published in the last 25 years. Moreover, several studies contain methodological flaws such as lack of rigorous definitions of the syndrome, failure to use direct methods for follow-up (postal and telephone enquiries yield inaccurate information), failure to trace enough patients, short duration of follow-up [relapses are common in anorexia nervosa and Morgan and Russell (1975) recommend a 4-year follow-up period], and inadequate outcome criteria. These can lead to false impressions about the usefulness of specific treatments and in determining important aetiological and prognostic factors.

Anorexia nervosa is a life-threatening disorder with a mortality rate of about 5%, with reports of death rates ranging from 0 to 21% in 25 studies from 1970. Specific dangers are electrolyte disturbances because of vomiting and use of purgatives, inanition, and suicide. Outcomes are normally assessed according to nutritional status, menstruation, eating problems, psychiatric status, sexuality, and social behaviour. Surprisingly few authors include body weight as a factor to be considered for outcome. Those who report on weight claim that 50–70% of patients recover, but often at weights below average. Whether weight restoration should be a crucial factor is unclear; thus, Goetz *et al.* (1977) report that 87% of their patients recovered normal body weight but only 60% were well adjusted psychosocially. Normalisation of menstrual function is found in 50–70% of patients and may be related to weight restoration. Longer follow-up periods are associated with reports of higher rates of normal menstrual function. Wide variations in the recovery of normal eating habits are reported (20–70%), and those who control weight by vomiting and purgative abuse have the most difficulty in regaining normal eating patterns.

It is difficult to formulate conclusions about the psychiatric outcome for anorectics, since patients in the acute stage of the illness can have various psychiatric symptoms including depression, obsessive–compulsive characteristics, and anxiety. There are wide variations in the reported incidence of psychiatric symptoms at follow-up, but "novel" symptoms are unusual, and the consensus is that the illness "breeds true". Many anorectics remain abnormal in psychosexual attitude and behaviour, and chronicity plays an important part (Hsu, 1980). But the future for the anorectic need not be entirely bad; marriage and childbearing is frequently reported in recovered anorectics. Frigidity and fear of pregnancy is found in some recovered anorectics, but how this compares with "normal" people is uncertain. Surprisingly, bulimic anorectics (and vomiters), whose general prognosis is poorer than the "restricter" type, appear more normal in psychosexual adjustment.

Recovery of normal patterns of social interaction is difficult to assess; scholastic and job performance can be measured objectively but quality of social contacts and family interactions are hard to judge. According to Steinhausen and Glanville (1983), in studies that grade recovery "good–fair–poor", the common estimate of recovery is 50–80%; younger patients recover best.

Dally and Sargant (1966) propose that anorexia should be considered chronic if it persists for more than 5 years despite treatment. The incidence of chronicity is probably below 20%, although the reported variation ranges from 0 to 79%; the latter was found by Beumont *et al.* (1976) in patients categorised as "vomiters and purgers".

Thus, many anorectics can establish a semblance of normal life, even if some will have persistent eating, psychiatric, and social problems. Indicators of poor prognosis include long duration of illness, older age at onset, severe weight loss, vomiting to control weight, purgative abuse and bulimia, being working class, being male, and acute body perception disturbance.

14 Conclusion

Anorexia nervosa is an enigmatic disorder; why it occurs and how to cure it remain unclear. The evidence on psychosocial factors in its aetiology is convincing, but there must be biological predispositions that make women more prone to it and specific individuals likely anorectics. Although bulimia nervosa and anorexia nervosa are related disorders, it is not clear why some women become bulimics and others anorectics. Perhaps personality factors, such as self-control or neurotic introversion, determine which will be contracted.

There are strong social pressures on women to be slim (and sexually attractive) which dispose them to diet. However, dieting for weight loss is harder for women than for men, since the former are biologically adapted for coping with conditions of famine. This probably arose because parturition and suckling impose severe metabolic demands that need to be met even when food is scarce (see Hoyenga and Hoyenga, 1982). In conditions of plenty, female mammals (including women) have a greater tendency to gain weight—store excess food as white fat—and then lose (use) this tissue in times of food drought. Consequently, slimming is more difficult for women than for men, since women are more efficient users of stored nutrients. To lose weight women must diet severely. For most women this will be an exercise that is limited by increasing hunger, or self-control, or because their idealised weight is easier to attain. For other women, dieting, or alternative means of weight control, such as vomiting after eating, will be excessive and result in either anorexia nervosa or bulimia nervosa.

A mathematical exposition for this view would probably be within the framework of catastrophe theory (see Zeeman, 1976, for a simplified account). Catastrophe theory was developed to deal with discontinuous behaviour, and it has been applied to diverse systems including earthquakes, animal behaviour, and the Wall Street crash. An example provided by Zeeman hypothesises a link between fear and agression: if aggression is strong, then attack occurs; if fear is strong, the creature avoids; but at certain intermediate amounts of fear and aggression the animal's behaviour can dramatically change from withdrawal to attack or vice versa. This occurs because of a "pleat" or "cusp" in the behavioural plane (a hypothetical construct within the theory). It is this "pleat" that provides the predictive power of catastrophe theory.

The causal factors in a modeling of anorectic behaviour are hunger and the desire to be slim, and behaviour would vary from starvation to gorging. For most people hunger will be sufficiently dominant to ensure adequate eating, but desire to be slim will reduce eating. The theory predicts, because of the pleat in the behavioural plane, that what might start as an understandable wish to reduce weight, with ensuing reduction in food consumption, could change suddenly into excessive dieting or starvation. In bulimia nervosa, the person's desires might cause her to be at a particular "pleat" region so that behaviour changes abruptly from gorging to food elimination. The characteristics of the "pleat" region, reflecting the effects of sexual selection and hormonal states, would differ between women and men. Thus, the difficulty women experience in regulating (and losing) body weight is embodied in the properties of the behavioural plane.

Although this is a loosely argued model, I think that an explanation drawing on sex selectional factors—because women are prone to eating disorders—and the power of catastrophe theory might help understand these so-far baffling eating disorders. Whether such a model has predictive power is yet to be investigated.

References

Abraham, S. F., and Beumont, P. J. (1982). How patients describe bulimia or binge eating. *Psychological Medicine*, **12**, 625–635.

Abraham, S. F., Beumont, P. J., and Cobbin, D. M. (1981). Catecholamine metabolism and body weight in anorexia nervosa. *British Journal of Psychiatry*, **138**, 244–247.

American Psychiatric Association (1980). "Diagnostic and Statistical Manual of Mental Disorders (DSM-III)." American Psychiatric Association, Washington, D.C.

Aono, T., Kinugasa, T., Yamamoto, T., Miyake, A., and Kurachi, K. (1975). Assessment of gonadotrophin secretion in women with anorexia nervosa. *Acta Endocrinologia*, **80**, 630–641.

Asberg, M., Thoren, P., Traskman, L., Bertilsson, L., and Rinberger, V. (1976). Serotonin depression: A biochemical subgroup within the affective disorders? *Science*, **191**, 478–480.

Askevold, F. (1975). Measuring body image. *Psychotherapy and Psychosomatics*, **26**, 71–77.

Bell, E. T., Harkness, R. A., Loraine, J. A., and Russell, G. F. M. (1966). Hormone assay studies in patients with anorexia nervosa. *Acta Endocrinologia*, **51**, 140–148.

Bemis, K. M. (1978). Current approaches to the etiology and treatment of anorexia nervosa. *Psychological Bulletin*, **85**, 593–617.

Ben-Tovim, D., Marilov, V., and Crisp, A. H. (1979). Personality and mental state (P.S.E.) within anorexia nervosa. *Journal of Psychosomatic Research*, **23**, 321–325.

Beumont, P. J. (1977). Further categorization of patients with anorexia nervosa. *Australian and New Zealand Journal of Psychiatry*, **11**, 223–226.

Beumont, P. J., and Abraham, S. F. (1981). Continuous infusion of luteinizing hormone releasing hormone (LHRH) in patients with anorexia nervosa. *Psychological Medicine*, **11**, 477–484.

Beumont, P. J., George, G. C. V., and Smart, D. E. (1976). 'Dieters' and 'vomiters and purgers' in anorexia nervosa. *Psychological Medicine*, **6**, 617–622.

Beumont, P. J. V., and Russell, J. (1982). Anorexia nervosa. *In* "Handbook of Psychiatry and Endocrinology" (Ed. G. D. Burrows), pp. 63–96. Elsevier Biomedical, Amsterdam.

Bhanji, S., and Thompson, J. (1974). Operant conditioning in the treatment of anorexia nervosa: A review and retrospective study of 11 cases. *British Journal of Psychiatry,* **124,** 166–172.

Biggs, S. J., Rosen, B., and Summerfield, A. B. (1980). Video-feedback and personal attribution in anorexic, depressed and normal viewers. *British Journal of Medical Psychology,* **53,** 249–254.

Blankenstein, J., Reyes, F. I., Winter, J. S. D., and Faiman, C. (1981). Endorphins and the regulation of the human menstrual cycle. *Clinical Endocrinology,* **14,** 287–294.

Bodner, R. J., Kelly, D. D., Spiaggia, A., and Glusman, M. (1978). Biphasic alterations of nociceptive thresholds induced by food deprivation. *Physiological Psychology,* **6,** 391–395.

Boyar, R. M., Hellman, L. D., Roffway, H., Katz, J., Zumoff, B., O'Connor, J., Barlow, H. L., and Fukoshima, D. K. (1977). Corticol secretion and metabolism in anorexia nervosa. *New England Journal of Medicine,* **296,** 190–193.

Brambilla, F., Cocchi, D., Nobile, P., and Muller, E. E. (1981). Anterior pituitary responsiveness to hypothalamic hormones in anorexia nervosa. *Neuropsychobiology,* **7,** 225–237.

Branch, C. H., and Eurman, L. J. (1980). Social attitudes towards patients with anorexia nervosa. *American Journal of Psychiatry,* **137,** 631–632.

Bremner, W. J., and Paulson, C. A. (1974). Two pools of luteinizing hormone in the human pituitary: Evidence from constant administration of luteinizing hormone releasing hormone. *Journal of Clinical Endocrinology and Metabolism,* **39,** 811–815.

Brown, G. M., Garfinkel, P. E., Jeuniewic, N., Moldofsky, H., and Stancer, H. C. (1977). Endocrine profiles in anorexia nervosa. *In* "Anorexia Nervosa" (Ed. R. A. Vigersky), pp. 123–136. Raven, New York.

Browning, C. H. (1977). Anorexia nervosa: Complications of somatic therapy. *Comprehensive Psychiatry,* **18,** 399–403.

Bruch, H. (1973). "Eating Disorders." Basic Books, New York.

Buhrich, N. (1981). Frequency of presentation of anorexia nervosa in Malaysia. *Australian and New Zealand Journal of Psychiatry,* **15,** 153–155.

Button, E. J., Fransella, F., and Slade, P. D. (1977). A reappraisal of body perception disturbance in anorexia nervosa. *Psychological Medicine,* **7,** 235–243.

Button, E. J., and Whitehouse, A. (1981). Subclinical anorexia nervosa. *Psychological Medicine,* **11,** 509–516.

Cabanac, J., and Duclaux, R. (1970). Obesity, absence of satiety aversion to sucrose. *Science,* **168,** 496–497.

Cantwell, D. P., Sturzenberger, S., Burroughs, J., Salkin, B., and Green, J. K. (1977). Anorexia nervosa: An affective disorder? *Archives of General Psychiatry,* **34,** 1087–1093.

Casper, R. C., Davis, J. M. and Pandey, G. N. (1977). The effect of nutritional status and weight changes on hypothalamic tests in anorexia nervosa. *In* "Anorexia Nervosa" (Ed. R. A. Vigersky), pp. 137–147. Raven, New York.

Casper, R. C., and Frohman, L. A. (1982). Delayed TSH release in anorexia nervosa following injection of thyrotropin releasing hormone (TRH). *Psychoneuroendocrinology,* **7,** 59–68.

Casper, R. C., Halmi, K. A., Goldberg, S. C., Eckert, E. D., and Davis, J. M. (1979). Disturbances in body image estimations as related to other characteristics and outcome in anorexia nervosa. *British Journal of Psychiatry,* **134,** 60–66.

Charcot, J. M. (1889). "Disorders of the nervous system." New Sydenham Society, London

Crisp, A. H. (1970). Anorexia nervosa: Feeding disorder, nervous malnutrition or weight phobia? *World Review of Nutrition and Diet,* **12,** 452–504.

Crisp, A. H. (1977). Diagnosis and outcome of anorexia nervosa. *Proceedings of the Royal Society of Medicine,* **70,** 464–470.

Crisp, A. H., and Fransella, F. (1972). Conceptual changes during recovery from anorexia nervosa. *British Journal of Medical Psychology,* **45,** 395–405.

Crisp, A. H., Harding, B., and McGuiness, B. (1974). Psychoneurotic characteristics of parents: Relationship to prognosis. *Journal of Psychosomatic Research,* **18,** 167–173.

Crisp, A. H., Hsu, L. K., and Hartshorn, J. (1980). Clinical features of anorexia nervosa: A study of a consecutive series of 102 female patients. *Journal of Psychosomatic Research,* **24,** 179–191.

Crisp, A. H., Jones, M. G., and Slater, P. (1978). The Middlesex Hospital Questionnaire: A validity study. *British Journal of Medical Psychology,* **51,** 269–280.

Crisp, A. H., and Kalucy, R. S. (1974). Aspects of the perceptual disorder in anorexia nervosa. *British Journal of Medical Psychology,* **47,** 349–361.

Crisp, A. H., Palmer, R. L., and Kalucy, R. S. (1976). How common is anorexia nervosa? A prevalence study. *British Journal of Psychiatry,* **128,** 549–554.

Dally, P., and Sargant, W. (1966). Treatment and outcome of anorexia nervosa. *British Medical Journal,* **ii,** 793–795.

Doerr, P., Fichter, M., Pirke, K. M., and Lund, R. (1980). Relationship between weight gain and hypothalamic–pituitary–adrenal function in patients with anorexia nervosa. *Journal of Steriod Biochemistry,* **13,** 529–537.

Donohoe, T. P. (1984). Stress-induced anorexia: Implications for anorexia nervosa. *Life Sciences,* **34,** 203–218.

Donohoe, T. P., and Stevens, R. (1981). Modulation of food intake by amygdaloid estradiol benzoate implants in female rats. *Physiology and Behavior,* **27,** 105–114.

Donohoe, T. P., and Stevens, R. (1983). Effects of ovariectomy, estrogen treatment and CI-628 on food intake and body weight in female rats treated neonatally with gonadal hormones. *Physiology and Behavior,* **31,** 325–329.

Drossman, D. A., Outjes, D. A., and Heizer, W. D. (1979). Anorexia nervosa. *Gastroenterology,* **77,** 1115–1131.

Dubois, A., Gross, H. A., Ebert, M. H., and Castell, D. O. (1979). Altered gastric emptying and secretion in primary anorexia nervosa. *Gastroenterology,* **77,** 319–323.

Eckert, E. D., Goldberg, S. C., Halmi, K. A., Casper, R. C., and Davis, J. M. (1979). Behaviour therapy in anorexia nervosa. *British Journal of Psychiatry,* **134,** 55–59.

Eckert, E. D., Goldberg, S. C., Halmi, K. A., Casper, R. C., and Davis, J. M. (1982). Depression in anorexia nervosa. *Psychological Medicine,* **12,** 115–122.

Eysenck, H. J., and Rachman, S. (1965). ''The Causes and Cures of Neurosis.'' Routledge & Keegan Paul, London

Feighner, J. P., Robins, E., Guze, S. B., Woodruff, Jr., R. A., Winokur, G., and Munoz, R. (1972). Diagnostic criteria for use in psychiatric research. *Archives of General Psychiatry,* **26,** 57–63.

Feldman, M. M. (1975). The body image and object relations: Exploration of a method utilizing repertory grid techniques. *British Journal of Medical Psychology,* **48,** 317–332.

Finkelstein, B. A. (1972). Parenteral hyperalimentation in anorexia nervosa. *Journal of the American Medical Association,* **219,** 217.

Fransells, F., and Crisp, A. H. (1979). Comparisons of weight concepts in groups of neurotic and anorexic females. *British Journal of Psychiatry,* **134,** 79–86.

Friedman, M. I., and Stricker, M. E. (1976). The physiological psychology of hunger: A phsyiological perspective. *Psychological Review,* **83,** 409–431.

Fries, H. (1974). Secondary amenorrhoea, self-induced weight reduction and anorexia nervosa. *Acta Psychiatrica Scandinavica Supplement,* **248.**

Fries, H. (1977). Studies on secondary amenorrhea, anorectic behavior and body image perception: Importance for the early recognition of anorexia nervosa. *In* ''Anorexia Nervosa'' (Ed. R. A. Vigersky). Raven, New York.

Frisch, R. E. (1972). Weight in menarche. *Pediatrics,* **50,** 445–450.

Frisch, R. E. (1977). Food intake, fatness and reproductive ability. In ''Anorexia Nervosa'' (Ed. R. A. Vigersky), Raven Press, New York.

Frisch, R. E., and McArthur, J. W. (1974). Menstrual cycles: Fatness as a determinant of minimum weight for height necessary for their maintenance or onset. *Science,* **185,** 949–951.

Garfinkel, P. E., Garner, D. M., and Moldofsky, H. (1977). The role of behavior modification in the treatment of anorexia nervosa. *Journal of Pediatric Psychology,* **2,** 113–121.

Garfinkel, P. E., Moldofsky, H., Garner, D. M., Stancer, H. C., and Coscina, D. V. (1978). Body awareness in anorexia nervosa: Disturbance in body image and satiety. *Psychosomatic Medicine,* **40,** 487–498.

Garner, D. M. (1981). Body image in anorexia nervosa. *Canadian Journal of Psychiatry,* **26,** 224–227.

Garner, D. M., and Garfinkel, P. E. (1979). The Eating Attitude Test: An index of symptoms of anorexia nervosa. *Psychological Medicine,* **9,** 273–279.

Garner, D. M., and Garfinkel, P. E. (1980). Socio-cultural factors in the development of anorexia nervosa. *Psychological Medicine,* **10,** 647–656.

Garner, D. M., Garfinkel, P. E., Stancer, H. C., and Moldofsky, H. (1976). Body image disturbances in anorexia nervosa and obesity. *Psychosomatic Medicine,* **38,** 323–337.

Gerner, R. H., and Gwirtsman, H. E. (1981). Abnormalities of dexamethasone suppression test and urinary MHPG in anorexia nervosa. *American Journal of Psychiatry,* **138,** 650-653.

Gerner, R. H., and Wilkins, J. N. (1983). CSF cortisol in patients with depression, mania, or anorexia nervosa and in normal subjects. *American Journal of Psychiatry,* **140,** 92–94.

Gillman, M. A., and Lichtigfeld, F. J. (1981). Naloxone in anorexia nervosa— the role of the opiate system. *Journal of the Royal Society of Medicine,* **74,** 631–632.

Glucksman, M. L., and Hirsch, J. (1969). The response of obese patients to weight reduction. III. The perception of body size. *Psychosomatic Medicine,* **31,** 1–7.

Goetz, P. L., Succop, R. A., Reinhart, J. B., and Miller, A. (1977). Anorexia nervosa in children: A follow-up study. *American Journal of Orthopsychiatry,* **47,** 597–603.

Gold, M. S., Pottash, A. L. C., Sweeney, D. R., Martin, D. M., and Davies, R. K. (1980). Further evidence of hypothalamic–pituitary dysfunction in anorexia nervosa. *American Journal of Psychiatry,* **137,** 101–102.

Goldberg, R. C., Halmi, K. A., Casper, R. C., Eckert, E. D., and Davis, J. M. (1977). Pretreatment predictors of weight gain in anorexia nervosa. *In* "Anorexia Nervosa" (Ed. R. A. Vigersky). Raven, New York.

Goldberg, R. C., Halmi, K. A., Casper, R. C., Eckert, E. D., and Davis, J. M. (1979). Cyproheptadine in anorexia nervosa. *British Journal of Psychiatry,* **134,** 67–70.

Gomez, J., and Dally, P. (1980). Psychometric rating in the assessment of progress in anorexia nervosa. *British Journal of Psychiatry,* **136,** 290–296.

Gull, W. W. (1874). Anorexia nervosa (apepsia hysterica, anorexia hysterica). *Transactions of the Clinical Society of London,* **7,** 22–28.

Gwirtsman, H. E., and Gerner, R. H. (1981). Neurochemical abnormalities in anorexia nervosa: Similarities to affective disorders. *Biological Psychiatry,* **16,** 991–995.

Halmi, K. (1974). Anorexia nervosa: Demographic and clinical features in 94 cases. *Psychosomatic Medicine,* **36,** 18–26.

Halmi, K. A. (1978). Anorexia nervosa: Recent investigations. *Annual Review of Medicine,* **29,** 137–148.

Halmi, K. A., Dekirmenjian, H., Davis, J. M., Casper, R., and Goldberg, S. (1978). Catecholamine metabolism in anorexia nervosa. *Archives of General Psychiatry,* **35,** 458–460.

Halmi, K., Eckert, E., and Falk, J. R. (1983). Cyproheptadine, an antidepressant and weight inducing drug for anorexia nervosa. *Psychopharmacology Bulletin,* **19,** 103-105.

Halmi, K. A., Goldberg, S. C., Casper, R. C., Eckert, E. D., and Davis, J. M. (1979). Preatment predictors of outcome in anorexia nervosa. *British Journal of Psychiatry,* **1134,** 71–78.

Halmi, K. A., Goldberg, S. C., and Cunningham, S. (1977). Perceptual distortion and body image in adolescent girls: Distortion of body image in adolescence. *Psychological Medicine,* **7,** 253–257.

Hauserman, N., and Lavin, P. (1977). Post-hospitalization continuation treatment of anorexia nervosa. *Journal Of Behavior Therapy and Experimental Psychiatry,* **8,** 309–313.

Hayward, C., Stevens, R., and Donohoe, T. P. (1984). Immobilization stress reduces food intake and influences the oestrogenic modulation of feeding in ovariectomized rats. *British Feeding Group Conference, Sussex University.*

Head, H. (1920). ''Studies in Neurology.'' Hodder and Stoughton, London.

Hollister, L. E., Johnson, K., Boukhabza, D., and Gillespie, H. K. (1981). Adverse effects of naltrexone in subjects not dependent on opiates. *Drug Alcohol Dependence,* **8,** 37–41.

Holt, S., Ford, M. J., and Heading, R. C. (1981). Abnormal gastric emptying in primary anorexia nervosa. *British Journal of Psychiatry,* **139,** 550–552.

Hoyenga, K. B., and Hoyenga, K. T. (1982). Gender and energy balance: Sex differences in adaptations for feast and famine. *Physiology and Behaviour,* **28,** 545–563.

Hsu, L. K. (1980). Outcome of anorexia nervosa: A review of the literature (1954 to 1978). *Archives of General Psychiatry,* **37,** 1041–1046.

Hsu, L. K., and Crisp, A. H. (1980). The Crown–Crisp Experiential Index (CCEI) in anorexia nervosa. *British Journal of Psychiatry,* **136,** 567–573.

Hsu, L. K. G., Crisp, A. H., and Harding, B. (1979). Outcome of anorexia nervosa. *Lancet,* **I,** 61–65.

Jennings, K. P., and Klidjian, A. M. (1977). Acute gastric dilation in anorexia nervosa. *British Medical Journal*, **2**, 477–478.

Johnson, C., and Larson, R. (1982). Bulimia: An analysis of mood and behavior. *Psychosomatic Medicine*, **44**, 341–351.

Kalucy, R. S., Crisp, A. H., and Harding, B. (1977). Prevalence and prognosis in anorexia nervosa. *Australian and New Zealand Journal of Psychiatry*, **11**, 251–257.

Katz, J. L.; Boyar, R., Roffwarg, H., Hellman, L., and Weiner, H. (1978). Weight and circadian luteinizing hormone secretory pattern in anorexia nervosa. *Psychosomatic Medicine*, **40**, 549–567.

Kaye, W. H., Pickar, D., Naber, D., and Ebert, M. H. (1982). Cerebrospinal fluid opioid activity in anorexia nervosa. *American Journal of Psychiatry*, **139**, 643–645.

Kellerman, J. (1977). Anorexia nervosa: The efficacy of behavior therapy. *Journal Of Behavior Therapy and Experimental Psychiatry*, **8**, 387–390.

Kendler, K. S. (1978). Amitryptyline-induced obesity in anorexia nervosa: A case report *American Journal of Psychiatry*, **135**, 1107–1108.

Knuth, V. A., Hull, M. G. R., and Jacobs, H. S. (1977). Amenorrhoea and loss of body weight. *British Journal of Obstetrics and Gynaecology*, **84**, 801–807.

Kolb, L. C. (1959). Disturbances of the body image. *In* "American Handbook of Psychiatry: Volume One" (Ed. S. Arieti), pp. 749–769. Basic Books, Inc., New York.

Lacey, J. H., Stanley, P. A., Crutchfield, M., and Crisp, A. H. (1977). Sucrose sensitivity in anorexia nervosa. *Journal of Psychosomatic Research*, **21**, 17–21.

Lasègue, E. P. (1873). De L'Anorexie Hysterique. *Archives of General Medicine*, **1**, 385.

Levine, A. S., Rogers, B., Kneip, J., Grace, M., and Morley, J. E. (1983). Effects of centrally administered corticotrophin releasing factor (CRF) on multiple feeding paradigms. *Neuropharmacology*, **22**, 337–339.

Lowenkopf, E. L. (1982). Anorexia nervosa: Some nosological considerations. *Comprehensive Psychiatry*, **23**, 233–240.

Luck, P., and Wakeling, A. (1982). Set-point displacement for behavioural thermoregulation. *Clinical Science*, **62**, 677–682.

Maas, J. W. (1976). Biogenic amines and depression. *Archives of General Psychiatry*, **32**, 1357–1361.

Macaron, C., Wilber, J. F., Green, O., and Freinkel, N. (1978). Studies of growth hormone (GH), thyrotropin (TSH) and prolactin (PRL) secretion in anorexia nervosa. *Psychoneuroendocrinology*, **3**, 181–185.

Maloney, M. J., and Farrell, M. K. (1980). Treatment of severe weight loss in anorexia nervosa with hyperalimentation and psychotherapy. *American Journal of Psychiatry*, **137**, 310–314.

Margules, D. L. (1979). Beta-endorhpin and endoloxone: Hormones of the autonomic nervous system for the conservation or expenditure of bodily resources and energy in anticipation of famine or feast. *Neuroscience and Biobehavioral Research,* **3,** 155–162.

Mawson, A. R. (1974). Anorexia nervosa and the regulation of intake: A review. *Psychological Medicine,* **4,** 289–308.

Mecklenberg, R. S., Loriaux, D. L., Thompson, R. H., Anderson, A. E., and Lipsett, M. B. (1974). Hypothalamic dysfunction in patients with anorexia nervosa. *Medicine,* **53,** 145–159.

Mills, I. H. (1976). Amitryptyline therapy in anorexia nervosa. *Lancet,* **ii,** 687.

Minuchin, S., Baker, L., Rosman, B. L., Liebman, R., Milman, L., and Todd, T. (1975). A conceptual model of psychosomatic illness in children. *Archives of General Psychiatry,* **32,** 1031–1038.

Minuchin, S., Rosman, B. L., and Baker, L. (1978). ''Psychosomatic families: Anorexia Nervosa in Context.'' Harvard University Press, Cambridge, Massachusetts.

Miyai, K., Yamamoto, T., Azukizawa, M., Ishibashi, K., and Kumahara, Y. (1975). Serum thyroid hormones and thyrotropin in anorexia nervosa. *Journal of Clinical Endocrinology and Metabolism,* **40,** 334–338.

Moldofsky, H., Jeuniewic, N., and Garfinkel, P. E. (1977). Preliminary report on metoclopramide in anorexia nervosa. *In* ''Anorexia Nervosa'' (Ed. R. A. Vigersky), pp. 373–375. Raven, New York.

Moore, D. C. (1977). Amitryptyline therapy in anorexia nervosa. *American Journal of Psychiatry,* **134,** 1303–1304.

Moore, R., Mills, I. H., and Forster, A. (1981). Naloxone in the treatment of anorexia nervosa: Effect of weight gain and lipolysis. *Journal of the Royal Society of Medicine,* **74,** 129–131.

Morgan, H. G., and Russell, G. F. M. (1975). Value of family background and clinical features as predictors of long-term outcome in anorexia nervosa: Four-year follow-up study of 41 patients. *Psychological Medicine,* **5,** 355–371.

Morley, J. E. (1980). The neuroendocrine control of appetite: The role of the endogenous opiates, cholecystokinin, TRH, gamma-amino-butyric acid and the diazepam receptors. *Life Sciences,* **27,** 355–368.

Morley, J. E., Levine, A. S., and Rowland, N. E. (1983). Stress-induced eating. *Life Sciences,* **32,** 2169–2182.

Moshang, T., and Utiger, R. D. (1977). Low triiodothyronine euthyroidism in anorexia nervosa. *In* ''Anorexia Nervosa'' (Ed. R. A. Vigersky), pp. 263–270. Raven, New York.

Moult, P. J. A., Grossman, A., Evans, J. M., Rees, L. H., and Besser, G. M. (1981). The effect of naloxone on pulsatile gonadotrophin release in normal subjects. *Clinical Endocrinology,* **14,** 321–324.

Needleman, H. L., and Waber, D. (1977). The use of amitryptyline in anorexia nervosa. *In* ''Anorexia Nervosa'' (Ed., R. A. Vigersky), pp. 357–362. Raven, New York.

Palazzoli, M. S. (1978). ''Self-Starvation: From Individual to Family Therapy in the Treatment of Anorexia Nervosa.'' Aronson, New York.

Palmer, R. L. (1979). The dietary chaos syndrome: A useful new term. *British Journal of Medical Psychology, 52,* 187–190.

Pertschuk, M. J., Forster, J., Buzby, G., and Mullen, L. (1981). The treatment of anorexia nervosa with total parenteral nutrition. *Biological Psychiatry, 16,* 539–550.

Piazza, E., Piazza, N., and Rollins, N. (1980). Anorexia nervosa: Controversial aspects of therapy. *Comprehensive Psychiatry, 21,* 177–189.

Pierloot, R. A., and Houbon, M. E. (1978). Estimation of body dimensions in anorexia nervosa. *Psychological Medicine, 8,* 317–324.

Pope, H. G., Hudson, J. I., and Yurgelun-Todd, D. (1984). Anorexia and bulimia among 300 suburban women shoppers. *American Journal of Psychiatry, 141,* 292–294.

Redmond, D. E., Huang, Y. H., Snyder, D. R., and Maas, J. W. (1977). Norepinephrine satiety in monkeys. *In* ''Anorexia Nervosa'' (Ed. R. A. Vigersky), pp. 81–96. Raven, New York.

Reitman, E. E., and Cleveland, S. E. (1964). Changes in body image following sensory deprivation in schizophrenic and control groups. *Journal of Abnormal and Social Psychology, 68,* 168–176.

Rosen, L. W. (1980). Modifications of secretive or ritualized eating behaviour in anorexia nervosa. *Journal Of Behavior Therapy and Experimental Psychiatry, 11,* 101.-104.

Russell, G. (1979). Bulimia nervosa· An ominous variant of anorexia nervosa. *Psychological Medicine, 9,* 429–448.

Russell, G. F. M. (1966). Acute dilation of the stomach in anorexia nervosa. *British Journal of Psychiatry, 112,* 203–207.

Russell, G. F. M. (1970). Anorexia nervosa: Its identity as an illness and its treatment. *In* ''Modern Trends in Psychological Medicine'' (Ed. J. G. Harding-Price), pp. 131–164. Butterworths, London.

Russell, G. F. M. (1977). The present status of anorexia nervosa. *Psychological Medicine, 7,* 363–367.

Saleh, J. W., and Lebwohl, P. (1979). Gastric emptying studies in patients with anorexia nervosa: Effects of metoclopramide. *Gastroenterology, 76,* 1233.

Salkind, M. R., Fincham, J., and Silverstone, T. (1980). Is anorexia nervosa a phobic disorder? *Biological Psychiatry,15,* 803-808.

Schilder, P. (1935). ''Image and Appearance of Human Body'' Kegan, Paul, Trench, Truber, & Co., London

Schildkraut, J. J., Keeler, B. A., and Papousek, M. (1973). MHPG excretion in depressive disorders. *Science, 181,* 762–764.

Schlemmer, Jr., R. F., Casper, R. C., Narasimhachari, N., and Davis, J. M. (1979). Clonidine induced hyperphagia and weight gain in monkey. *Psychopharmacology, 61,* 133–134.

Schwabe, A. D., Lippe, B. M., Chang, J., Pops, M. A., and Yager, J. (1981). Anorexia nervosa. *Annals of Internal Medicine,* **94,** 371–181.

Schwartz, D. M., and Thompson, M. T. (1981). Do anorectics get well: Current research and future needs. *American Journal of Psychiatry,* **138,** 319–323.

Scobie, B. A. (1973). Acute gastric dilation and duodenal ileus in anorexia nervosa. *Medical Journal of Australia,* **2,** 940–942.

Sherman, B. M., and Halmi, K. A. (1977). Effect of nutritional rehabilitation on hypothalamic–pituitary function in anorexia nervosa. *In* "Anorexia Nervosa" (Ed. R. A. Vigersky), pp. 211–224. Raven, New York.

Silverman, A. (1977). Anorexia nervosa: Clinical and metabolic observations in a successful treatment plan. *In* "Anorexia Nervosa" (Ed. R. A. Vigersky), pp. 331–340. Raven, New York.

Silverstone, J. T., and Russell, G. F. M. (1967). Contractions in anorexia nervosa. Gastric "hunger" contractions in anorexia nervosa. *British Journal of Psychiatry,* **113,** 257–263.

Slade, P. (1982). Towards a functional analysis of anorexia nervosa and bulimia nervosa. *British Journal of Clinical Psychology,* **21,** 167–179.

Slade, P. D., and Russell, G. F. M. (1973). Awareness of body dimension in anorexia nervosa: Cross-section and longitudinal studies. *Psychological Medicine,* **3,** 188–199.

Slater, E., and Roth, M. (1969). "Mayer-Gross Slater and Roth Clinical Psychiatry" (3rd. ed.). Baillerie, Tindall and Cassell, London.

Small, A. C., Madero, J., Gross, H., Tegano, L., Leib, J., and Ebert, M. (1981). A comparative analysis of primary anorexics and schizophrenics on the MMPI. *Journal of Clinical Psychology,* **37,** 733–736.

Steinhausen, H. C. and Glanville, K. (1983). Follow-up studies of anorexia nervosa: A review of research findings. *Psychological Medicine,* **13,** 239–249.

Sternbach, H. A., Annitto, W., Pottash, A. L. C., and Gold, M. S. (1982). Anorexic effects of naltrexone in man. *Lancet,* **8268** (Vol 1 for 1982), 388–389.

Stonehill, E., and Crisp, A. H. (1977). Psychosomatic characteristics of patients with anorexia nervosa before and after treatment and at follow-up 4-7 years later. *Journal of Psychosomatic Research,* **21,** 187–193.

Strober, M. (1980). Personality and symptomatological features in young non-chronic anorexia nervosa patients *Journal of Psychosomatic Research,* **24,** 353–359.

Strober, M. (1981a). The relation of personality characteristics to body image disturbance in juvenile anorexia nervosa: A multivariate analysis. *Psychosomatic Medicine,* **43,** 323–330.

Strober, M. (1981b). The significance of bulimia in juvenile anorexia nervosa: An exploration of possible etiological factors. *International Journal Of Eating Disorders,* **1,** 28–43.

Strober, M., and Goldenberg, I. (1981). Ego boundary disturbance in juvenile anorexia nervosa. *Journal of Clinical Psychology,* **37,** 433–438.

Strober, M., Goldenberg, I., Green, J., and Saxon, J. (1979). Body image disturbance in anorexia nervosa during the acute and recuperative phase. *Psychological Medicine,* **9,** 695–701.

Trygstad, O., Foss, I., Edminson, P. D., Johansen, J. H. and Reichelt, K. L. (1978). Humoral control of appetite: A urinary anorexigenic peptide. Chromatographic patterns of urinary peptides in anorexia nervosa. *Acta Endocrinologia,* **89,** 196–208.

Vigersky, R. A. (Ed.). (1977). "Anorexia Nervosa." Raven, New York.

Vigersky, R. A., and Loriaux, D. L. (1977). The effect of cyproheptadine in anorexia nervosa: A double-blind trial. *In* "Anorexia Nervosa" (Ed. R. A. Vigersky), pp. 349–356. Raven New York.

Vigersky, R. A., Loriaux, D. L., Andersen, A. E., Mecklenberg, R. S., and Vaitukaitus, J. L. (1976). Delayed pituitary hormone response to LRF and TRF in patients with anorexia nervosa and with secondary amenorrhoea associated with simple weight loss. *Journal of Clinical Endocrinology and Metabolism,* **43,** 893–906.

Wagner, E. E., and Wagner, C. F. (1978). Similar Rorschach patterning in three cases of anorexia nervosa. *Journal of Personality Assessment,* **42,** 426–432.

Wakeling, A., De Souza, V. F. A., and Beardwood, C. J. (1977). Assessment of the negative and positive feedback effects of administered oestrogen on gonadotrophin release in patients with anorexia nervosa. *Psychological Medicine,* **7,** 397–405.

Wakeling, A., De Souza, V. F. A., Gore, M. B. R., Sabur, M., and Kingstone, D. (1979). Amenorrhoea, body weight and serum hormone concentrations, with particular reference to prolactin and thyroid hormones in anorexia nervosa. *Psychological Medicine,* **9,** 265–272.

Wakeling, A., Marshall, J. C., Beardwood, C. J., De Souza, V. F. A., and Russell, G. F. M. (1976). The effects of clomiphene citrate on the hypothalamic–pituitary–gonadal axis in anorexia nervosa. *Psychological Medicine,* **6,** 371–380.

Walsh, B. T. (1982). Endocrine disturbances in anorexia nervosa and depression. *Psychosomatic Medicine,* **44,** 85–91.

Walsh, B. T., Katz, J. L., Levin, J., Kream, J., Fukushima, D. K., Hellman, L. D., Weiner, H., and Zumoff, B. (1978). Adrenal activity in anorexia nervosa. *Psychosomatic Medicine,* **40,** 499–506.

Walsh, B. T., Katz, J. L., Levin, J., Kream, J., Fukushima, D. K., Weiner, H., and Zumoff, B. (1981). The production rate for cortisol declines during recovery from anorexia nervosa. *Journal of Clinical Endocrinology and Metabolism,* **53,** 203–205.

Warren, M. P., Jewelewicz, R., Dyrenfurth, I., Ans, R., Khalef, S., and Wiele,

R. L. Vande (1975). The significance of weight loss in the evolution of pituitary response to LH–RH in women with secondary amenorrhea. *Journal of Clinical Endocrinology and Metabolism,* **40,** 601–611.

Weller, R. A., and Weller, E. B. (1982). Anorexia nervosa in a patient with an infiltrating tumor of the hypothalamus. *American Journal of Psychiatry,* **139,** 824–825.

Willi, J., and Grossman, S. (1983). Epidemiology of anorexia nervosa in a defined region of Switzerland. *American Journal of Psychiatry,* **140,** 564–567.

Wingate, B. A., and Christie, M. J. (1978). Ego strength and body image in anorexia nervosa. *Journal of Psychosomatic Research,* **22,** 201–204.

Winokur, A., March, V., and Mendels, J. (1980). Primary affective disorder in relatives of patients with anorexia nervosa. *American Journal of Psychiatry,* **137,** 695–698.

Wolpe, J. (1975). Behavior therapy in anorexia nervosa and in general. *Journal of the American Medical Association,* **233,** 317–318.

Yager, J. (1982). Family issues in the pathogenesis of anorexia nervosa. *Psychosomatic Medicine,* **44,** 43–60.

Yates, A., Leehey, K., and Shisslak, C. M. (1983). Running—An analogue of anorexia? *New England Journal of Medicine,* **308,** 251–255.

Yen, S. S. C. (1977). Neuroendocrine aspects of the regulation of cyclic gonadotrophin release in women. *In* "Clinical Endocrinology" (Ed. G. M. Besser), pp. 175–196. Academic Press, New York.

Yoshikatsu, M., Yutaka, S., Shigeru, M., and Hiroo, I. (1978). Triidothyronine immunoassay using polyethylene glycol to precipitate antibody-bound hormone. *Japanese Journal of Medicine,* **17,** 15–21.

Zeeman, E. C. (1976). Catastrophe theory. *Scientific American,* **234,** 65–83.

7 Sleep and Its Disorders

J. A. C. EMPSON

Department of Psychology,
The University,
Hull, England

1 Introduction

Psychophysiological measures have been so enormously successful in the study of sleep that they are now used to define sleep states, rather than merely to describe them. Aserinsky and Kleitman (1953) first reported the regularly occurring periods of eye movements with low-voltage electroencephalography (EEG), in both infants and adults, and Berger (1961) discovered the loss of tonus in extrinsic laryngeal muscles which accompanies these episodes. These two findings formed the basis of the recording and scoring methods for humans now in use all over the world, and which have been definitively summarised by Rechtschaffen and Kales (1968).

Figure 1 shows good examples of the psychophysiology associated with relaxed wakefulness and five internationally recognised stages of sleep—four slow-wave sleep (SWS) stages, numbered 1–4, and stage REM (rapid eye movement) sleep, which is associated with dreaming.

Figure 2 illustrates the typical patterning of sleep through the night, as shown by a healthy adult. On going to sleep, all normal people start with slow-wave sleep, and do not have any REM sleep until at least 45 minutes have elapsed. There is then an alternation between slow-wave sleep and REM sleep, with REM sleep recurring about every hour and a half. The first REM sleep period is usually shorter than the subsequent ones—about 15 minutes in adults, as against later periods of about half an hour. Deep slow-wave sleep (stage 4) predominates in the first half of the night.

Both REM sleep and stage 4 sleep are "fragile" in the sense that systematic disruption of sleep can cause their replacement by light slow-wave sleep (stages 1 and 2). Dement (1960) and Agnew *et al.* (1964) have shown that both REM sleep and stage 4 sleep, respectively, can be displaced in their entirety, and that there is a specific "rebound" phenomenon on recovery nights, so that up to 50% of the REM or stage 4 sleep "lost" is made up.

Aspects of Consciousness
Volume 4. Clinical Issues

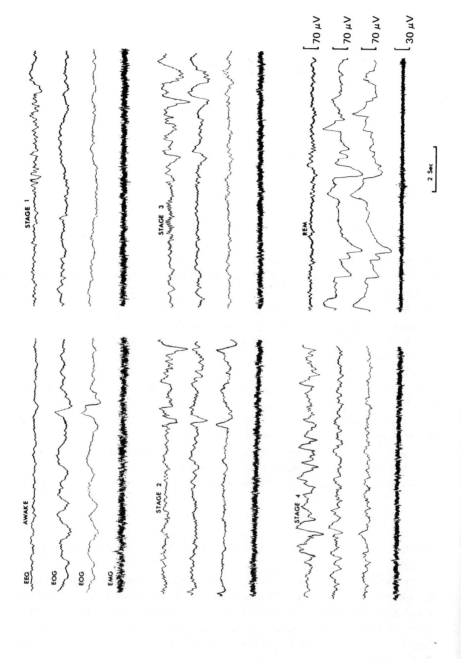

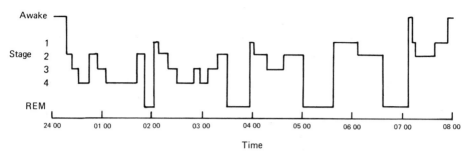

FIG. 2. A typical night's sleep for a young adult.

Table 1 shows norms for sleep parameters over a range of ages. These data have been derived from the percentages given by Williams *et al.* (1974) and are based on about 20 subjects in each age group. They confirm the general findings of previous studies based on fewer subjects (e.g., Roffwarg *et al.*, 1966; Feinberg, 1968.

The youngest subjects (3–5 year olds) slept about 10 hours, compared to the adults' 7, and the additional 3 hours were made up almost entirely of REM sleep (twice as much) and stage 4 (50% more than in adults). Theories relating sleep functions to anabolic processes and growth (Roffwarg *et al.* 1966, Oswald, 1969) have relied heavily on this evidence for increased levels of sleep being correlated with the periods of maximum growth. REM sleep quantity seems to be well correlated with brain weight increase in the early years, and Oswald (1969) hypothesised that brain protein synthesis is elevated during REM sleep. Adam (1980) has pointed out that the time required for protein synthesis is too long to allow for the completion of significant amounts during the short REM periods of some small mammals. It could be, however, that processes initiated in early phases of REM are completed in REM sleep later in the night. Recent be-

---

FIG. 1. Examples of sleep stages as defined by EEG (Channel 1), EOG (Channels 2 and 3), and submental EMG (Channel 4). Waking: EEG, low-voltage, mixed frequency, or with alpha rhythms (8–12 H$_z$). EOG, saccades and blinks predominate, even when eyes are shut; EMG, high tonic activity in neck and laryngeal muscles. Stage 1: EEG, low-voltage, mixed frequency, with some theta rhythms (3–7 Hz). Occasional vertex waves; EOG, rolling eye movements. EMG, slightly lowered tonic activity. Stage 2: EEG, K complexes and/or spindles (12–15 Hz) as phasic events. Tonic activity low voltage, mixed frequency, similar to 1; EOG, eyes still, but EEG manifestations of stage 2 normally predominate, as both K complexes and spindles occur frontally on the scalp; EMG, tonic activity maintained. Stage 3: EEG, slow waves (<2 Hz) occupy 20–50% of the record, intermixed with K complexes and spindles; EOG, dominated by EEG; EMG, tonic activity maintained. Stage 4: EEG, slow waves (< Hz) occupy over 50% of the record; EOG, dominated by slow-wave activity from the scalp; EMG, very low—can be as low as in REM sleep. REM: EEG, low voltage, mixed frequency—very similar to stage 1; EOG, phasic rapid eye movements; EMG, no tonic activity measurable.

TABLE 1
Sleep Achieved by Subjects of Different Ages[a]

Age group	Total sleep time (min/night)	Sleep latency	Sleep stages					Wakenings	Number of subjects
			1	2	3	4	REM		
3–5	594	14	12	276	18	102	186	1	21
6–9	581	12	12	280	17	99	163	1	22
10–12	560	17	17	267	23	97	153	1	24
13–15	484	16	20	230	25	83	127	3	20
16–19	451	18	18	224	27	78	101	2	23
20–29	425	14	17	205	26	60	116	2	21
30–39	424	8	22	237	26	30	108	2	20
40–49	407	9	29	278	25	13	106	4	21
50–59	410	11	25	250	21	13	93	5	23
60–69	406	13	40	243	13	8	97	6	21
70–79	393	24	41	248	14	9	92	7	21

[a]After Williams *et al.*, 1974.

havioural evidence (Empson *et al.*, 1981) suggests that the consolidation of memories during sleep relies on an orderly sequence of REM sleep periods, in that the beneficial effect of REM sleep later in the night seemed to be dependent on the uninterrupted completion of a short period of REM sleep early in the night.

Stage 4 sleep does not develop until about 6 months postpartum, but then and thereafter the quantity taken is well correlated with bodily growth in the juvenile. The nocturnal secretion of growth hormone (which stimulates protein synthesis and cell growth and repair) is actually dependent on uninterrupted stage 4 slow-wave sleep (Sassin *et al.*, 1969). In adulthood, a chronic lack of stage 4 sleep is found in sufferers from fibrositis, and the disturbance of stage 4 sleep in healthy volunteers actually causes the symptoms of fibrositis to appear (Moldofsky *et al*, 1975). All this evidence is consistent with a general anabolic function for sleep; REM sleep subserving brain growth, repair, and memory functions, and slow-wave (stage 4) sleep promoting bodily growth and repair.

Sleep is an unusually stereotyped activity, both behaviourally and physiologically. Every human being goes through the same rough pattern of electrophysiological changes almost every night of the year. Although predictably affected by age and to some extent by drugs, diet, and exercise, sleep still seems a largely autonomous process relatively impervious to the vicissitudes of life. The parallel to processes essential to metabolism, such as respiration and digestion, is obvious. The difference is that we understand the role these play in metabolism, as well as the mechanisms, or drives, regulating breathing, eating, and drinking, while the functions of sleep remain mysterious.

Comparative studies with animals have shown that all vertebrates sleep. The orthodox view of the origins of sleep has been that slow-wave sleep developed first, and paradoxical sleep (as REM sleep is called in animals) evolved in warm-blooded animals. Jouvet (1967), for instance, says "it is at least clear that in the course of evolution slow wave sleep preceded paradoxical sleep. The latter seems to be a more recent acquisition." Hennevin and Leconte (1971) say that "Paradoxical sleep does not exist in fishes, reptiles , or amphibians. . . . It has been recorded in birds (the chicken, the pigeon), but its proportion is less then 0.3% of orthodox sleep . . . except among predatory birds. . . in fact, paradoxical sleep does not appear with all its characteristics except in mammals" (my translation). This has been consistent with the idea that REM sleep is concerned with protein synthesis in the central nervous system (Oswald, 1969) or with memory processes or the elaboration of fixed, instinctive response repertoires (Jouvet, 1963, 1978) in that, obviously, mammals have much better developed nervous systems than reptiles.

Systematic comparisons of different animals with respect to sleep length, metabolic rate, life span, brain weight, and other relevant variables, made initially by Zepelin and Rechtschaffen (1974), have shown that there is a strong relationship between metabolic rate and total sleep taken over 53 mammalian species. This has been interpreted both in terms of sleep as a mechanism for reducing energy consumption, in animals with high metabolic rates, at times when activity is not essential but a certain level of reactivity of stimuli is necessary (Walker and Berger, 1980), and in terms of sleep as a period of recuperation, with high levels of metabolism demanding longer periods of sleep (Oswald, 1980). Oswald has also pointed out that long sleepers amongst humans have higher body temperatures than short sleepers (Taub and Berger, 1976), suggesting that longer sleep may be associated with higher metabolic rates even within a species.

Theorizing about the evolution of both sleep and temperature regulation is necessarily quite speculative, based mainly on considerations of habit and extrapolations from the fossil evidence relating to population parameters, for instance, in relation to homeothermy. It can be argued that REM sleep in humans is more similar to reptilian sleep than SWS, and therefore that REM sleep evolved first. This would explain the anomaly of the appearance of REM sleep before SWS in the foetus (when in embryological ontogeny normally follows phylogeny) and the loss of thermoregulation in paradoxical sleep in mammals (Heller and Glotzbach, 1977). There are problems, however, with this analysis in that birds (which show unequivocal SWS) are conventionally viewed as having evolved along with dinosaurs and pterosaurs in parallel to the evolution of mammals from a common primeval reptile. Thus, as Meddis (1983) says, "the stem reptiles ancestral to birds, mammals, turtles and crocodiles must have been pre-adapted to develop this kind of sleep pattern (SWS) under certain conditions (such as homeothermy).'' If we follow Desmond (1977) in accepting the persuasive evidence for dinosaurs having been warm-blooded animals, then perhaps this problem could be rationalised by hypothesising a common warm-blooded ancestor, showing SWS, to mammals, dinosaurs, and birds, which diverged from the reptilian stem in prehistory. It seems that in this area one man's speculation is as good as another's.

More seriously, actual evidence about the nature of modern reptilian sleep is by no means unambiguous. Most laboratory studies of the EEG of the reptile have shown few signs of slow waves in their periods of quiescence. Meglasson and Huggins (1979), however, found clear evidence of EEG slow waves in 8-month-old crocodiles who were allowed to sunbathe, and they offer the explanation that thermoregulatory behaviour (increasingly recognised as being a major determinant of the temperature of "cold-blooded" animals) may be necessary for the production of slow-wave sleep, and that this may be common to all reptiles, including the ancestral stem reptiles from which birds, mammals, dinosaurs, and modern reptiles evolved. This is a more parsimonious explanation than the ones involving either multiple stem "ancestors" or "pre-adaptations." So far as the contradictory laboratory evidence goes, as recently as 1971 it was claimed on the basis of EEG recordings that cattle did not sleep at all (Merrick and Scharp, 1971). The experimenters had wired up three steers in individual pens and not one had shown any signs of sleep for 3 days. Any cowman could have told them that cattle hate to sleep alone, and that in a herd there is always one individual awake and standing. Properly conducted experiments subsequently have shown that cattle, like all other mammals, show both REM and slow-wave sleep. It seems likely that reptiles are similarly disposed to sleep only when conditions are entirely to their liking, and, therefore, we must wait for more evidence on reptilian sleep before reaching any firm conclusions.

The suggestion that sleep is a period of enforced inactivity, reducing metabolic demands and keeping the organism out of trouble during periods of the day when other essential needs have been satisfied, has been followed up by Meddis (1977, 1983) with the suggestion that it has no other function, is an evolutionary vestige in humans, and is mediated through instinctual mechanisms. Meddis argues that sleep evolved in the same way as instincts controlling courtship and mating in birds and fish. He does not explain how these instincts no longer control mammalian behaviour in quite the same stereotyped way, while the sleep instinct does. Nor can he explain why every known mammal shows the same patterning of sleep (despite large variations in the total quantity taken). Preventing the expression of some instincts (such as by crowding chickens in small cages) does not result in death, but may produce faster growth and egg laying. Interfering with sleep, however, is a much more serious matter.

Direct experiment has shown that animals entirely deprived of food for twenty days, and which have then lost more than half their weight, may yet escape death if fed with precaution—that is to say, in small amounts often repeated. On the other hand, I found by experimenting on ten puppies that the complete deprivation of sleep for four or five days (96 to 120 hours) causes irreparable lesions in the organism, and in spite of every care the subjects of these experiments could not be saved. Complete absence of sleep during this period is fatal to puppies in spite of the food taken during this time, and the younger the puppy the more quickly he succumbed. Manaceine (1897)

This work was subsequently confirmed by Kleitman (1927) using 12 puppies deprived of sleep from 2 to 7 days. Unlike Manaceine, Kleitman gives full details of the methods he used to enforce wakefulness, stressing the importance he attached to avoiding any physical damage being inflicted on his dogs. A slight pull on the chain and a short walk would result in wakefulness persisting for some time. Control puppies (allowed ad-lib sleep) were introduced to play with the experimental puppies, and this often banished somnolence entirely. Despite this relatively gentle regime, two of the puppies died, and all showed a marked drop in red blood cells (apart from obvious signs of sleepiness, photophobia, and some viciousness).

Meddis argues that the amount of sleep taken by different species of mammal is related to life-style rather than phylogeny. However, it could be put slightly differently, that *despite* enormous differences in life-style, *all* mammals have to find time for a minimum amount of sleep. Thus, the porpoise has evolved a system of sleeping with the two sides of the brain alternately (Mukhametov and Poliakova, 1981). If there were no other evidence for the absolute necessity of sleep, this would be eloquent enough.

Clearly, therefore, sleep has acquired an essential role in physiology, whatever the evolutionary pressures which led to its appearance in primeval reptiles. There is, however, no physiological process that can be identified that is unique to sleep, so whatever essential role sleep has must be in the interaction of known existing proceses, or their coordination. As Oswald (1980) has pointed out, the hormone patterns during wakefulness promote catabolism, while sleep seems necessary for the pattern promoting anabolic processes at night. The impulse to ascribe a functional role to sleep will obviously not be satisfied until we have a clearer understanding of the interactions of the slow neurophysiological swings which punctuate our circadian cycle. The contention that sleep serves no function at all has only been useful insofar as it has forced us critically to examine our preconceptions and assumptions about the role of sleep.

2 Insomnia and the Sleeping Pill Habit

Sleep disturbance is extremely common. Bixler *et al.* (1979), in a survey of over 1000 households in Los Angeles, found 38% of their adult respondents complaining of some sleep disorder. As in a British survey of comparable size

(McGhie and Russell, 1962), dissatisfaction with sleep increased with age, especially among women. Bixler *et al.* also considered the general and mental health correlates of sleep disorder and found that over 50% of people complaining of insomnia had other recurring health problems. They were also significantly more likely to complain of tension, loneliness, depression, and the need for help with emotional problems, but were not more likely than others to have made any use of mental health facilities. The general picture is thus of sleep disturbance being related to unhappiness, anxiety, and poor health, but not necessarily mental instability.

Assessment of the prevalence of use of hypnotics in the general population in Great Britain relies on statistics for the number of prescriptions for various preparations and on a certain amount of guesswork—firstly as to the purpose for which the tablets were prescribed, and secondly as to the proportion actually ingested. At the time of McGhie and Russell's survey in Dundee and Glasgow (1961) the sedatives normally prescribed were barbiturates, and their respondents reported increasing dependence on them with age, especially among women, so that over 25% of women aged 45 and over were in the habit of taking a sedative, while only about 15% of 45-year-old men did so. Recent estimates of consumption levels (e.g., Williams, 1983) reflect a very marked change in prescribing habits over the past 20 years—of 14 million prescriptions for hypnotics in 1960, all were for barbiturates, while in 1973 the proportion of nonbarbiturate hypnotics prescribed had increased to almost half the total, and by 1978 the barbiturate prescriptions were less than half. A continuing survey of the prescribing habits of all 859 doctors who entered general practice in the year 1969/1970 clearly shows that by 1976 barbiturates were prescribed essentially only to patients who had become dependent on them, by these recently qualified GPs, and practically all new prescriptions for hypnotics are of the nonbarbiturate variety (Birmingham Research Unit, 1978).

Patterns of prescribing of particular preparations can also be gauged from a survey of the medical response of five GPs at the Aldermoor Health Centre, attached to the Southampton University Medical School, to 250 patients presenting with "insomnia" (Freeman, 1978). Only four prescriptions for barbiturates were given, and the most popular drugs were nitrazepam (Mogadon), diazepam (Valium), and other benzodiazepines. However, almost half the prescriptions for the under-14-year-old patients were for antihistamines, and almost a third of those for the over-65-year-old patients were for chlormethiazole, a powerful barbituratelike sedative. (It is known that some milder drugs such as nitrazepam can cause confusion and dementia in the elderly, so these rather potent sedatives represent the lesser of two evils for these patients.) Chloral derivatives and antidepressants were also given quite often, the former mainly to patients under 14.

No definable class of pharmacological preparations can therefore be classed as

TABLE 2

Estimates of Frequency of Prescription of Classes
of Benzodiazepine in Britain[a]

	Benzodiazepines: millions of prescriptions		
Year	Marketed as hypnotics: nitrazepam flurazepam temazepam triazolam[b]	Marketed as anxiolytics	
		Diazepam[c]	Others[d]
1975	9.8	10.9	5.9
1977	11.7	11.2	6.8
1979	13.4	10.5	7.0
1981	13.8	8.0	7.6

[a]Based on a sample of 1 in 200 prescriptions in England and Wales and 1 in 100 in Scotland—dispensed in contracting chemist's establishments (including drug stores) and by appliance contractors. Data supplied by DHSS Statistical and Research Division.
[b]E.g., Mogadon, Dalmane, Cerepax, Halcion.
[c]E.g., Valium, Tensium, Evacalm, Atensine.
[d]E.g., Librium, Tranzene, Ativan.

"hypnotics" anymore, since doctors obviously attempt to match prescriptions to patients' specific symptoms and to make use of a wide variety of drugs. Data for the number of prescriptions of particular classes of preparation (such as those presented in Table 2) must be interpreted with some caution. Over the past 5 years the number of prescriptions for benzodiazepines has stabilized at about 30 million, for Great Britain, with about 13 million being accounted for by those marketed as hypnotics. An unknown number of the remaining 17 million "anxiolytics" will have been prescribed as hypnotics, and, of course, the use that patients make of these drugs is also obscure.

It thus seems that official statistics on prescribing levels cannot provide more than a very rough guide to the prevalence of people taking "sleeping pills." A survey of psychotropic drug consumption in the general population carried out in 1977 (Murray *et al.*, 1981) found that only 11% of adults had taken "sedatives" in a 2-week period, the same percentage as that found 8 years previously by Dunnell and Cartwright (1972), despite a large increase over the same period in the number of prescriptions. Cartwright (1980) suggests that there has been a decline in the proportion of patients taking the drugs prescribed to them, and also the development of a degree of skepticism of medical authority between 1969 and 1977, so that patients now take drugs as they feel the need for them, rather than as the doctor ordered. Despite the lower than expected levels of consumption, however, Murray *et al.*'s survey confirmed previous British and American evidence (McGhie and Russell, 1962; Bixler *et al.*, 1979) that women are very much more likely than men to take hypnotics, and that this difference increases with age. Interestingly, the proportion of women taking other psychotropic drugs actually decreased with age.

3 The Sleep of Insomniacs

Electrophysiological studies of the sleep of insomniacs—that is, of people who complain of sleeping badly—have consistently shown that self-report of sleep quality does not predict quantity or quality of sleep as assessed in the laboratory at all well. Most people overestimate the time it takes to get to sleep (Lewis, 1969). Insomniacs tend to have longer latencies to sleep onset and do achieve less overall sleep than normal controls (Monroe, 1967; Karacan *et al.*, 1971).

However, their complaints of lack of sleep or of failure to get to sleep may often seem out of proportion to the psychophysiological evidence, and some insomniacs will even report wakefulness when roused from slow-wave sleep (Rechtschaffen and Monroe, 1969). Recent work (Hauri and Olmstead, 1983) has shown that the best estimate of an insomniac's definition of sleep onset is the beginning of the first 15 minutes of uninterrupted stage 2 sleep, rather than stage 2 sleep onset per se, which they confirmed as being the best estimate of subjective sleep onset in normals. Insomniacs, therefore, not only suffer less or worse sleep than normals, but their perception of it exacerbates the problem. Some people demanding sedatives may not be deprived of sleep at all, but only of the experience of unconsciousness. Many "normals" have less sleep than most "insomniacs," without complaint. Gaillard (1975) expressed this fourfold typology very neatly in a diagram (See Fig.3).

4 Disorders of Initiating Sleep

Almost half of the people in Bixler's survey who reported insomnia had difficulty in falling asleep. Normal levels of anxiety and stress do not seem to have any simple effect on sleep latency in the laboratory (Haynes *et al.*, 1981; Freedman and Sattler, 1982). Rosa *et al.* (1983), in a study of subjects selected for the presence of anxiety, found them to sleep slightly less, more lightly, and with fewer wakenings than a control group. Sleep latency was unaffected. Priest (1978) suggests that strong emotions of resentment or anger will more commonly prevent sleep, and that in persistent cases attention should be directed at sources of conflict, rather than any resulting sleep problems. Obviously, very high levels of anxiety or worry can also prevent sleep, and sleep always suffers during

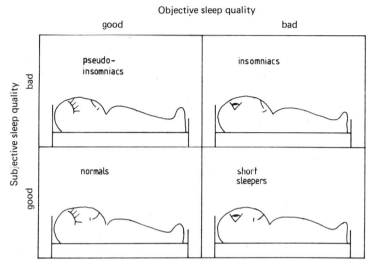

FIG. 3. Types of sleepers. Satisfaction with sleep need not correlate well with objectively determined sleep quality. (From Gaillard, 1975.)

psychiatric crises, but the relationship between sleep and arousal is not simple, and can be paradoxical. Oswald (1959) pointed out how bodily restraints and rhythmic stimulation can induce "animal hypnosis" in a variety of species, and that this was known to be accompanied by EEG signs of sleep. His own experiments on human volunteers confirmed that sleep could be induced in conditions that could otherwise be described only as highly arousing. All this is consistent with the Pavlovian notion that impossible tasks or very disagreeable conditions can result in "inhibitory experimental neuroses"—including withdrawl and sleep. A similar explanation, applied to infantile sleep behaviour by Harry Stack Sullivan, is that of the "dynamism of somnolent detachment."

A recent, and most helpful, interpretation of the aetiology of sleep onset insomnia has been Weitzman's suggestion that it is caused by a disturbance of biological rhythm. The cure proposed for patients with a chronic inability to fall asleep at a particular clock time ("chronotherapy") is to reset their circadian rhythms with a progressive phase delay of bedtime by 3 hours each week until the desired bedtime is arrived at (Weitzman, 1981).

5 Disorders of Maintaining Sleep

Almost three-quarters of Bixler *et al.*'s insomniacs reported difficulty in staying asleep, and just under half reported early wakening. These two symptoms both increased in frequency with age, especially the latter. Wakenings and arousals to light stage 1 sleep typically occur at the end of REM sleep periods in normals (Langford *et al.*, 1972) but are not usually remembered because they are brief. Persistent maintenance insomnia is commonly associated with affective illness, drug or alcohol abuse, respiratory impairments, or periodic movements during sleep. Lightened sleep and relatively early wakenings are normal features of old age and are not normally associated with daytime sleepiness.

Both monopolar and bipolar affective disorders are associated with shortened REM latency (time between sleep onset and the first REM sleep period) and reduced stages 3 and 4. Monopolar depression is also associated with reduced sleep, repeated wakenings, and early arousal (Kupfer, 1976; Gillin *et al.*, 1979). The classic relationships between endogenous depression and early wakening, and exogenous depression with failure to initiate sleep, have never been confirmed, despite the fact that these considerations have presumably been taken into account whenever these sorts of diagnoses have been made (Costello and Selby, 1965; Mendels and Hawkins, 1967). Monoamine oxidase inhibitors actually abolish REM sleep as they take effect on the patient's mood, and it has even been proposed (Dunleavy and Oswald, 1973; Vogel *et al.*, 1975) that it is the deprivation of REM sleep that brings the therapeutic effect. The tricyclic antidepressants depress REM sleep, but adaptation occurs over a few nights, and REM returns to normal levels.

A minority of patients complaining of insomnia actually suffer from "alpha–delta" sleep (Hauri and Hawkins, 1973) in which the EEG patterns of wakefulness (the 10-Hz alpha rhythm) persist during slow-wave sleep, and the 12- to 15-Hz spindling of stage 2 sleep is superimposed on the low-voltage mixed frequency EEG of stage REM sleep. These patients report not having slept at all, and feel that they derive little benefit from sleep, although they regularly sleep uninterruptedly for 6 hours or more.

Alcoholics drying out and suffering from delirium tremens will have fitful sleep, with 50–100% REM hallucinatory dreams, for 6 to 8 days (Allen *et al* 1971). Disturbances of sleep will continue for up to 6 months after the first "good night's sleep," however, with delayed sleep onset and multiple wakenings through the night. Essentially similar symptoms result from withdrawal from the barbiturates (Oswald and Priest, 1965). Kales *et al.* (1969) have argued that tolerance to central nervous system (CNS) depressants produces a syndrome of its own—drug dependency insomnia—and any beneficial sleep-inducing properties of, for instance, barbiturate hypnotics are lost after a few weeks of use.

Drugs taken initially to deal with transient sleep problems (such as sleep onset insomnia caused by some life crisis) can thus become the mainstay of a drug-dependent pattern of sleep.

The routine use of a measure of respiration in the nighttime assessment of the sleep of patients complaining of maintenance insomnia led Guilleminault, *et al.*

1973) to discover that the causation of insomnia in a few of them was entirely respiratory. Not only that, but this fact was unknown to them or their doctors, and, typically, they had a lengthy history of taking a variety of hypnotics which only exacerbated their problems. These people suffer from sleep apnoea, in which respiration ceases during sleep until the buildup of carbon dioxide in blood causes them to wake up gasping for air. Peripheral airway obstruction can be implicated as the primary cause in a minority of patients, and these persons can be cured entirely by surgery. No cure can be suggested at present for central sleep apnoeas, but hypnotics are obviously no help, and can gradually be withdrawn.

Lastly, maintenance insomnia may be caused by periodic movements in Ekbom's "restless legs syndrome." These occur every 20–30 seconds during slow-wave sleep, disrupting sleep onset, and causing disturbance throughout the night. There is no known cure for this condition and, as with sleep apnoea, heavy sedation is not beneficial.

6 Disorders of Arousal

Broughton (1968) has suggested that somnambulism, enuresis, and night terrors are all disorders of autonomic arousal associated with deep slow-wave sleep. Sleepwalking is fairly common. Anders and Weinstein (1972) report that 15% of all children have had at least one episode, and between 1 and 6% suffer from frequent attacks. Typically, the subject sits up in bed, or gets up, in stage 3 or 4 sleep, following some particularly large paroxysmal slow waves in the EEG (Kales *et al.*, 1966). Generally the episode lasts less than 15 minutes, and after some apparently nonpurposive, often repetitive activity the subjects either go back to sleep—often in their own beds—or wake up. There is anecdotal evidence that this disorder runs in families. A student who consulted me about problems caused by sleepwalking in her hall of residence, for instance, revealed that the whole of her family had once awakened in the early hours of the morning seated around the kitchen table where they had all happened to congregate in their sleep. Anders and Weinstein (1972) suggest that enuresis, night terrors, as well as somnambulism, may be genetically associated.

Enuresis is, of course, invariable in babies. "Primary" enuresis is defined as the persistence of bed-wetting into childhood and "secondary" enuresis as its reappearance after a period of successful bladder continence. Broughton (1968) estimates that 10–15% of "nervous" children and 30% of institutionalized children wet their beds and cites evidence indicating that 1% of U.S. naval recruits are enuretic (despite screening for this amongst other disorders), as are 24% of naval recruits discharged on psychiatric grounds. Anders and Weinstein (1972) confirm, as these figures would suggest, that enuresis is associated with emotional stress, and often reappears as late as adolescence. Enuresis typically occurs after a period of deep slow-wave sleep (Broughton, 1968) and is preceded by an increasingly strong series of bladder contractions (which could also be stimulated by clicks, handclaps, or other noises) quite unlike the pattern of bladder pressures recorded in normal controls. These excessive bladder contractions did not always result in bed-wetting, but invariably preceded those episodes that were recorded, which also always occurred during slow-wave arousals.

Nightmares should be distinguished from night terrors, in that they consist of a frightening dream concerning some anxiety-laden topic and normally occur during REM sleep. Waking up from an anxiety nightmare of this sort can be just as frightening as from a night terror, with the difference that reassurance is possible, as the fear is caused by the subject matter and plot of the dream. With night terrors it seems that the fear comes first, with no "supporting" dream scenario. Typically, a child wakes its parents with an ear-splitting scream, and remains inconsolably terrified for 10 or 15 minutes before falling back again into a deep sleep. Next morning only the parents can remember the incident. Adults can also suffer from night terrors, although less commonly and less spectacularly.

Another related disorder of arousal is sleep paralysis, in which the flaccid paralysis of REM sleep intrudes into wakefulness. Attacks last up to 10 minutes, and can occur at sleep onset or during the night's sleep at the end of a REM period. Sleep paralysis can in itself be very frightening especially if accompanied by hallucinations or preceded by a nightmare. The idea of pressure on the chest, of immobility, implied in the notions of *incubus* and *cauchemar* , which signify being lain upon, and pressing down upon, respectively, must surely refer to sleep paralysis rather than the other two varieties of nightmare. It is, of course, very common indeed in patients suffering from narcolepsy (one of the symptoms associated with this disorder) but is also relatively common in normal adolescence. Goode (1962) found that 5% of a sample of medical and nursing students reported sleep paralysis as having occurred at least once in the past year. People who regularly suffer from attacks may gain some "lucidity," so that they recognise what is happening to them and wait for the resumption of control over their bodies in relative tranquility (Hishikawa, 1976).

7 The Hypersomnias

Excessive daytime sleepiness can simply be caused by the lack of sleep at night, caused, for example, by sleep apnoea. Most patients studied by Guilleminault *et al.* suffering from sleep apnoea indeed complained of sleepiness during the day.

Narcolepsy itself is characterised by a tetrad of symptoms—sleep attacks and daytime somnolence, cataplexy, hypnagogic hallucinations, and sleep paralysis. The sleep of narcoleptics is essentially normal, with the important difference that they can typically go straight from wakefulness to REM sleep (Rechtschaffen *et al.*, 1963). The tendency to do this is more marked in subjects who also complain of cataplexy, and is common to daytime sleep attacks and nighttime sleep onset.

Cataplexy is an extreme form of the helplessness that can be induced in anybody laughing hilariously, or being "tickled to death." Any extreme of emotion causes narcoleptics to fall down with flaccid paralysis of all muscles except the respiratory and extraocular ones, just as in REM sleep. Hypnagogic hallucinations, and visual and auditory images that many people experience with the onset of sleep, are always reported by narcoleptics. Sleep paralysis, as noted above, is common in adolescence, but persists throughout life in patients suffering from narcolepsy, and is a wakening in which the flaccid paralysis of REM sleep is maintained.

8 The Effects of Hypnotic Drugs

The dramatic change in prescribing habits in hypnotics in the late 1960s was due not only to the toxicity of the barbiturates and the availability of acceptable alternatives, but also to advances in understanding of their precise effects on sleep, and their addictiveness. Oswald and Priest (1965) showed that barbiturates reduce the amount of REM sleep when first taken, like many other drugs. As tolerance develops over a few days, the level of REM sleep returns to normal, but on withdrawal the habitual barbiturate user will experience vivid dreams and nightmares, with frequent nighttime wakenings caused by a massive REM sleep rebound with double the usual amount of REM sleep lasting for 5 or 6 weeks.

Chlordiazepoxide (a benzodiazepine) increases the time spent asleep without reducing REM sleep (Hartmann, 1968). It has also been found to reduce the amount of deep slow-wave sleep (stage 4), and over long periods there is evidence that REM sleep may be reduced (Hartmann, 1976), although after a month of drugged sleep no strong evidence of REM rebound could be found in a recovery month.

Chloral hydrate, like the barbiturates, suppresses REM sleep initially, and causes a massive rebound on withdrawl (Hartmann, 1976). It is, however, rapidly metabolised, unlike either the benzodiazepines or barbiturates, whose half-lives in the body are between 14 and 30 hours.

Amitriptyline is an antidepressant frequently prescribed to patients presenting with sleep problems. It has been shown to slightly increase total sleep time, to reduce REM sleep time with no adaptation over a 30-day period, and to cause a relatively short-lived REM sleep rebound on withdrawl (Hartmann, 1976).

Most hypnotics have a long half-life in blood, so that their effects are not confined to the night, if taken in the evening. Walters and Lader (1971) have shown that both a benzodiazepine and a barbiturate can depress performance on simple psychomotor tasks on the day following administration, not surprisingly, perhaps, in the case of the barbiturate, but somewhat unexpectedly in the benzodiazepine, which is supposed to tranquillise without sedating.

9 Sleep Disorder Clinics

It has already been pointed out that people are not very accurate in their recollections of wakenings during the nights, or the delay to sleep onset, or of whether they were asleep (according to EEG criteria) or awake. Even the most conscientious physician is therefore at a disadvantage when attempting to make a diagnosis of primary insomnia on the basis of a patient's self-report.

In the United States a number of sleep disorder clinics have been founded, offering routine polysomnographic assessment, and their collective experience has been summarised in a systematic classification of sleep disorders (Association of Sleep Disorders Centers, 1979). Ancoli-Israel *et al.* (1981) report on the effects of referral to such a clinic of 170 consecutive patients. One hundred seventeen of them were deemed to require polysomnographic assessment. Fifty-one of these were found to have sleep apnoea, which was obstructive in origin in 37. Patients with apnoea were significantly older than those without (51.6 years compared to 41.5) and a good number of them were obese. Nine were treated with tracheostomy, which was successful in eight of them. Eight patients were admitted and treated with a strict reducing diet, and three of the four who did achieve normal weights had fewer apnoeic attacks. The seriousness of this condition is demonstrated by the fact that two of these patients died in their sleep, one of them at the age of 47 with no other medically recognised disease. Twelve patients assessed in the clinic suffered from uncomplicated nocturnal myoclonus (Ekbom's syndrome). Twenty-nine other patients were given specific diagnoses of sleep disorders related to depression, drug abuse, organic brain disease, or factitious complaints.

In summing up the benefits of the clinic, Ancoli-Israel *et al.* stress the importance of discouraging unnecessary referrals, and limiting polysomnography to those patients "for whom a clinical indication is strong," and ascribe their success in achieving specific diagnoses in 90% of the patients recorded to this selectivity. Several of the patients suffering from sleep apnoeas or narcolepsy were able to resume work, with treatment appropriate to their conditions. None of the patients actually given treatments died in the course of the study, while five of the untreated patients died. It is clear that a few patients can benefit enormously from this sort of assessment, and after a lifetime of taking inappropriate but highly potent drugs can at last be given some real relief from their symptoms.

Rather mysteriously, the incidence of sleep apnoea in the United Kingdom is extremely low (Shapiro *et al.*, 1981). Since it is only in the apnoeic syndromes that polysomnographic evidence is crucial in making a diagnosis, this could be taken as an argument for not pursuing this sort of assessment, which is both costly and laborious. However, in view of the prevalence of the suffering caused by sleep disorders, and the widespread use of hypnotics, it could be argued that some relatively inexpensive system of recording EEG, electrocardiogram, electromyogram, and respiration at home would improve both the accuracy of diagnosis and the suitability of prescribing in those patients who seem to be chronically in need of sedatives. This could be a service provided by psychologists attached to group practices or health centres. A postal survey of all the general practioners in the Hull area in 1979 showed there was firm support for a proposed service like this amongst a sizable majority of the respondents, and that a referral rate of three or four patients per year could be expected from each of these doctors.

Enough is now known about the aetiology of sleep disorders to show that the palliatives offered in the past have been ineffective, and in some cases positively harmful. While there have certainly been great pharmacological improvements, in that modern sedatives are rarely lethal in overdose and are nonaddictive, relatively little has been done to develop polysomnography and provide ordinary clinicans with understandable information about the sleep of their patients.

Acknowledgement

I would like to thank Ray Meddis for carefully reading an early draft of this chapter and for being very helpful with the section on sleep functions.

References

Adam, K. (1980). Sleep as a restorative process and a theory to explain why. *Progress in Brain Research,* **53,** 289–306.

Agnew, H., Webb, W. and Williams, R. (1964). The effect of stage four sleep deprivation. *EEG Journal,* **17,** 68–70.

Allen, R. P., Wagman, A., Faillace, L. A., and McIntosh, M. (1971). EEG sleep recovery following prolonged alcohol intoxication in alcoholics. *Journal of Nervous and Mental Disease,* **152,** 424–433.

Ancoli-Israel, S., Kripke, D. F., Menn, S. J. and Messin, S. (1981). Benefits of a sleep disorders clinic in a veterans administration medical center. *Western Journal of Medicine,* 14–18.

Anders, T. F., and Weinstein, P. (1972). Sleep and its disorders in infants and children—in a review. *Pediatrics,* **50,** 312–324.

Aserinsky, E., and Kleitman, N. (1953). Regularly occurring periods of eye motility, and concomitant phenomena, during sleep. *Science,* **118,** 273–274.

Association of Sleep Disorders Centers, (1979). Diagnostic classification of sleep and arousal disorders. *Sleep,* **2,** 1–137.

Berger, R. J. (1961). Tonus of extrinsic laryngeal muscles during sleep and dreaming. *Science,* **134,** 840.

Birmingham Research Unit of the Royal College of General Practitioners (1978). Practice activity analysis 4. Psychotropic drugs. *Journal Royal College of General Practice,* **28,** 122–124.

Bixler, E. O., Kales, A., Soldatos, C. R., Kales, J. D., and Healey, S. (1979) Prevalence of sleep disorders in the Los Angeles metropolitan area. *American Journal of Psychiatry,* **136,** 1257–1262.

Broughton, R. J. (1968). Sleep disorders: Disorders of arousal? *Science,* **159,** 1070–1078.

Cartwright, A. (1980). Prescribing and the patient–doctor relationship. *In* "Essays on Doctor–Patient Communication" (Ed. J. Hasler, and D. Pendleton. Academic Press, London.

Costello, C. G., and Selby, M. M. (1965) The relationship between sleep patterns and reactive and endogenous depressions. *British Journal of Psychiatry,* **111,** 497–501.

Dement, W. C. (1960). The effect of dream deprivation. *Science,* **131,** 1705–1707.

Desmond, A. J. (1977). "The Hot-Blooded Dinosaurs." Futra, London.

Dunleavy, D. L. F., and Oswald, I. (1973). Phenelzine, mood response and sleep. *Archives of General Psychiatry,* **28,** 353-356.

Dunnell, K., and Cartwright, A. (1972). "Medicine Takers, Prescribers and Hoarders." Routledge and Kegan Paul, London.

Empson, J. A. C., Hearne, K. M. T., and Tilley, A. J. (1981). REM sleep and reminiscence. *In* "Sleep 1980: Circadian Rhythms, Dreams, Noise and Sleep, Neurophysiology, Therapy" (Ed. W. P. Koella). Karger, Basel.

Feinberg, I. (1968). The ontogenesis of human sleep and the relationship of sleep variables to intellectual function in the aged. *Compr. Psychiatr.* **9,** 138–147.

Freeman, R. R., and Sattler, H. L. (1982). Physiological and psychological factors in sleep-onset insomnia. *Journal of Abnormal Psycholgy,* **91,** 380–389.

Freeman, G. K. (1978). Analysis of primary care prescribing—a 'constructive' coding system for drugs. *Journal Royal College of General Practitioners,* **28,** 547–551.

Gaillard, J-M. (1975). Temporal organization of sleep stages in man. Paper presented at the 2nd International Sleep Research Congress, Edinburgh, Scotland.

Gillin, J. C., Duncan, W., Pettigrew, K. D., Frankel, B. L., and Snyder, F. (1979). Successful separation of depressed, normal and insomniac subjects by EEG sleep data. *Archives of General Psychiatry,* **36,** 85–90.

Goode, G. B. (1962). Sleep paralysis. *Archives of Neurology,* **6,** 228–234.

Guilleminault, C., Eldridge, F. L., and Dement, W. C. (1973). Insomnia with sleep apnea: A new syndrome. *Science,* **181,** 856–858.

Hartmann, E., (1976). Long-term administration of psychotropic drugs: effects on human sleep. *In* "Pharmacology of Sleep," (Eds. R. L. Williams, and I. Karacan), pp. 211–223. Wiley, New York.

Hauri, P., and Olmstead, E. (1983). What is the moment of sleep onset for insomniacs? *Sleep,* **6,** 10–15.

Hauri, P., and Hawkins, D. R. (1973). Alpha–delta sleep. *EEG Journal,* **34,** 233–237.

Haynes, S. N., Adams, A., and Franzen, M. (1981). The effects of presleep stress on sleep-onset insomnia. *Journal of Abnormal Psychology,* **90,** 601–606.

Heller, H. C. and Glotzbach, S. F. (1977). Thermo-regulation during sleep and hibernation. Environmental Physiology II. *International Review of Physiology,* **15,** 147–188.

Hennevin, E. and Leconte, P. (1971). La fonction du sommeil paradoxal. *L'Annee Psychologique,* **71,** 489–519.

Hishikawa, Y. (1976). Sleep paralysis. *In* "Narcolepsy" (Eds. C. Guilleminault, W. C. Dement, and P. Passouant), pp. 97–124. Spectrum, New York.

Jouvet, M. (1963). The rhombencephalic phase of sleep. *Progress in Brain Research,* **1,** 406–424.

Jouvet, M. (1967). Neurophysiology of the states of sleep. *Physiology Review,* **47,** 117–177.

Jouvet, M. (1978). Does a genetic programming of the brain occur during paradoxical sleep? *In* "Cerebral Correlates of Conscious Behavior"(Eds. P. Buser, and A. Buser-Rougeul), pp. 245-261. Elsevier/North Holland.

Kales, A., Jacobson, A., Paulson, M J., Kales, J. D., and Walter, R. D. (1966). Somnambulism: psychophysiological correlates. *Achives of General Psychiatry,* **14,** 586–594.

Kales, A., Malmstrom, E. J., Scharf, M. B., and Rubin, R. J. (1969). Psychophysiological and biochemical changes following use and withdrawl of hypnotics. *In* "Sleep Physiology and Pathology" (Ed. A. Kales), pp. 331–343. Lippincott, New York.

Karacan, I. *et al.* (1971). New approaches to the evaluation and treatment of insomnia. *Psychosomatics,* **12,** 81–88.

Kleitman, N. (1927). Studies on the physiology of sleep. V. Some experiments on puppies. *American Journal of Physiology,* **84,** 386–395.

Kupfer, D. J. (1976). REM latency: A psychobiologic marker for primary depressive disease. *Biological Psychiatry,* **11,** 159.

Langford, G. W., Meddis, R. and Pearson, A. J. D. (1972). Spontaneous arousals from sleep in human subjects. *Psychonom. Sci.,* **28,** 228–230.

Lewis, S. A. (1969). Subjective estimates of sleep: An EEG evaluation. *British Journal of Psychology,* **60,** 203–208.

McGhie, A., and Russell, S. M. (1962) . The subjective assessment of normal sleep patterns. *Journal of Mental Science,* **8,** 642–654.

Manaceine, M. de (1897). ''Sleep: Its Physiology, Pathology, Hygiene and Psychology.'' Scott, London.

Meddis, R. (1977). ''The Sleep Instinct.'' Routledge and Kegan Paul, London.

Meddis, R. (1983). The evolution of sleep. *In* ''Sleep in Animals and Man ''(Ed. A. Mayes). Van Nostrand Reinhold, London.

Meglasson, M. D., and Huggins, S. E. (1979). Sleep in a crocodilian, *Caiman sclerops. Comparative Biochemistry and Physiology,* **63A,** 561–567.

Mendels, J. and Hawkins, D. R. (1967). Sleep and depression. *Archives of General Psychiatry,* **16,** 344–354.

Merrick, A. W., and Scharp, D. W. (1971). Electroencephalography of resting behavior in cattle, with observations on the question of sleep. *American Journal of Veterinary Research,* **32,** 1893–1897.

Moldovsky, H., Scarisbrick, P., England, R., and Smythe, H. (1975). Musculoskeletal symptoms and non-REM sleep disturbance in patients with ''fibrositis syndrome'' and healthy subjects. *Psychsomatic Medicine,* **37,** 341–351.

Monroe, L. J. (1967). Psychological and physiological differences between good and bad sleepers. *Journal of Abnormal Psychology,* **72,** 255–264.

Mukhametov, L. M. and Poliakov, I. G. (1981). EEG investigations of the sleep of porpoises, *Phocoena phocoena. Zhurnal Vysshei Nervnoi Deyatel'nosti,* **31,** 333–339.

Murray, J., Gunn, G., Williams, P., and Tarnopolsky, A. (1981). Factors affecting the consumption of psychotropic drugs. *Psychology Medicine,* **11,** 551–560.

Oswald, I. (1959). Experimental studies of rhythm, anxiety and cerebral vigilance. *Journal of Mental Science,* **105,** 269–294.

Oswald, I. (1969). Human brain protein, drugs and dreams. *Nature,* **223,** 893–897.

Oswald, I. (1980). Sleep as a restorative process: Human clues. *Progress in Brain Research,* **53,** 279–288.

Oswald, I., and Priest, R. G. (1965). Five weeks to escape the sleeping-pill habit. British Medical Journal, **2,** 1093–1099.

Priest, R. G. (1978). Sleep and its disorders. *In* ''Current Themes in Psychiatry'' (Eds. R.N. Gaind, and B.L. Hudson), pp. 83–93. Macmillan: London.

Rechtschaffen, A., and Kales, A. (Eds). (1968). "A Manual of Standardized Terminology, Techniques and Scoring System for Sleep Stages of Human Subjects." Public Health Service, U.S. Govt Printing Office, Washington, D.C.

Rechtschaffen, A., *et al.* (1963) Nocturnal sleep of narcoleptics. *EEG Journal,* **15,** 599–609.

Roffwarg, H., Muzio, J., and Dement, W. C. (1966). Ontogenetic development of the human sleep-dream cycle. *Science,* **152,** 604–619.

Rosa, R. R., Bonnet, M. H., and Kramer, M. (1983). The relationship of sleep and anxiety in anxious subjects. *Biological Psychology,* **16,** 119–126.

Sassin, J. F., *et al.* (1969). Effects of slow wave sleep deprivation on human growth hormone release in sleep: Preliminary study. *Life Science,* **8,** 1299–1307.

Shapiro, C. M., Catteral, J. R., Oswald, I., and Flenley, D. C. (1981). Where are the British sleep apnea patients? *Lancet,* **2**(8245), 523.

Taub, J. N., and Berger, R. J. (1976). Effects of acute sleep pattern alteration depend on sleep duration. *Physiology and Psychology,* **4,** 412–420.

Vogel, G. W. *et al.* (1975). REM sleep reduction effects on depression syndromes. *Archives of General Psychiatry.* **32,** 765–780.

Walker, J. N., and Berger, R. J. (1980). Sleep as an adaptation for energy conservation functionally related to hibernation and shallow torpor. *Progress in Brain Research,* **53,** 255–278.

Walters, A. J., and Lader, M. H. (1971). Hangover effects of hypnotics in man. *Nature,* **229,** 637–638.

Weitzman, E. D. (1981). Sleep and its disorders. *Annual Review of Neuroscience,* **4,** 381–417.

Williams, P. (1983). Psychotropic drug prescribing. *The Practitioner,* **227,** 77–81.

Williams, R. L., Karacan, I., and Hursch, C. J. (1974). "Electroencephalography of Human Sleep: Clinical Applications." Wiley, New York.

Zepelin, H., and Rechtschaffen, A. (1974). Mammalian sleep, longevity, and energy metabolism. *Brain Behavior and Evolution,* **10,** 425–470.

8 Consciousness and Deafness

DAVID WOOD

Department of Psychology,
Nottingham University,
Nottingham, England

1 Introduction

Two competing images of prelingually deaf people have provided the major impetus to research, argument, and educational debate. The first holds that the deaf are fundamentally similar to the hearing in their intellectual capacities. The most widely known exponent of this view is Hans Furth (1966, 1971). Working within the framework of Piagetian theory, Furth's studies explored the capacities of deaf children in tasks demanding concrete and formal operational thinking. His main conclusion is that profound, prelingual deafness does not inhibit the development of rational thinking. Although deaf people are usually delayed in the achievement of logical thought, they eventually reach the same stages of development as the hearing. Contingent upon this conclusion, within Piagetian theory, is the corollary that language is not a basis for the development of thought. As one system within the semiotic function, it is an articulation of structures developed through action in the world. Actions, and the systems of operations to which they lead, constrain all representational functions; the operative dictates the figurative.

In opposition to the notion of universals is the view that deaf people display a "special" psychology. This view is best represented in the theorising of Myklebust (1964). His wide-ranging studies of deaf subjects—including motor development, language acquisition, and thinking—led him to conclude that the absence (not simply loss) of one sensory modality influences the general course of growth and development. Deafness affects not only linguistic functioning, but also occasions an "organismic shift." The absence of sound entails the development of conceptual frameworks that are qualitatively different from those that emerge in the sensorily intact organism.

Although "consciousness" has seldom been a focus in the comparative study of deaf and hearing people, research into the development of language, thinking, and personality in the deaf is clearly relevant to a discussion of this topic. A

Aspects of Consciousness
Volume 4. Clinical Issues

useful scheme for relating research in deafness to general approaches to the study of consciousness is provided by Lunzer (1979) (Volume 1, this treatise). He proposes distinctions between three different usages of the term. Before considering research findings in detail, the major implications of Lunzer's distinctions for deafness will be explored.

2 Consciousness I

Consciousness I "includes all differential reactions" and holds that "an organism is conscious of an aspect of its environment if it reacts differentially with respect to variation within that aspect." It is the most "rudimentary" form of consciousness.

Even at this basic level one is invited to consider possible differences in the conscious experiences of the deaf and hearing. If, for example, speech is conceived of as an auditory signal alone, one composed simply of segmental and suprasegmental elements that are imperceptible to the deaf, then they can never be deemed "conscious" of spoken language. However, one can respond to this commonsense view with the observation that only a tiny minority of the deaf are completely insensitive to sound, given the highest levels of amplification available. The speech signal is also highly redundant. For example, auditory information about certain consonant clusters might occur at frequencies high in the speech range that are imperceptible to the deaf, but if these covary systematically with auditory information at lower (perceived) frequencies, the deaf person might have enough audiological stimulation to develop a model of the speech signal which is functionally equivalent to that perceived by the normally hearing person.

Even if no perfect correspondence exists between all distinctive features in the normally perceived speech signal and the distorted or attenuated version perceived by the deaf person (which is certainly the case), does some form of "top-down" processing enable "gaps" in the signal to be inferred by interpolation? That such processes occur in normally hearing people attending to speech in high noise levels, and in those who go progressively deaf after having developed language, seems certain. Whether and to what extent it is possible for the pre-lingually deaf person to develop higher order structures or rules to infer lower order constituents, when those constituents have never been heard, is a more difficult question. However, I shall argue later that this seems to be the case.

Consider too that in face-to-face interactions the auditory signal does not occur in a vacuum. Paralinguistic, nonverbal, and contextual cues are also in evidence and, plausibly, covary systematically with elements of the auditory message. Thus, lip movements, facial expression, posture, deliberate and spontaneous gesture, together with a range of contextual cues accompany acts of communication. The description of each of these dimensions is still sketchy and the interrelationships between them poorly understood. Hence, our knowledge of their potential involvement in the deaf person's attempts to understand speech remains sparse.

Such complexities, technical and conceptual, in developing an understanding of Consciousness I in the deaf are also contingent on any attempt to understand the deaf person's awareness of "sound" in general. Nonspeech sounds also covary with visual elements of experience. The movements of objects relate lawfully to the sounds they occasion. How, if at all, do the concomitants of sound enter into the conscious experience of the deaf? Is sound for the deaf, perhaps, akin to our own concept of the square root of minus 1—a "structural" concept that takes meaning and significance because of the power it gives in developing models of the world but never, itself, part of sensory or empirical experience in any concrete sense?

Whilst such issues defy any convincing resolution at present, they are amenable to empirical enquiry and theoretical formulations. In the following pages, discussions of language development and cerebral organisation in the deaf are particularly relevant.

3 Consciousness II

Lunzer, by way of an approximation, defines Consciousness II as existent "if an organism is capable of responding differentially to the same elements (perceptual cues from the environment or, alternatively, verbal or quasi-imaginal determinants in its own mentation) in different contexts and hence with different behaviours. . . [and] if different complexes of cues, often corresponding to the same definable object, elicit similar differential behaviours." Thus, the organism classifies immediate stimulation according to some system of equivalence classes or concepts. Consciousness I demands a receptive capacity that differentiates experiences, that is, "detection," whereas Consciousness II involves a capacity to abstract critical or distinctive features that transcend those aspects of stimulation attributable to transient changes in the organism–object relationship, for example, relative position or illumination.

The notion of Consciousness II raises questions about the spontaneous, "intuitive," or personal concepts developed by the deaf before self-consciousness and linguistic interactions begin to transform these into Consciousness III. How does the absence of sound dictate not only what will or will not be detected and differentiated but also how it is analysed and classified? How, if at all, is the progressive discovery of those features of the world that offer stability in the face of constant flux affected by lack of hearing?

4 Consciousness III

Consciousness III implies that "the object of cognition can be attended to by the subject and can therefore become an object for voluntary representation or for verbal communication." Unlike the organism at level of Consciousness II, who cannot "turn around on (his own) schema," the individual at level III is able to focus on, inspect, and judge the determinants of his own response.

The distinction between Consciousness II and III introduces important methodological problems in the study of deafness. Piaget, particularly in his later writings, laid considerable stress on the distinction between success and understanding in the performance of any given task. His experimental method examines not only a subject's success or failure in solving problems, but also his ability to provide rational and compelling accounts of and for his judgements. These provide the main basis for inferences about his mental abilities.

Soliciting such accounts from deaf people is often impossible. The linguistic rules demanded for comprehension and production of complex conditional clauses, for example, are simply beyond most of them. So far as I know, no one has attempted to solicit such accounts using sign language with the deaf, so the matter remains open. This issue raises fundamental questions about the relationships between cognitive abilities and the acquisition of linguistic structures. Is the failure to comprehend attributable to a lack of linguistic facility, or is the incapacity to acquire certain linguistic rules the result of a failure of the preverbal understanding that enables the function of those rules to be recognised? This issue also occupies our attention later.

5 Language and Deafness: Speaking, Reading, and Writing

In this section, I first examine some of the main findings of research into the (oral) linguistic abilities of deaf children to explore the questions raised under the heading "Consciousness I." I also try to identify some of the specific features of oral language (and I shall be talking almost entirely about English) that create particular problems for the deaf. This, in turn, leads to a brief review of research on sign language to see how far it is possible to draw parallels between the syntactic structure of sign languages and those features of spoken English that create problems for the deaf. The rationale for this undertaking is to explore the question of a "special" psychology of deafness from a linguistic perspective. To the extent that parallels can be established, it is possible to support the contention that languages acquired largely or wholly through vision (whether of signs or lipreading) of necessity display qualitatively different organisations from those acquired aurally.

Early studies of deaf children's language soon established a controversy between those, like Heider and Heider (1940), who argued that deaf children resemble younger or less mature hearing children and others, for example Fusfield (1955), who contended that the written language of deaf children constituted a "tangled web of expression in which words . . . do not align themselves in an orderly array." According to one school of thought, deaf children acquire language more slowly than the hearing but generate similar structures; for the other, deaf children develop no systematic grammar at all. Contingent on the latter view is the conclusion that the lack of access to sound leaves no systematic basis for the development of linguistic structure.

More recent research, however, enables us to reject the second of these conclusions. More sensitive and detailed systems of analysis made available by the development of Chomsky's theory of generative grammar have enabled researchers to identify systematic patterns underlying both reading and writing in deaf children (Ivimey, 1976; Wilbur and Quigley, 1975). The most extensive studies along these lines have been undertaken by Quigley and his colleagues at the University of Illinois in the United States (e.g., Quigley *et al.*, 1976a, 1976b; Quigley *et al.*, 1978; Wilbur *et al.*, 1976). This group has looked in detail at deaf children's capacities to handle several different syntactic "environments." These include question formation, negation, pronominalisation, complement structures, and various aspects of verb processes. Their studies revealed (1) that deaf children show some command of syntactic structures in English, (2) that many of their "errors" or deviations from standard English are systematic and common to the deaf population, (3) that such deviations change with age (at least up to age 18 years) and develop towards standard forms, albeit very slowly, (4) that some deviations parallel those found in the language of much younger hearing children, and (5) that other deviations do not and constitute, in Myklebust's terminology, "deafisms."

One pervasive feature of the reading and writing of deaf children is particularly significant. They tend both to read sentences and to write spontaneously as though structures in English follow the subject–verb–object rule (S–V–O) (which, of course, many do). Thus, given a sentence "The boy hit the girl," the meaning deaf children infer is almost certain to reflect the true deep structure of the sentence. However, if given the passive construction, "The girl was hit by the boy," they are likely to decide that the girl is the deep subject and the boy the object of the utterance (thus, that the girl does the hitting). This same rule is consistent with errors made in other syntactic environments.

This pattern of deviation is interesting because sign languages do not generally follow the S–V–O pattern (e.g., Brennan, 1981). Many other spoken languages also capitalise on a different ordering, thus such an ordering is arbitrary whether viewed in relation to signed or spoken languages. Here, then, is at least one aspect of the structure of deaf children's grammar that must be derived from spoken (or written) English. Whether or not deaf children are conscious of speech sounds (Consciousness I), there is evidence that they develop some basis for top-down linguistic processing, with the implications drawn out above.

One interpretation of this result, however, is that such regularities are formally taught and learned, not acquired as is usually the case (Kyle, 1981). Thus viewed, they do not represent a "natural" linguistic development. However, there is another feature of the Illinois results that is difficult to reconcile with this view. Although Quigley *et al.* do not identify this feature in their results, there is another aspect of deaf children's deviations which is both common to the earlier language of hearing children and compatible with a variety of errors that they make in almost all the syntactic environments studied. This is the "minimum distance principle" (MDP) (Chomsky, 1969; Bowerman, 1979).

In many English utterances, such as "John promised Mary to leave" two or more words may "agree" with and "compete" for another—both John and Mary are potential "leavers." If one examines the data of Quigley *et al.* with this principle in mind, then in virtually all contexts where two nouns, for example, compete for a verb in this way, children follow the MDP—that is, they alway choose the competing word which is closest to the word competed for in the surface structure. This produces systematic errors of interpretation in sentences such as "Mummy told John that she would feed the dog" and "Mary kicked the dog and ran away"—when John would be seen to feed the dog and the dog would be expected to run away from Mary. It seems unlikely that such principles are formally taught. Indeed, in our own research (which has involved some 40 or so teachers and around 300 deaf children from many schools) we have never encountered a single example of instruction along such lines. This is not to say that there are no environmental factors associated with this feature of deaf children's grammar (for example, people may not often use such complex forms in talking to deaf children), but whatever these may be, it seems unlikely that the MDP is a product of formal instruction. We are left, then, with the conclusion that this aspect of deaf children's language is acquired spontaneously from exposure to spoken or written language, and it is an aspect that parallels the deviations from English found in the language of hearing children around 5 years of age.

Quigley's group also identified several "deafisms"—errors, often systematic, produced by deaf children that are never found in the language of the hearing. However, given that the deaf child or adolescent is employing at least some of the syntactic rules evidenced in the language of much younger hearing children at a time when they are mentally more mature, the problem of identifying specific deafisms becomes complex (Wood, 1982). They may be attempting to convey much more difficult ideas than the younger hearing child while employing similar grammatical devices. This would produce utterances that are semantically more complex than the hearing child's and which, in consequence, look "odd" or are extremely difficult to comprehend.

However, there are areas of production and comprehension that do not parallel those found in hearing children's development of standard English (e.g., Ivimey, 1976). The important point, however, is the conclusion that deaf children do develop grammatical rules about spoken English which parallel those found in the hearing. I shall return to this point later.

Another way of looking at the data of Quigley and his colleagues is from a more "cognitive" orientation. Deaf children comprehend and produce language conforming to the "simple–active–affirmative–declarative" register. In English (though not in all languages) these also involve the least complex linguistic constructions. To move beyond this register—for instance, to talk about the past or future or to entertain the conditional, negative, passive, or interrogative—it is necessary to exploit additional rules. Thus, there is a clear confounding of cognitive and linguistic complexity. Within all existing developmental theories, consciousness of the here and now, the concrete and ongoing, precedes awareness of negation, the absent, past, future, hypothetical, and so on. Each of these steps demands some degree of "decontextualisation" (Bruner, 1966, Donaldson, 1978), decentration (Piaget, 1960), or "semiotic extension" (McNeill, 1979). But each, in English, also demands the acquisition of additional syntactic rules.

We may, then, view the linguistic problems of deaf children from two different points of view. We could argue that the linguistic system embodies a natural, hierarchical structure that imposes a clear path of "privilege of occurrence." Some rules must be acquired before others can be. Alternatively, one could agrue that the acquisition of such rules follows a systematic sequence imposed by relative degrees of cognitive complexity. In each case, the difficulties encountered by the deaf would follow a similar general path to that briefly outlined above.

Studies of oral language alone will not resolve this issue. But there are several other ways of exploring it. First, one might examine nonverbal cognitive functioning in the deaf to see if they can handle tasks in nonverbal form that display similar underlying structures to those failed when presented in largely verbal forms. This, of course, rests on the validity of the epistemological system used to provide structural descriptions.

If, as several linguists and psychologists believe, sign language is the "natural" language of the deaf, then any purely linguistic barrier to the articulation of cognition should disappear in children raised in signing environments. Furthermore, if linguistic reasons exist for the delay, arrest, or deviations in deaf children's language development, it might prove possible to identify processes or mechanisms underlying this phenomenon. For instance, the development of linguistic structures of increasing complexity, generally speaking, involves the use of increasing numbers of words. Negative interrogatives about past events delivered in the passive voice (e.g., "Was Mary not being hit by Peter?") are generally longer than either the passive, interrogative, past, or negative alone. If, as some research suggests, the capacity of the deaf to hold sequences of words in memory is limited in comparison to that of the hearing (e.g., Conrad, 1979), then there may be some fundamental sensory constraints acting on language development. Furthermore, if this limitation is bound up with the deaf acquiring language by eye rather than by ear, then we might establish links between differences found in patterns of information processing in audition and vision on the one hand, and specific problems in the acquisition of language on the other.

6 Consciousness of Speech

The vast majority of deaf people exhibit some degree of residual hearing. Few of them fail to respond to sound at some frequency or other (almost always in the lower speech frequencies) given substantial amplification in formal audiometric assessments. However, many severely and profoundly deaf people (with losses greater than 85–90 dB average in their better ear) do not respond to naturally occurring sounds even when wearing their hearing aids—though the reasons for this are a matter of debate. The less than perfect predictive power of methods of audiometric assessment for auditory function, coupled with a limited knowledge of speech processing, means that models of the auditory experiences of deaf people are very poor. Thus, the problem of deciding just which aspects of speech a given deaf person perceives and how he or she perceives them remains unsolved.

In this section, I shall begin with the simplifying assumption that such deaf people perceive no speech sounds, qualifying this later in the face of contradictory evidence. I shall also concentrate on indirect behavioural measures of auditory capacity—for example, speech intelligibility and subvocalisation.

Theoretically, it is possible to conceive of a deaf person developing a functional model of the phonemic structure of a spoken language through articulation. If auditory feedback from one's own voice is not a necessary condition for developing articulation, then it is possible that a deaf person could learn to talk intelligibly. Feedback in this case would have to be provided in some other way, for example, through formal instruction of some kind. Similarly, at least some aspects of speech comprehension could develop through lipreading, facial expressions, and so on. Although some phonemic distinctions are largely "invisible" (e.g., cat, rat) it is still possible that some visual model of the speech system could be developed—albeit, perhaps, an incomplete one. The obvious test for the development of such a system would be through measures of lipreading ability, speech intelligibility, and, arguably, reading.

In a comprehensive survey of hearing-impaired and deaf children leaving school in England and Wales in 1974–1976, Conrad (1979) examined their performance on tests of lipreading, speech intelligibility, and reading. His work confirmed findings from less comprehensive studies performed in many other countries. He found, for example, that lipreading skill, the capacity to speak intelligibly to a stranger, and reading ability were very poor. In the group with severe to profound losses, scores were particularly low. The average reading age over the sample as a whole was around 8 years.

What such studies show is that while many deaf children may develop a knowledge of some aspects of the grammar of English, these do not meet the demands of everyday life (e.g., talking to and understanding strangers, reading newspapers, television subtitles, or instructions).

An original feature of Conrad's work was the incorporation of a test of "inner speech" designed to measure the extent to which an individual utilises auditory "imagery" when reading and remembering lists of words. Normally hearing children of the age tested find the task of reading and remembering lists of "pseudohomophones" (e.g., few, zoo, pew) more difficult than lists of non-homophones, implying that verbal coding, rehearsal, or both create greater inter-ference for words with similar sounds, leading to poorer retention. By expressing the number of items successfully recalled in homophonic and nonhomophonic conditions as a ratio, Conrad created his measure of inner speech (Inner Speech Ratio or ISR). When this same test was administered to the deaf sample, he found that ISRs generally approached unity. This he took as evidence that the deaf children were unlikely to be using phonemic encoding. The explanatory power of this measure was revealed by significant correlations between the ISR and measures of reading, speech intelligibility, and lipreading skill. As might be expected, it also correlated with degree of hearing loss and, less powerfully, with nonverbal intelligence. Thus, Conrad concluded that increasing deafness, partic-ularly if coupled with low intelligence, systematically reduces the probability that a child will evidence inner speech or think in word sounds.

How, then, do such deaf children manage to read, lipread, or speak at all? One possibility is that they read by a direct visual route, so features of word shapes in text and also, presumably, on the lips, access meaning directly. More recent research has provided some support for this hypothesis (Kyle, 1980), although it must be admitted that the relationships between articulation, auditory storage, and visual features in the reading of normally hearing people still leave open the question of the role of such direct access in skilled readers (e.g., Underwood, 1979; Briggs, 1983).

While clearly important, these results leave several questions unanswered. Although the correlations between ISR and linguistic measures were significant, most of the variance in such measures was unaccounted for. This technique only examines retention of "disconnected" words. If one assumes that all linguistic processing by the deaf is "bottom-up"—from single words to larger units, for example—then a measure of performance with words alone might well suffice. However, there are several reasons to believe that other aspects of language are involved in determining reading and lipreading abilities. Some profoundly deaf people with losses above 100 dB do perceive aspects of speech (e.g., Risberg,

1976). They may, for example, be able to differentiate tape recordings of questions from declaratives. Whilst not hearing segmental sounds, for example consonant clusters, they may hear suprasegmental features, for example intonation. This seems to make sense audiologically, since a good deal of information about features such as intonation, rhythm, and stress is carried at low frequencies, which is the most likely field of residual hearing to remain with severe to profound losses.

Risberg's audiological studies parallel recent findings of our own. We have found, for example, that severely and profoundly deaf children can discriminate different types of utterances in natural conversation. They differentiate questions from statements, and also discriminate between questions demanding a forced-choice response from different ''Wh''-type questions (i.e., who, what, when, where, why) (Wood *et al.*, 1982). Clearly, in natural discourse many nonverbal cues are also likely to differentiate such linguistic forms (slight movements of the head; movements of the eyebrows, etc.), so the child may or may not be conscious of any audiological distinctions. However, they do differentiate some linguistic forms and this, coupled with Quigley's data that show some sentential processing by the deaf, suggests that they have some form of conceptual framework for top-down processing. This conclusion is strengthened by more recent research in our group. We have found, for example, that children's verbal responses to different linguistic forms are correlated with reading ability (Griffiths, 1983). More specifically, the child's ability to follow a teacher's Wh-type questions with long answers correlates with measures of his reading ability. Furthermore, the syntactic accuracy of his spontaneous speech correlates with the accuracy of his writing, which correlates with his language in response to teacher, and his reading age. All the children in this study were severely or profoundly deaf, thereby adding weight to the conclusion that they can and do process higher order structures in spoken and written language, and posses a generative (albeit limited) linguistic system.

In part, such results complement those of Conrad, in that children who say more in discourse are also, one suspects, those most likely to develop some inner speech. However, they extend his analysis in demonstrating competence beyond the word level. This leaves open the issue of how far and in what ways top-down processes are involved in the determination of linguistic ability.

Moving on from this conclusion to develop testable models of what and how deaf children process in language is difficult. However, there are some lines of evidence that are relevant. These hinge on the role of visuospatial information in language development of the deaf, to which we turn next.

7 Sign Language and the Psychology of Deafness

The systematic description of sign language is a new undertaking. The study of sign language in use and the relationships between it and aspects of cognitive functioning are even more recent in origin. The aim of this section is not to attempt a comprehensive review of these topics but to consider their contribution to the various issues already introduced.

Most systems for describing the structure of sign languages are based on the analysis developed by Stokoe (1960, 1978) for American Sign Lanugage (ASL). In such systems, language is analysed in terms of the permissible combinations of hand shape, orientation, movement, and location in the formation of signs. The analyses show that, within a given language, the concatenation of these dimensions is rule governed, since, as in spoken languages, it is possible to generate inadmissible strings that a native speaker would reject as ungrammatical. There are several important differences in the structure of signed and spoken languages. In the latter, concatenation of elements (ignoring intonation) is serial. In sign language, however, the parameters are largely simultaneous. A given sign includes information about hand shape, location, orientation, and movement in parallel. This invites a clear distinction between languages acquired by vision, which capitalise on spatial information, and those acquired by ear, which are more temporally organised (e.g., word order, prefixes, and suffixes).

Work has also begun on the exploration of syntactic structures in sign language. As with morphemic processes, sign language exploits visuospatial information and displays different principles of organisation from spoken language. Consider, for example, "aspectual" information in sign and English. Aspect subsumes distinctions such as progressive and perfective verb processes. In English, we can talk about an event located in the past, future, or present as being in progress (e.g., he was watching), as completed (he watched), or as habitual (he watches or he is a watcher), exploiting auxiliary verbs and inflexions together with adverbs of frequency, duration, degree, and so on to convey such aspectual distinctions. In sign language (e.g., British Sign Language, or BSL), however, much of this information is conveyed in the verb form itself (Brennan, 1981); for example, a sign may be repeated several times to convey repetition or habituality, or may be performed once, but sustained, to indicate duration. This phenomenon is a familiar feature of sign languages. Because information is conveyed by movement, position, facial expression, hand shape, and so forth, it can (and often must) be produced in parallel. Thus, the visual nature of signs imposes quite different constraints on the "design" features of the language from those operative on aural languages.

Such marked differences in the structures of signed and spoken languages, some linguists argue, indicate different processes underlying language learned by ear and eye. Some (e.g., Tervoort, 1975) contend that whether the deaf child is learning spoken language by lipreading or sign language, the process of acquisition, rooted in visuospatial structures, is qualitatively different from that followed by the hearing child acquiring language by ear. Intriguing and important though this hypothesis is, the evidence in support of it is not definitive, and attempts to test it in formal experimental situations have proved inconclusive. In part, this results from considerable methodological problems in testing deaf children's oral language abilities for sign language structure. In one study, for example, Dawson (1981) presented deaf and hearing children with sentences written in standard English syntax, "deaf" English syntax, and BSL syntax. She discovered, amongst other things, that deaf children found it easier to recall the latter, whereas hearing children did better with standard English. However, there is no written form of BSL, it is a nonliterate language. Thus, information about aspect, for example, was not conveyed in the written signing. Other words, like prepositions, were also omitted from the signed version. Consequently, this was structurally simpler and almost always of shorter length than the English version. Thus, the sign syntax might be easier because it corresponds more closely to the English grammar of the deaf and omits difficult structures or, as Dawson concludes, its simplicity could be due to "interference" from sign syntax. The matter is not resolved.

The most systematic observational studies in this area to date have examined the emergence of signs and early sign combinations in deaf babies of deaf parents whose mother tongue is American Sign Language. These stress the similarities in the development of language in deaf and hearing children (Schlesinger, 1978). They pass through similar stages and, current evidence suggests, deaf infants do so at a somewhat *earlier* age than hearing children. Bonvillian (1983) argues that such findings are in contradiction with Piagetian views on the emergence of symbolism, since the explanation for age of emergence in hearing children within Piaget's theory is that it coincides with the development of the object concept at the end of the sensorimotor stage. The issue is complex, however, since reliable systems for differentiating deferred imitation and the gestures to which this leads from "true" words have not been formulated. Until they are, and are applied to young hearing babies, it is not clear whether the same criteria for symbolic processes are being used in the studies of deaf and hearing.

Whatever the status of such differences, the main import of these studies for the present discussion is the finding that communication, symbolic functioning, and at least the early stages of syntactic development follow similar paths in deaf and hearing children. This contradicts any notion that sound is necessary for the emergence of symbolic thought and the view that deaf children are cognitively retarded, at least in the early stages. More work along these lines, on the later stages of linguistic development, may well answer questions about the nature of language acquisition by eye for more complex structures. Except for Tervoort's pioneering observations, such evidence has not been forthcoming.

Another line of attack on the same set of questions has begun in research on language and memory, with attempts to study similarities and differences in the retention of information from signed and spoken languages. However, such studies are complicated because deaf children as a population (and even as individuals) are exposed to a range of different sign systems not all of which are "true" languages (Jensema and Trybus, 1978). Some schools, for example, use one-handed or two-handed finger spelling, systems of hand shapes with a one-to-one correspondence with the English alphabet. Studies of children exposed to these and other systems show that they can and do use them as mnemonic aids (e.g., Dornic *et al.*, 1973). More interesting, however, are questions about the structural characteristics of memory based on such different coding systems. Some work shows, for example, that the semantic structure of memory for signs has similar hierarchical characteristics to those found in spoken language (e.g., Kyle, 1981). But recent work in this field also presents some puzzling results and suggests basic differences in the relationships between signed and spoken languages and memory.

In a series of studies, Kyle (1981) examined deaf and hearing people's recall of information under various conditions of presentation. For example, they were shown words and signs and asked to recall them. He found that (hearing) bilingual sign speakers, hearing people who were fluent in signs, and others who were inexperienced users, recalled more words than signs. The deaf people showed no difference. More surprising was the finding that whilst concurrent vocalisation of words read improves recall in hearing people, concurrent signing by the deaf interferes with recall for signs. One might argue that this shows direct, visual lexical access with no "inner signing." Thus, the role of articulation in the reading of both signs and words by the deaf remains unclear. "Direct" visual coding seems to be involved in both.

One final line of research also generates some interesting but puzzling results. A general assumption pervading linguistics, following in part on Chomsky's theory, is that no language is inherently more complex or better formed than any other. In opposition to the Whorfian hypothesis, it is also widely held that any concept or idea can be expressed in any language, albeit, perhaps, with varying degrees of ease (e.g., Hockett, 1954). However, Schlesinger (1971) has found that deaf people using Israeli Sign Language failed several communication tests where one signer had to describe a picture of a nonsensical event to another whose task was to select the picture from an array (e.g., a bear is giving a boy doll to a girl). They were unable to disambiguate aspects of the message such as direct and indirect object. One might argue on this basis that signed communication usually involves a great deal of pragmatic knowledge in its interpretation, since the pictures used were deliberately bizarre.

In other studies (reported in Quigley and Kretschmer, 1982) another apparent limitation in signed communication emerges. When deaf subjects are asked to draw inferences from a series of propositions (e.g., if the blanket is under the bed; the cat is on the blanket; the cat is white—where is the cat?) they do poorly in comparison to hearing people, and they are more likely to draw inferences from a written English than a signed presentation. Why should the deaf perform better in a written version of a second or foreign language than with their own mother tongue? Do these results imply that written language is the deaf person's most effective mode of communication? This seems highly unlikely since signing was presumably the preferred (and, hence, most effective) mode of communication for subjects in all these studies. It might imply, however, that the pragmatic and contextual basis of sign language is far more important in communication than is the case for (literate) users of spoken language. Sign language, by its nature, is used in face-to-face situations when many contextual and pragmatic cues are available. Does this mean that the rules for conveying information are less formalised in the deaf, that syntactic rules designed for communication out of direct visual contact are not needed and have not evolved? Such a characterisation of sign language, which parallels Bernstein's (1960) description of a "restricted code," runs directly counter to most contemporary thinking in linguistics. Certainly, it is not a hypothesis that is being entertained in work on sign language. However, such a view is compatible with several generalisations often made about the concrete, context dependent, egocentric, and impulsive functioning of the deaf. But are such phenomena linguistic, cognitive, or, perhaps, attributable to social experience? Such questions draw the study of linguistic capacities in the deaf into a consideration of cognition, to which we now turn.

8 Cognition and Deafness

It is easy to identify significant differences in the performances of deaf and hearing people on many formal cognitive tasks, although the deaf's performance (as a population) on some tests of nonverbal IQ are normal or only 5 IQ points below that of the hearing (e.g., Anderson and Sisco, 1977). However, on all measures of academic achievement, even in areas which appear largely nonverbal, such as mathematical computation, deaf children lag behind hearing peers (Wood *et al.*, 1983).

In a variety of (modified) Piagetian tasks such as the achievement of conservation of number, weight, amount, and quantity, deaf people do achieve success, although estimates of their "delays" vary from study to study (e.g., Oleron, 1977; Furth, 1971). Does this imply, as Furth argues, that deaf children develop through exactly the same stages as hearing children but at a slower rate because of "experiential deficits," or is retardation attributable to qualitative differences in their developmental processes?

The problem in achieving a definitive answer to this general question is that all major theoretical frameworks admit both similarities and differences in performance. What is lacking in all these theoretical accounts are principles that are detailed and general enough to specify before any study exactly what differences and similarities will be found.

Concerning Furth's arguments about universal stages in development, several problems can be identified that greatly limit the predictive and explanatory power of his position. In the first place, the notion of "experiential deficit," which is the key to the explanation of delay and apparent failures in competence, is not formulated in any detail. It is recruited post hoc as an explanation for lack of success. It appeals to the commonsense notion that poor communication inhibits the range and rate of experience but provides no explicit guidelines as to how such factors can be identified or quantified. Second, his studies fail, by Piagetian criteria, to discriminate between success and understanding. Special experimental procedures can solicit successful performance from deaf subjects, showing that their reasoning processes may be formally similar to those of the hearing. However, it is also possible that different processes underly such success and mask a limited understanding of logical necessity per se. Indeed, this is one major line of criticism levelled by Piagetians against attempts to demonstrate "precocious" logical understanding in "preoperational" hearing children. This, in turn, raises a fundamental epistemological question that can be phrased in several ways. For example, in many situations where deaf children are asked to draw inferences, perceive analogies, or generalise principles "spontaneously," they fail. By manipulating instructions to make task structure more obvious and more accessible visually and kinaesthetically, Furth has shown that success can be engineered. It could be argued that this overcomes performance limitations caused by poor communication, so revealing true competence. Alternatively, one might argue that the experimenter has taken over control of processes of task analysis or decentration that are hallmarks of sophisticated thinking. In other words, only by supplementing the subject's limited powers of understanding and competence can joint success be achieved.

Further, research into the linguistic capacities of the deaf shows that they cannot validly be regarded as nonlingual controls; they do not lack linguistic competence. To explain success or failure, then, it is necessary to formulate more precise relationships between linguistic and cognitive functioning. If we are to gain insights into the role of language in cognition through comparative studies of deaf and hearing subjects, then it is necessary to complement measures of cognitive functioning with reliable measures of language ability. Even here, however, correlations between linguistic and cognitive abilities must be treated with caution. Any relationship might be attributable to the causal influence of language on thought—showing, perhaps, that linguistic operations are fundamental to the achievement of given types of reasoning. Alternatively, the connection could be more indirect. Language might correlate with measures of cognitive abilities because it either facilitates the transmission of knowledge through instruction or makes the task of assessing competence in experiments and tests more straightforward, or both.

Finally, research by Bryant (1974), amongst others, provides an alternative explanation to Piaget's of the relationships between operativity and perception.

His studies show that young children's performances on tasks such as seriation and judgements of relative size can be explained by perceptual organisation and memory. This greater emphasis on perceptual organisation, not mediated by Piagetian operations, provides another way of explaining the cognitive abilities of the deaf. Here the emphasis lies neither on action in the world nor on language but on principles of organisation operating in visuospatial perception.

A theoretical scheme which places instruction and language at the heart of intellectual development also provides the beginnings of an explanatory framework for similarities and differences in the cognitive abilities of deaf and hearing people. This is the theory developed by Luria. The basic divide between Piagetian theory and Soviet psychology is revealed in a single sentence from Luria and Yudovich (1971), p. 23, who write "it would be mistaken to suppose that verbal intercourse with adults merely changes the content of the child's conscious activity without changing its form". Language involves much more than the articulation of structures or concepts previously established through sensorimotor development. Even at the level of word acquisition, the Soviet psychologists argue for a qualitative shift in consciousness from that before acquisition.

The word has a basic function not only because it indicates a corresponding object in the external world, but also because it abstracts, idealises, isolates, the necessary signal, generates perceived signals and relates them to certain categories [what we have called Consciousness II] introducing forms of analysis and synthesis into the child's perception which he would be unable to develop by himself. (p.23)

Thus, the word not only articulates the "object" concept, it is a sociohistorical "tool" that, in its relationships to other categories, embodies the development of many past generations. It is because of the long, complex history of the word that the individual child cannot develop it by himself, within a single, limited life span. Thus, the word "deepens and immeasureably enriches his direct perception, forms his consciousness."

The effect of language on consciousness is to free the individual from the dictates of the "first signal system"; from responding simply to the immediate conditions of stimulation. Language arises in social interaction and, progressively, the child internalises such dialogue to recall, guide, and plan his own activities. Lacking speech, the deaf-mute

does not possess all those forms of reflection of reality which are realised through verbal speech. The deaf mute who has not been taught to speak indicates objects or actions with a gesture; he is unable to abstract the quality or action from the actual object, to form abstract concepts, to systematise the phenomena of the external world with the aid of abstracted signals furnished by language but which are not natural to visual, practically acquired experience. (Luria and Yudovich, 1971)

Given this analysis, we would expect deaf children to be limited in their capacities to transcend the dictates of immediate experience. They should be context bound (concrete), lack the ability to take account of the needs and perspectives of others (egocentric), unable to inhibit the dictates of immediate stimulation (impulsive), and lack the capacity mentally to represent future possibilities and, hence, to exhibit choice (rigidity). Furthermore, they should display, as children, primitive levels of play, evidencing no planning or thematic coherence in what they do. Their capacity for social interaction should be limited, particularly their ability to display attention to the narrative of others (and, hence, should show poor development in the foundations of literacy). Finally, since the theoretical account of language development is closely tied to a model of neurological functioning, we would also expect differences in cerebral organisation.

Each of these predictions can be supported by empirical and clinical studies of the deaf. Investigations of personality, cognitive style, interpersonal relationships, play, reading, and so forth, can be found which are consistent with this view (see Meadow, 1980).

The matter does not end there, however. In the first place, the Soviet psychologists admit the possibility that language can be "taught" to the deaf. Thus, any effects of deafness are likely to be in degree and not of kind and will vary as a product of educational experience. Although there is some evidence to show that social and educational factors do influence performance in language (e.g., Breslaw *et al.*, 1981; Quigley and Kretschmer, 1982), no strong empirical links have, as yet, been established between such factors and the quality of instruction, although some work along these lines is being undertaken (e.g., Wood and Wood, 1984). At the moment, it is not possible to test the theory directly nor to produce detailed predictions about individual differences in the deaf population.

Another problem with the Soviet account concerns the limited view it offers of nonverbal communication. The theory does not specify that all instruction takes place verbally, but, on several occasions, Luria makes it clear that language is the major force behind development and that he equates language with speech. It would be interesting to hear his reactions to recent studies of sign language. In their absence, we can only guess at his position. First, can a sign language present a second signal system? The evidence reviewed above indicates that signs are true symbols, not simply gestures tied to a given object or context. They are, in part at least, arbitrary, and belong to a generative linguistic system. Looked at in this way, they seem to fulfill the criteria for a second signal system.

Notwithstanding these developments in our understanding of sign language since Luria talked of context-tied "gestures," I suspect that Luria's analysis of the relationships between language and thought would still lead him to conclude that sign language leads to qualitative differences in the conscious experiences of hearing and (nonspeaking) deaf people. His emphasis on the sociohistorical nature of language and his view that language does not simply express but also restructures thought takes him close to Whorf's (1952) position.

Sign language has a different sociocultural history from spoken language. Thus, what it passes on to children will differ from that communicated by a spoken language, although the two will intersect in varying degrees depending on the overlap in their evolutions. Because, in the Soviet view, language exerts an influence on the content and structure of consciousness, a different language entails a different psychology.

Thus, where Furth points to deaf children's successes and takes these as evidence of a general competence limited only by performance and communication factors, Luria interprets those same examples of success as the outgrowth of successful instruction, and failure as incompetence. By making problems more accessible, visible, and practical for the deaf, Furth, in this view, has taken responsibility for solving problems associated with the second signal system, allowing the child to operate at a lower level. Viewed as instruction, such experiments may help to develop children's competence further through problem solving, but they cannot be treated as equivalent to that of a person who spontaneously solves the problems of task analysis and generalisation on his own.

9 The "Organismic Shift" Hypothesis

Furth's theory assumes that deafness has little effect on the development of understanding and rationality. Luria sees deafness as a barrier to the inheritance of culture, but seems to view the deaf not so much as different from the hearing, but as merely facing special problems of spoken communication which, if overcome by effective oral instruction, will lead to similar patterns of cognitive function as those of hearing people. Both theories, then, share the basic image of the deaf as psychologically similar to the hearing.

One theoretical approach which works with the view that deaf people display some important qualitative differences from the hearing is that put forward by Myklebust (1964). The emphasis in his "special psychology" of deafness is not simply on the barrier to speech created by deafness, but on the importance of sound in general. As I have already argued, visually based communication demands the transmission of linguistic information in parallel while speech exploits temporal organisation. There are other aspects of deafness that demand a more "serial" organisation in consciousness. Whereas, for example, a hearing child may monitor speech whilst maintaining visual attention, for example on the thing being talked about, profoundly deaf children—whether lipreading or sign reading—must distribute their visual attention sequentially between the act of communication and its referent. This leads to additional demands on the deaf child in communication situations (Wood, 1980). He must attend to and integrate two or more loci of information, whereas the hearing child can maintain his visual attention on one source while someone else takes responsibility for timing the act of communication to fit his ongoing activity. Thus, the structure of interactions in general and the process of instruction in particular are organised somewhat differently for the deaf and the hearing. Furthermore, as Myklebust argues, sound often serves to distract or redirect attention in unpredictable ways. Sudden sounds, changes in speaker, noises accompanying the unforeseen consequences of an action occurring out of the immediate sphere of consciousness, often serve to expand or relocate the field of conscious awareness. Lacking access to these adventitious sources of information, the deaf individual is more likely to be "locked" into his own projects or plans; to display a necessary or structural egocentrism.

Several connections can be made between such aspects of intersensory functioning and specific problems in the development of knowledge and language. Transcending the here-and-now—that which is located in immediate awareness—is more difficult when one lacks the conceptual underpinnings that sound and speech make possible. Communicating about the past, future, hypothetical, and so on, is inhibited when interaction tends to be en face, supported by paralinguistic and extralinguistic cues tied to the immediate context (Howarth and Wood, 1977).

A variety of sources of evidence could be cited to add credibility to this view of deafness and cognition—linguistic problems, personality characteristics such as egocentrism and impulsivity, difficulties in making inferences, and so forth. However, attempts to establish clear-cut relationships between deafness and such fundamental aspects of cognitive functioning in controlled empirical studies have failed to provide strong support for this view.

In one study, for example, Norden (1975) compared deaf and hearing adolescents on 36 different tasks involving measures of both linguistic and non-linguistic abilities. The nonlinguistic battery included tests of mathematical reasoning and computation, sequencing skills, tests of field dependence–independence, embedded figures, and formal tests of nonverbal intelligence. She found no evidence that the deaf are necessarily more "illogical," egocentric, or field dependent than the hearing. However, there was a wider range of individual differences in the deaf than the hearing. She also found subgroups of deaf children who seemed unable to "decentre," that is, to take two or more aspects of a problem into account simultaneously, suggesting that some deaf adolescents had not achieved concrete operational thinking. However, the incidence of other problems (associated, for example, with cause of deafness) was also high in this subgroup, underlining the danger of generalisations from this heterogeneous population. Norden's sample is not atypical in this respect. All major surveys report an abnormally high incidence of children with more than one handicap in deaf samples (e.g., CEC, 1979; Wood, in press).

The great variance in the performances of the deaf points to the danger of single-factor explanations of deaf–hearing differences. An important finding, however, is that deafness per se does not, of necessity, lead to egocentric, illogical, or impulsive task performances. Despite the heterogeneity of the deaf sample, a high proportion of the "merely" deaf performed within the normal range on a variety of nonverbal tasks, ruling out any strong theoretical connection between sound and fundamental aspects of nonverbal intelligence. Norden concludes that the low performances of the deaf on tests of scholastic knowledge do not reflect fundamental cognitive deficits on their part, but specific educational problems caused by poor communication.

In a recent study of mathematical abilities in deaf children, we came to a similar conclusion. Although deaf children are retarded in mathematical attainment, there is no evidence of deviance. They tend to get the same pattern of right and wrong answers as hearing children of similar maths ages, and their error patterns are virtually indistinguishable (Wood, *et al.*, 1983). Furthermore, their test performance produced evidence that, like hearing children, they were selective in the test items attempted. They tended to bypass problems that gave a low conditional probability of success whilst attempting those that gave a high probability, which is difficult to reconcile with theories predicting generalised impulsivity or a lack of self-awareness.

Other studies comparing the performances of deaf and hearing children on tests demanding spatiotemporal coding suggest that deaf children face specific problems. On nonverbal IQ tests they score less well on tasks demanding sequencing or rearrangement, such as the Picture Arrangement subscale of the WISC. Such results are compatible with Myklebust's theory, in that rearrangements demand that a child transcend the immediate spatial array to impose an alternative structure on what is seen. O'Connor and Hermelin (1978) have also produced evidence showing that deaf children are less successful than hearing peers in recalling the temporal as opposed to spatial arrangement of a series of objects. For example, if three objects are put down in the temporal sequence 1–2–3 to occupy a spatial sequence 3–1–2, deaf subjects are more likely than hearing ones to recall the spatial order. However, in some task situations deaf subjects do recall temporal sequences. This leads Hermelin and O'Connor to conclude that deaf and hearing people display a different hierarchy of strategies in such tasks. However, the deaf find ways of attending to and recalling spatiotemporal information.

The introduction of "strategies" into a discussion of cognitive performance transforms the debate. If one accepts that similar performances can be generated from qualitatively different cognitive processes, and there is ample evidence for this (see Wood, 1969, 1978; Simon, 1975), then simply examining the incidence of success in a given situation is unlikely to yield useful insights into cognitive performance. As I have already pointed out, soliciting introspective accounts and justifications from deaf subjects is a complex, difficult, and often impossible task. This means that inferences about differential strategies must come from detailed analyses of performance in a variety of situations, when patterns of differences and similarities may be used to infer underlying processes. At the moment, the evidence available is not robust enough to enable the development and evaluation of any general models along these lines. Deafness may well affect the basic structure of experience in the ways envisaged by Myklebust. If so, however, the performance of deaf people in a range of tasks underlines the versatility and plasticity of human capacities, in that they appear to overcome their limited sensory resources to achieve comparable performance in a wide range of situations. At some level of functioning, the resources exist for overcoming the limitations imposed by "peripheral" damage, even when such damage is to a system so seemingly central to our experiences as that of hearing.

10 Deafness and Cerebral Specialisation

Hypotheses about the greater reliance of the deaf on visuospatial organisation raise specific questions about differential neurological organisation in deaf and hearing people. It is widely accepted (e.g., Springer and Deutsch, 1981) that within a large sample of (hearing) individuals there will be evidence of hemispheric specialisation. The left hemisphere is regarded as being more involved in linguistic function and the right in visuospatial functioning. It has also been argued that sequential–temporal functioning is more characteristic of the left hemisphere with the right exhibiting more holistic, less analytic modes of function. It is not a long step from the formulation of generalisations about the differential nature of conscious experience in deaf and hearing people to the suggestion that there may be different patterns of asymmetry in the two populations.

For example, sign language takes place in the visual modality and is organised spatially. Does it follow that processing of signs by the deaf is largely carried out in the right hemisphere? Some evidence suggests that it is (Poizner and Lane, 1979), other evidence that it is not (e.g., McKeever *et al.*, 1976). Even if the results of such studies were unequivocal, which they are not, they do not tease apart the linguistic and visuospatial aspects of sign. Right hemisphere superiority might mean that visuospatial functioning takes place in that location, or that linguistic functioning does, or that both do. If language is largely processed in the right hemisphere of the deaf and the left hemisphere of the hearing, then it could follow that the different structures of signed and spoken languages and the specific problems that the deaf have with spoken and written language are causally related to the differential functioning of the left and right hemispheres. Such an argument is consistent with recent theorising by Chomsky (1981) who argues that aspects of syntactic processing are located in the left hemisphere. Without normal left hemisphere function, he suggests, specific syntactic rules (such as the passive voice in English) cannot be acquired.

But these implications only follow if the deaf can be shown to display language processing in the right hemisphere. Attempts have been made to tease apart the linguistic and visuospatial aspects of sign language processing. For example, if the deaf also show a right hemisphere advantage for English words, this would suggest a generalised right hemisphere involvement in linguistic function. Here too, experiments produce conflicting results. Some researchers, using tachistoscopic presentation of English words (McKeever *et al.*, 1976), report a significant RVF (left hemisphere) advantage for the deaf, suggesting that sign stimuli are processed in the right hemisphere because of spatiotemporal and not linguistic factors. Coupled with evidence suggesting right hemisphere involvement in the deaf for nonlinguistic visuospatial stimuli, such findings imply that cerebral organisation of deaf and hearing people is similar. If so, linguistic and spatiotemporal problems must have other causes. However, other research refutes the findings of left hemisphere specialisation in language function, finding significant RVF advantage for hearing subjects with stimuli such as words and letters but no evidence for such specialisation in the deaf (e.g., Kelly and Tomlinson-Keasey, 1981). Yet other studies report *reversed* asymmetry in the deaf, supporting the view that signs (and written language) are represented in the right hemisphere (Ross *et al.* 1979).

The empirical evidence is, then, somewhat confused, and offers no grounds for firm statements about neurological organisation nor for implications about "natural" neurological barriers to the achievement, say, of normal reading ability in the deaf (see Conrad, 1979; Arnold, in press, for examples of the debate in this area).

There are many potential reasons for this confused picture. As already argued, experiments with the deaf are always hazardous. Coupled with this are wide individual differences within the deaf population associated with aetiology of the handicap and with educational and familial experiences. Phippard (1977) claims, for example, that educational history is correlated with patterns of asymmetry, with orally taught deaf children showing greater left hemisphere involvement in processing written letters than children taught through a combination of sign and speech. Another problem is that experiments with deaf children, where responses are to be made in non-oral modalities, introduce issues about differences from the hearing caused not by perception and encoding but by response mode.

Clinical studies of the effects of brain damage on congenitally deaf people for whom sign language is the "mother tongue" are less equivocal. Kimura (1981, p. 309), reviewing relevant case histories, reports that "in right handers, signing is typically disturbed after left hemisphere lesions . . . It appears that within the left hemisphere, posterior damage may be sufficient to produce a manual signing disorder". She goes on to argue that signing disorders in these cases are based on "manual apraxia"—on difficulty in selecting correct movements *whether they have or do not have linguistic content.* Furthermore, the effect of such lesions on sign *comprehension* is not marked.

Comparing the pattern of symptoms of deaf and hearing people with similar, posterior, left hemisphere damage, she argues that both result in similar effects. Manual signing and vocal aphasias can be regarded as subcategories of apraxia, each caused by damage to the same region of the left hemisphere. This evidence is consistent with the view (Kimura, 1979) that the primary specialisation of the left hemisphere is not for language as such but has to do with the organisation and control of complex sequences of movements. This evidence also points to the essential similarity in specialisation of function in deaf and hearing people, though it does not, of course, address the issue of where any specialised functioning for language *is* for both groups.

Other paradigms have also been employed to try to locate specific centres of functioning in the brains of hearing and deaf people, but, here too, the evidence is equivocal (Ashton and Beasley, 1982).

One final line of evidence relevant to the issue of cerebral specialisation comes from comparative studies of the relationships among sex, language, and cognition in deaf and hearing people. There is some evidence for such specialisation in hearing subjects (Moore, 1967), suggesting that whilst linguistic ability in females is predictive of aspects of nonverbal functioning it is not for males. Similar results have been found for the deaf (e.g., Norden, 1975). These are particularly interesting since the actual levels of performance, whilst significantly different and favouring males in the hearing, are not significantly different in deaf samples (Wood *et al.*, 1983). Thus, whilst deafness attenuates sex differences in level of performance, it results in similar patterns of association among sex, linguistic ability, and mathematical achievements.

One might argue from such findings for a genetically based link among sex, cognition, and language mediated by differential neurological organisation in male and female populations (Hutt, 1972). Current evidence suggests somewhat greater degrees of lateralisation for spatial and linguistic function in males than females. If these differences are causally related to differential functioning in visuospatial, mathematical, and linguistic tasks and to different interrelationships between these in males and females, then the somewhat similar results from the deaf suggest that the underlying neurological organisation might well be similar in deaf and hearing people.

Such results, though clearly too confused to permit selection amongst the various competing theories outlined above, do illustrate how, in the longer term, comparative studies of neurological functioning in the deaf may help to shed light onto the relationships between behaviour, cortical organisation, and consciousness in both deaf and hearing people. Reviewing the studies in this area (Poizner, 1979) does lead, on balance, to the judgement that cerebral asymmetry of functioning in the deaf is less marked than in the hearing. This, too, may appear somewhat paradoxical if one takes a simpleminded view of the relationships between asymmetry of function and behaviour. In hearing people, less marked asymmetry of function in females is, if anything, associated with superior spoken linguistic ability. This can hardly be claimed for the deaf. Clearly, the development of a useful model of the relationships between asymmetry of function and differential abilities in deaf and hearing people is some way off.

11 Conclusions

Three competing images of deafness and its effects on the psychology of the individual have been explored in the light of recent research on deafness. Each has motivated important studies into the effects of deafness on mental life, but none accounts adequately for the data generated by these. The view promoted by Furth, which portrays the deaf individual as cognitively normal but linguistically incompetent, must be revised in the light of research into the symbolic and linguistic abilities of the deaf. They can no longer be viewed as alingual controls for studies in language and cognition. Myklebust's ''special psychology'' of deafness also leads to untenable generalisations about the egocentric, impulsive, and context-dependent intellectual style of the deaf. A good deal of evidence reviewed in this chapter is inconsistent with a strong empirical link between deafness and fundamental differences in the structure of consciousness. Luria's analysis was formulated in the context of his views about the symbolic and generative character of sign languages, leading to predictions about the cognitive capacities of the deaf which do not always stand up to empirical scrutiny.

Whilst research suggests that there are no such inevitable, general consequences of deafness, it has identified differences in rates of development between deaf and hearing children and has shown that the deaf person is more likely to display a rather context-dependent style of thinking. The reasons for such differences are still not clear. If they are not, as I have argued, an inevitable correlate of profound, prelingual deafness, reasons must be sought in terms of individual differences that are either constitutional in nature (related, perhaps, to aetiological factors) or attributable to differential social and educational experiences. Although individual differences have been explored to some extent, we do not have sufficient evidence to formulate any general models of their precise nature nor of their ontogenesis. The wide range of variability in this population warns against generalisations in terms of *the* deaf.

More positively, research has shed considerable light onto the nature of linguistic ability and its development in the deaf, inviting the formulation of more precise models of the relationships between languages acquired by ear or eye and specific cognitive abilities. The issues involved in such formulations have not been resolved, but they are amenable to future enquiry.

Above all, to my mind, research has helped to tarnish that image of the deaf as underdeveloped or inadequate hearing people. Although the theory that their consciousness is structurally different from our own is still arguable, the view that it is somehow inevitably limited or less well developed becomes increasingly untenable.

References

Anderson, R. J., and Sisco, F. H. (1977). "Standardisation of the WISC-R Performance Scale for Deaf Children." Office of Demographic Studies, Gallaudet College, Washington, D.C.

Arnold, P. (in press). Oralism and the deaf child's brain: a reply to Dr. Conrad. *International Journal of Otorhinolaryngology.*

Ashton, R., and Beasley, M. (1982). Cerebral laterality in deaf and hearing children. *Developmental Psychology,* **18**(2), 294–390.

Bernstein, B. (1960). Language and social class. *British Journal of Sociology,* **11,** 271–276.

Bonvillian, J. (1983). Early sign language acquisition and cognitive development. *In* "Acquisition of Symbolic Skills" (Eds. R. D. Rogers and J. A. Sloboda). Plenum Press, New York and London.

Bowerman, M. (1979). The acquisition of complex sentences. *In* "Language Acquisition" (Eds. P. Fletcher and M. Garman). Cambridge University Press, Cambridge.

Brennan, M. (1981). Grammatical processes in British Sign Language. *In* "Perspectives on British Sign Language and Deafness" (Eds. B. Woll, J. Kyle, and M. Deuchar), pp. 120–135. Croom Helm, London.

Breslaw, P. I., Griffiths, A. J., Wood, D. J., and Howarth, C. I. (1981). The referential communication skills of deaf children from different educational environments. *Journal of Child Psychology and Psychiatry,* **22**(3), 269–282.

Briggs, P. (1983). "Phonological Coding in Good and Poor Readers." Ph.D. thesis, University of Nottingham.

Bruner, J. (1966). "Toward a Theory of Instruction." Norton, New York,

Bryant, P. (1974). "Perception and Understanding in Young Children." Methuen, London.

Commission of the European Communities (1979). "Childhood Deafness in the European Community." ECSC-EEC-EAEC, Brussels and Luxemburg.

Chomsky, C. S. (1969). "The Acquisition of Syntax in Children from 5 to 10." M.I.T. Press, Cambridge, Mass.

Chomsky, N. (1981). "Rules and Representations." Basil Blackwell, Oxford.

Conrad, R. (1979). "The Deaf School Child." Harper and Row, London.

Dawson, E. (1981). Psycholinguistic processes in prelingually deaf adolescents. *In* "Perspectives on British Sign Language and Deafness" (Eds. B. Woll, J. Kyle, and M. Deuchar), pp. 43–70. Croom Helm, London.

Donaldson, M. C. (1978). "Children's Minds." Fontana and Croom Helm, London.

Dornic, S., Hagdahl, R., and Hanson, G. (1973). "Visual Search and Short Term Memory in the Deaf" (Reports from the Institute of Applied Psychology, No. 38). University of Stockholm, Sweden.

Furth, H. G. (1966). "Thinking without Language." Free Press, New York.

Furth, H. G. (1971). Linguistic deficiency and thinking: Research with deaf subjects 1964–1969. *Psychology Bulletin* **76**(1), 58–72.

Fusfield, I. S. (1955). The academic program of schools for the deaf. *Volta Review,* **57,** 63–70.

Griffiths, A. J. (1983). "The Linguistic Competence of Deaf Primary-School Children." Ph.D. thesis, University of Nottingham.

Heider, F., and Heider, G. M. (1940). A comparison of sentence structure of deaf and hearing children. *Psychology Monograph,* **52**(1 Whole no. 232), 42–103.

Hutt, C. (1972). "Males and Females." Penguin, Harmondsworth.

Hockett, C. (1954). Chinese vesus English: An exploration of the Whorfian thesis. *In* "Language in Culture" (Ed. H. Hoijer). University of Chicago Press, Chicago.

Howarth, C. I., and Wood D. J. (1977). A research programme on the intellectual development of deaf children. *Teacher of the Deaf,* **1**(1), 5–12.

Ivimey, G. P. (1976). The written syntax of an English deaf child; an exploration in method. *British Journal Dis. Comm.* **11**(2), 103–120.

Jensema, C. J., and Trybus, R. J. (1978). "Communication Patterns and Educational Achievement of Hearing Impaired Students" (Series T No. 2) Office of Demographic Studies, Gallaudet College, Washington, D.C.

Kelly, R. R., and Tomlinson-Keasey, C. (1981). The effect of auditory input on cerebral laterality. *Brain and Language,* **13,** 67–77.

Kimura, D. (1979). Neuromotor mechanisms in the evolution of human communication. In "Neurobiology and Social Communication in Primates" (Eds. H. D. Steklis and M. J. Raleigh). Academic Press, New York.

Kimura, D. (1981). Neural mechanisms in manual signing. *Sign Language Studies,* **33,** Winter ed., 291–312.

Kyle, J. G. (1980). Reading development of deaf children. *Journal Research Read.* **8**(2), 127–134.

Kyle, J. (1981). Signs and memory: The search for the code. *In* "Perspectives on British Sign Language and Deafness" (Eds. B. Woll, J. Kyle, and M. Deuchar). Croom Helm, London.

Lunzer, E. A. (1979). The development of consciousness. *In* "Aspects of Consciousness. Vol. 1, Psychological Issues" (Eds. G. Underwood and R. Stevens). Academic Press, London.

Luria, A. R., and Yudovich, F. (1971). "Speech and the Development of Mental Processes in the Child." Penguin, Harmondsworth.

McKeever, W. F., Hoemann, H. W., Florian, V. A., and VanDeventer, A. D. (1976). Evidence of minimal cerebral asymmetries for the processing of English words and American Sign Language in the congenitally deaf. *Neuropsychology,* **14,** 413–423.

McNeill, D. (1979). "The Conceptual Basis of Language." Erlbaum, Hillside, New Jersey.

Meadow, K. P. (1980). "Deafness and Child Development." Arnold, London.

Moore, T. (1967). Language and intelligence: A longitiudinal study of the first eight years. *Human Development* **10**, 88–106.

Myklebust, H. R. (1964). "The Psychology of Deafness: Sensory Deprivation, Learning and Adjustment" (2nd ed.). Grune and Stratton, New York.

Norden, K. (1975). "Psychological Studies of Deaf Adolescents." Studia Psychologica et Paedagogica, Series Altera XXIX, CWK, Gleerup, Sweden.

O'Connor, N., and Hermelin, B. (1978). "Seeing and Hearing and Space and Time." Academic Press, London.

Oleron, P. (1977). "Language and Mental Development." Erlbaum, New Jersey.

Phippard, D. (1977). Hemifield differences in visual perception in deaf and hearing subjects. *Neuropsychology,* **15**, 555–562.

Piaget, J. (1960). "Play, Dreams and Imitation in Childhood." Basic Books, New York.

Poizner, H. (1979). Hemispheric specialisation in the deaf. *In* "The Science of Deaf Signing" (Ed. B. Frokjaer-Jensen). Copenhagen Univeristy.

Poizner, H., and Lane H. (1979). Cerebral asymmetry in the perception of American Sgin Language. *Brain and Language,* **7**, 210–226.

Quigley, S. P., and Kretschmer, R. E. (1982). "The Education of Deaf Children. Issues, Theory and Practice." Arnold, London.

Quigley, S. P. Montanelli, D. S., and Wilbur, R. B. (1976a). Some aspects of the verb system in the language of deaf students. *Journal of Speech and Hearing Research,* **19**, 536–550.

Quigley, S. P., Steinkamp, M. W., Power, D. J., and Jones, B. W., (1978). "The Test of Syntactic Abilities." Dormac, Beaverton, Oregon.

Quigley, S. P., Wilbur, R. B., and Montanelli, D. S. (1976b). Complement structures in the language of deaf students. *Journal of Speech and Hearing Research,* **19**, 448–457.

Risberg, A. (1976). IV. Speech and hearing defects and aids. A diagnostic rhyme test for speech audiometry with severely hard of hearing and profoundly deaf children. *STL-QPSR,* 2–3.

Ross, P., Perganent, L., and Anisfeld, M. (1979). Cerebral lateralisation of deaf and hearing individuals for linguistic comparison judgements. *Brain and Language,* **8**, 69–80.

Schlesinger, H. S. (1978). The acquisition of signed and spoken language. In "Deaf Children: Developmental Perspectives" (Ed. L. S. Liben). Academic Press, New York.

Schlesinger, I. M. (1971). The grammar of sign language and the problems of language universals. *In* "Biological and Social Factors in Psycholinguistics" (Ed. J. Morton). Logos, Plainfield, N.J.

Simon, H. A. (1975). The functional equivalence of problem solving skills. *Cognitive Psychology,* **7**, 268–288.

Springer, S. P., and Deutsch, G. (1981). "Left Brain, Right Brain." Freeman, San Francisco.

Stokoe, W. C. (1960). Sign language structure: An outline of the visual communication systems of the American deaf. *Studies in Linguistics: Occasional Papers 8.*

Stokoe, W. C. (1978). "Sign Language Structure: The First Linguistic Analysis of American Sign Language." Linstock, Silver Spring, Maryland.

Tervoort, B. T. (1975). Bilingual interference between acoustic and visual communication. *In* "The Proceedings of the International Congress of Education of the Deaf" (pp. 319–322). August 25–28, Tokyo.

Underwood, G. (1979). Memory systems and the reading process. *In* "Applied Problems in Memory" (Eds. M. M. Gruneberg and P. E. Morris). Academic Press, London.

Whorf, B. L. (1952). "Collected Papers in Metalinguistics." Wiley, New York.

Wilbur, R. B., and Quigley, S. P. (1975). Syntactic structures in the written language of deaf children. *Volta Review,* **77,** 194–205.

Wilbur, R. B., Montanelli, D. S. and Quigley, S. P. (1976). Pronominalization in the language of deaf students. *Journal of Speech and Hearing Research,* **19,** 120–140.

Wood, D. J. (1969). Approach to the study of human reasoning. *Nature,* **223,** 101–102.

Wood, D. J. (1978). Problem solving: The nature and development of strategies. *In* "Strategies of Information Processing" (Ed. G. Underwood). Academic Press, London.

Wood, D. J. (1980). Teaching the young child: Some relationships between social interaction, language and thought. *In* "The Social Foundations of Language and Thought" (Ed. D. Olson). Norton, New York.

Wood, D. J. (1982). The linguistic experiences of the prelingually, hearing-impaired child. *Teacher of the Deaf,* **6**(1), 86–93.

Wood, D. J. (in press). Social and educational adjustment in deaf children in relation to mental retardation. "Scientific Studies in Mental Retardation." McMillan, London.

Wood, D. J., and Wood, H. A. (1984). An experimental investigation of five styles of teacher conversation on the language of hearing-impaired children. *Journal of Child Psychology and Psychiatry,* **25**(1), 45–62.

Wood, D. J., Wood, H. A., Griffiths, A. J., Howarth, S. P., and Howarth, C. I. (1982). The structure of conversations with 6–10 year old deaf children. *Journal of Child Psychology and Psychiatry* **23**(3), 295–308.

Wood, D. J., Wood, H. A., and Howarth, S. P. (1983). Mathematical abilities of deaf school-leavers. *British Journal of Development Psychology* **1**(1), 67–74.

Index